KCET

Previous Years Solved Papers

KCET

Previous Years Solved Papers

Jeevitha Murugesh
3rd Rank Achiever
KCET-2010

Editor-in-Chief
Narendranatha Reddy P MDS
Founder-Director
Brihaspathi Academy
Bengaluru

CBS

CBS Publishers & Distributors Pvt Ltd

New Delhi • Bengaluru • Pune • Kochi • Chennai

Disclaimer
Science and technology are constantly changing fields. New research and experience broaden the scope of information and knowledge. The authors have tried their best in giving information available to them while preparing the material for this book. Although, all efforts have been made to ensure optimum accuracy of the material, yet it is quite possible some errors might have been left uncorrected. The publisher, printer and the authors will not be held responsible for any inadvertent errors or inaccuracies.

KCET
Previous Years Solved Papers

ISBN: 978-81-239-2043-6

First Edition: 2011

Published by Satish Kumar Jain and produced by Vinod K. Jain for
CBS Publishers & Distributors Pvt Ltd
4819/XI Prahlad Street, 24 Ansari Road, Daryaganj,
New Delhi 110 002, India.
Ph: 23289259, 23266861, 23266867
Fax: 011-23243014

Website: www.cbspd.com
e-mail: delhi@cbspd.com
cbspubs@airtelmail.in.

Branches

- Bengaluru: Seema House 2975, 17th Cross, K.R. Road, Banasankari 2nd Stage, Bengaluru 560 070, Karnataka
  Ph: +91-80-26771678/79 Fax: +91-80-26771680 e-mail: bangalore@cbspd.com
- Pune: Bhuruk Prestige, Sr. No. 52/12/2+1+3/2 Narhe, Haveli (Near Katraj-Dehu Road Bypass), Pune 411 051, Maharashtra
  Ph: 020-64704058, 64704059, 32342277 Fax: +91-020-24300160 e-mail: pune@cbspd.com
- Kochi: 36/14 Kalluvilakam, Lissie Hospital Road, Kochi 682 018, Kerala
  Ph: +91-484-4059061-65 Fax: +91-484-4059065 e-mail: cochin@cbspd.com
- Chennai: 20, West Park Road, Shenoy Nagar, Chennai 600 030, Tamil Nadu
  Ph: +91-44-26260666, 26208620 Fax: +91-44-45530020 email: chennai@cbspd.com

Printed at Somya Printers, Delhi 110053

to

Parents

From the Editor-in-Chief

I had been dreaming of two initiatives — ① establishing a premier coaching institution and ② providing a concise standard conceptual synopsis along with authenticated previous years solved papers — so that one can experience a high standard coaching with a superior quality study material to prepare for the MDS entrance examinations.

The first one came into reality on 19th May 2008 in the form of *Brihaspathi Academy* at Bengaluru. Since then the Academy has been flourishing day-by-day with the increased success sagas with just a fistful of students. Academy is backed by a group of 50 excellent academicians as well as the state-of-the-art library of over 200 volumes with the audio-video equipment.

Now, 2011 has given me an opportunity to fulfill the other dream in the form of the book now you are holding.

This series is followed by

COMEDK Previous Years Solved Papers,
Medical MCQs for Dental AIPG, AIIMS, COMEDK & KCET,
Complete Synopsis for all the Subjects and Quick Review for MDS Entrance Exam.

This book holds a complete set of authentic MCQs of KCET Previous Years Papers from 2003 to 2011 with 100% TEXTBOOK REFERENCES along with EXPLANATORY ANSWERS wherever necessary.

I request the readers to come up with their feedback on this initiative.

Wishing You All the Best for the Exams

Narendranatha Reddy P MDS
Founder-Director
Brihaspathi Academy
Bengaluru

If you have any doubt?
or a query?
mail to
support@brihaspathionline.com
or
post at
www.ask.brihaspathionline.com

Preface

Recently the competition for entrance exams has increased more than ever. Over the years MCQs have become tougher and confusing to answer correctly. No matter a share of new questions appear every year. The importance of diligent reading from standard textbooks is very important. But it is tough to deny that every year we see a bunch of questions from the previous years question papers. So students must be thorough with these questions before they attempt to solve new questions

This book presents year-wise solved question papers of KCET (2003–2011). The answers carry short crisp explanations in the form of tables, charts and points wherever necessary. This book is designed to aid in revision of the previous question papers. An endeavour has been made to provide 100% textbook references so that the student feels confident about each answer.

Best efforts have been put in to make the book student-friendly. If this goal is achieved, then it gives me an immense pleasure as this book will contribute to the success of many who are aspiring to get a MDS seat.

We have made sincere efforts to minimize errors. However, any suggestions to improve the book are always welcome.

Jeevitha Murugesh

Acknowledgements

This book owes its existence to many people. It gives me a great pleasure to thank all of them.

First and foremost I would like to thank Dr Narendranatha Reddy P, Founder-Director, Brihaspathi Academy, Bengaluru, for his strong support and encouragement. He has worked tirelessly for endless hours for the completion of this book. I find it hard to express my thanks in words.

My sincere thanks to Dr Asha and Dr Ajith of Brihaspathi Academy, Bengaluru, for their painstaking proofreading work of the book. Also Ms Chitra and Ms Shwetha of the Brihaspathi Academy for their untiring efforts in preparing the typescript.

I would like to thank my family and friends for their constant support and encouragement.

A special debt of thanks to CBS Publishers & Distributors particularly Mr YN Arjuna, Senior Director, Editorial and Publishing, and Mr SK Jain, Managing Director, for their endless support, and other staff of the publishing/production departments for their patience and efforts.

My sincere prayer of gratitude to the Almighty for giving me this opportunity.

Jeevitha Murugesh

Contents

Subjectwise Weightage Analysis

SUBJECT	TOTAL NUMBER OF MCQS APPEARED								
	2003	2004	2005	2006	2007	2008	2009	2010	2011
Anatomy	8	6	5	8	6	5	8	6	5
Physiology	6	4	7	7	8	4	4	5	7
Biochemistry	3	6	4	4	4	7	6	4	3
General Pathology	6	8	8	1	5	2	6	7	6
Microbiology	6	7	6	8	8	11	9	5	6
Pharmacology	7	6	5	8	7	7	8	6	7
General Medicine	11	10	15	13	9	11	9	8	11
General Surgery	9	6	8	6	9	7	7	8	11
Dental Materials	11	12	13	13	12	11	13	16	11
DADH	6	8	6	4	4	5	2	5	10
Oral Pathology & Oral Medicine	21	28	19	28	25	29	25	35	18
Oral Radiology	5	5	6	4	6	5	3	4	6
Orthodontics	15	14	19	14	16	12	11	11	12
Pedodontics	2	11	8	8	5	12	15	15	14
P & SD	16	15	15	15	17	16	17	15	15
Prosthodontics	16	15	13	11	16	16	15	14	14
Periodontics	16	14	14	16	14	17	20	15	15
Cons & Endo	13	11	15	18	16	14	13	9	14
Oral Surgery	15	14	15	14	13	9	9	12	15

List of Reference Textbooks Followed

Subject	Title of the Book	Author
Anatomy	Anatomy for Dental Students	BD Chaurasia
	Human Embryology	Arushi/Indu Khurana
	Textbook of Embryology	Inderbir Singh
	Di Fiore's Atlas of Histology	Victor P. Eroschenko
	Oral Anatomy	Sicher & Du Brul
	Atlas of Human Anatomy	Frank & Netter
	Manual of Practical Anatomy	Cunningham
	Anatomical Basis of Dentistry	Bernard Liebgott
	Textbook of Anatomy	AK Datta
	Osteology for Dental Students, 2e	Nafis Ahmad Faruqi
Physiology	Textbook of Medical Physiology	Guyton
	Textbook of Physiology for Dental Students, 2e	Marya/Marya
	Medical Physiology, 3e	RK Marya
	Essentials of Medical Physiology	Sembulingam
	Medical Physiology	A B Mahapatra
	Understanding Medical Physiology – A Textbook for Medical Students	RL Bijlani
Biochemistry	Textbook of Biochemistry with Biomedical Significance	PP Gupta
	Textbook of Biochemistry	U. Sathyanarayana U.Chakrapani
Pathology	Essential Pathology for Dental Students	Harsh Mohan
	Robbin's Pathologic Basis of Disease	Kumar, Abbas & Fausto
Microbiology	Textbook Microbiology for Dental Students, 3e	Arora
	Textbook of Microbiology	Ananthanarayan & Panicker
Pharmacology	Medical Pharmacology, 3e	Padmaja Udaykumar
	Essentials of Medical Pharmacology	KD Tripathi
	Pharmacology and Pharmacotherapeutics	R S Satoskar
General Medicine	Principles and Practice of Medicine	Sir Stanley Davidson
	Manipal Manual of Medicine for Dental Students	Shastry
	Principles of Internal Medicine	Harrison
	Pediatric Ophthalmology	Robison. D Harley

Contd...

Contd...

Subject	*Title of the Book*	*Author*
General Surgery	Manipal Manual of Surgery for Dental Students	Shenoy
	A Concise Textbook of Surgery	S Das
	Short Practice of Surgery	Bailey & Love
	General Surgery for Dental Students	Sukumar
Dental Materials	Craig's Restorative Dental Materials	John.M Powers & Ronald Sakaguchi
	Phillip's science of Dental Materials	Anusavice
	Dental Materials and their Selection	William O. Brien
	Science of Dental Materials: Clinical Applications	Sham Bhatt
	Basic Dental Materials	John Manappallil
Dental Anatomy	Wheeler's Dental Anatomy, Physiology and Occlusion	Ash & Nelson
Oral Histology	Ten Cate's Oral Histology Development, Structure and Function	Antonio Nanci
	Oral Anatomy, Histology and Embryology	Berkovitz Holland
	Oral Histology and Embryology	Orban
Oral Microbiology	Textbook of Oral Microbiology	KMK Masthan & N Arvindha Babu
Oral Pathology	Textbook of Oral Pathology	Shafer, Hine & Levy
	Oral and Maxillofacial Pathology	Neville, Damm & Allen
Oral Medicine	Burket's Oral Medicine, Diagnosis and Treatment	Greenberg
	Clinical Manual for Oral Diagnosis	Beena Varma
Oral Radiology	Oral Radiology—Principles and Interpretation	White & Pharoah
	Fundamentals of Dental Radiology	Vimal K Sikri
	Concise Oral Radiology	HR Umarji
Orthodontics	Orthodontics – The Art & Science	Bhalaji
	Contemporary Orthodontics	William.K.Proffit
	Textbook of Orthodontics	Gurkeerat Singh
	Current Orthodontic Concepts and Techniques	Graber & Vanarsdall
	Textbook of Orthodontics	Sameer. C. Bishala
Pedodontics	Textbook of Pedodontics	Shobha Tandon
	Dentistry for the Child & Adolescent	McDonald & Avery
	Pediatric Dentistry – Infancy through Adolescence	Pinkham
Preventive and Social Dentistry	Textbook of Community Medicine, 2e	Sunder Lal, Adarsh & Pankaj
	Public Health Dentistry	Poonam Sikri
	Textbook of Preventive Medicine	Park
	Essentials of Preventive and Community Dentistry	Soben Peter

Contd...

Contd...

Subject	*Title of the Book*	*Author*
	Dental Public Health: An introduction to Community Dental Health	Geoffrey. L Slack & BrianA Burt
	Common law tort and contract	Thomas Lundmark
	A Textbook of Children and Young People's nursing	Edward Vollen Gasper and Jim Richardson
	Community Dental Health	Anthony Jong
	Textbook of Preventive and Community Dentistry	Joseph John
Prosthodontics	Textbook of Prosthodontics	Nallasamy
	Textbook of Removable Partial Prosthodontics	Sharad Gupta
	Contemporary Fixed Prosthodontics	Rosensteil
	Prosthodontic Treatment for Edentulous Patients	Zarb and Bolender
	McCracken's Removable Partial Prosthodontics	McGivney & Castleberry
	Syllabus of Complete Dentures	Heartwell
	Essentials of Complete Denture Prosthodontics	Winkler
Periodontics	Glickman's Clinical Periodontology	Fermin A Carranza
Conservative Dentistry	Operative Dentistry, Modern Theory and Practice	Marzouk
	Pre-Clinical Conservative Dentistry	Vimal K Sikri
Operative Dentistry	Art and Science of Operative Dentistry	Sturdevant
	Textbook of Operative Dentistry, 2e	Vimal K Sikri
Endodontics	Endodontic Practice	Grossman
	Pathways of Pulp	Cohen
	Endodontics	Ingle & Backland
Oral Surgery	Textbook of Oral and Maxillofacial Surgery	Neelima Malik
	Practical Guide to Oral and Maxillofacial Surgery	Chandrakant P Taware
	Outline of Oral Surgery	Killey & Kay
	Textbook of Oral and Maxillofacial Surgery	Laskin
	Local Anaesthesia	Malamed
	Medical Emergencies in Dental Office	Malamed
	Local Anaesthesia	Monheim
	Minor Oral Surgery	Geoffrey.P.Howe
	Principles of Oral and Maxillofacial Surgery	Peterson
	Textbook of Oral and Maxillofacial Surgery	Kruger

1

KCET 2003

HUMAN ANATOMY

1. The only fixed cell of the connective tissue

A. Histiocyte
B. Lymphocyte
C. Polymorphs
D. Mast cell

2. Mature bone is otherwise called as

A. Woven bone
B. Lamellar bone
C. Irregular bone
D. Resorbing bone

3. The nerve supply of buccinator

A. The facial nerve
B. Mandibular nerve
C. Maxillary nerve
D. Auriculo temporal nerve

4. The weakest part of pharynx is

A. Sinus of Morgagni
B. Between thyropharyngeal and crico-pharyngeal sphincter
C. Piriform fossa
D. Pharyngeal recess

5. Thyroid gland develops from

A. Laryngo-tracheal diverticulum
B. Rathke's pouch
C. Buccinator muscle
D. Orbicularis oris muscle

6. Oral diaphragm is formed by

A. Mylohyoid muscle
B. Genioglossus muscle
C. Buccinator muscle
D. Orbicularis oris muscle

7. Supra–meatal triangle externally represents

A. Transverse sinus
B. Promontory of middle ear
C. Internal acoustic meatus
D. Mastoid antrum

8. Part of vertebral artery is related to

A. Superior cervical ganglion
B. Middle cervical ganglion
C. Stellate ganglion
D. Ciliary ganglion

PHYSIOLOGY

9. Percentage of body water is greater in

A. Females than in males
B. Children than in adults
C. Old than in young objects
D. Obese than in lean individuals

10. Sensitivity to local anesthetics is greater in

A. Type B fibers
B. Type C fibers
C. Type A delta fibers
D. Fibers supplying the muscle spindles

11. Deficiency of vitamin K leads to decreased activity of

A. Platelets
B. Coagulation factors II, V and VIII
C. Coagulation factors VII, IX and X
D. Fibrinolytic system

12. At high altitude the following changes take place EXCEPT

A. Increase in respiratory rate
B. Increase in depth of respiration

C. Increase in oxygen carrying capacity of blood
D. Increase in partial pressure of carbondioxide

13. Glucocorticoids have all the following actions EXCEPT
A. Increase in blood glucose level
B. Increase in protein catabolism
C. Anti-insulin action in peripheral tissues
D. Decreased glucose uptake by the Heart

14. Albumin is synthesized by
A. Liver
B. Muscle
C. Kidney
D. Spleen

BIOCHEMISTRY

15. Coenzyme A contains which of the following vitamin
A. Biotin
B. Pyridoxine
C. Pantothenic acid
D. Acetyl CoA

16. The amino acid from which niacin is synthesized
A. Tyrosine
B. Threonine
C. Tryptophan
D. Glucuronic acid

17. Bilirubin is conjugated with which of the following?
A. Glycine
B. Glutamine
C. Acetyl CoA
D. Glucuronic acid

GENERAL PATHOLOGY

18. Caseating granuloma is commonly seen in
A. Viral infections
B. Tuberculosis
C. Typhoid
D. Amoebiasis

19. The most definite feature of a malignant tumour is
A. Hemorrhage
B. Increased mitosis
C. Metastasis
D. Necrosis

20. Frozen sections can be used for the Demonstration of
A. Fat
B. Mucin
C. Cartilage
D. Iron

21. Increased proliferation of cells is called
A. Hypertrophy
B. Atrophy
C. Hyperplasia
D. Metaplasia

22. 'Nutmeg liver' is a term used to denote
A. Edema
B. Shock
C. Thrombosis
D. Chronic venous congestion

23. The increase in size of individual cells is referred to as
A. Hypertrophy
B. Hyperplasia
C. Anaplasia
D. Aplasia

MICROBIOLOGY

24. Sterilization of liquid paraffin is done by
A. Autoclaving
B. Hot air oven
C. UV radiation
D. Incineration

25. Multiple drug resistance of bacteria depends on which of the following
A. Resistance transfer factor (rtf)
B. Colicigenic factor (col)
C. Fertility factor (f)
D. All of the above

26. Both intranuclear and intracytoplasmic inclusion are present in which of the following

A. Pox virus
B. Measles virus
C. Hepatitis B virus
D. HIV

27. Afflatoxins are produced by

A. Aspergillus niger
B. Aspergillus fumigatus
C. Aspergillus flavus
D. All of the above

28. Which of the following is enrichment medium?

A. Blood agar
B. Selenite F broth
C. MacConkey agar
D. Nutrient broth

29. The most common organism related to dental caries is

A. Borrelia vincenti
B. Streptococcus mutans
C. *E. Coli*
D. Bacilli

PHARMACOLOGY

30. Ivermectin is indicated in

A. Scabies
B. Intestinal nematode infection
C. Filariasis
D. All of the above

31. Antibiotic of choice prior to dental procedure for the prophylaxis of endocarditis in adults is (Note: Patient is allergic to Penicillin and he is not able to take oral medicine)

A. Clarithromycin 500 mg 1 hour before dental procedure
B. Cephalexin 2 g 1 hour before dental procedures
C. Cefadroxil 2 g 1 hour before dental procedure
D. Clindamycin 600 mg 30 min before dental procedures

32. INFLIXIMAB (systemic treatment) is used in

A. Crohn's disease
B. To reduce the number of draining sinuses with enterocutaneous fistula in patients with fistulizing Crohn's disease
C. Rheumatoid arthritis (treatment)
D. All of the above

33. Triflusal

A. Anti-inflammatory drug
B. Antibiotic
C. Anti-arthritic drug
D. Anti platelet drug

34. Which of the benzodiazepine (BDZ) is comparatively safe in pregnancy

A. Alprazolam
B. Zolpidem
C. Lorazepam
D. None of the above

35. What is a suitable alternative antibiotic when a child is sensitive to penicillin?

A. Tetracycline
B. Erythromycin
C. Sulfanilamide
D. Ampicillin

36. Which of the following drugs CANNOT reduce the salivary secretion?

A. Amitriptyline
B. Disopyramide
C. Atenolol
D. Neostigmine

GENERAL MEDICINE

37. Malignant pustule is referred to

A. Facio–cervical actinomycosis
B. Cutaneous anthrax
C. Infected squamous cell carcinoma
D. None of the above

38. For diagnosis of acute rheumatic fever, essential feature is

A. Prior history of rheumatic fever
B. Recent sore throat infection
C. 1 major and 2 minor criteria
D. Erythema marginatum

39. **Petechiae in scurvy are due to**
   A. Platelet dysfunction
   B. Thrombocytopenia
   C. Endothelial disintegrity
   D. Erythrocyte margination

40. **Infective endocarditis is least likely to occur in**
   A. VSD
   B. ASD
   C. Tetralogy of fallot
   D. Coarctation of aorta

41. **Cardiac massage is usually done in the**
   A. Middle of sternum
   B. Lower 1/3 of sternum
   C. Manubrium
   D. Xiphisternum

42. **Most common opportunistic infection in AIDS is**
   A. Cryptococcosis
   B. Tuberculosis
   C. Candidiasis
   D. Aspergillosis

43. **Bleeding time is prolonged in**
   A. Hemophilia
   B. Von Willebrand's
   C. Henoch schonlein purpura
   D. Telengiectasia

44. **All of the following can be transmitted through blood transfusion EXCEPT**
   A. Malaria
   B. Leukemia
   C. Hepatitis
   D. AIDS

45. **Most important triad of symptoms in portal hypertension is**
   A. Splenomegaly, hepatomegaly and ascitis
   B. Splenomegaly, oesophageal varices and ascitis
   C. Piles, splenomegaly and general anasarca
   D. Oesophageal varices, piles and general anasarca

46. **Bone changes in hyperparathyroidism include**
   A. Generalized demineralization
   B. Brown tumor
   C. Cystic changes
   D. All of the above

47. **Serum alkaline phosphatase is elevated in all EXCEPT**
   A. Obstructive jaundice
   B. Heart disease
   C. Rickets
   D. Pregnancy

GENERAL SURGERY

48. **All the following nerves may be injured while doing excision of submandibular salivary gland EXCEPT**
   A. Lingual nerve
   B. Spinal accessory nerve
   C. Mandibular branch of facial nerve
   D. Hypoglossal nerve

49. **Sistrunk's operation is done for**
   A. Thyroglossal cyst
   B. Thyroglossal fistula
   C. Both of the above
   D. None of the above

50. **The ideal time for repair of cleft lip is**
   A. At birth
   B. Between 3–6 months of age
   C. At 1½ years of age
   D. At 1½ to 2 years of age

51. **The ideal time of repair of cleft of hard palate is**
   A. At birth
   B. Between 3–6 months of age
   C. Between 12–15 months of age
   D. After 2 years of age

52. **Lucid interval is characteristically seen in**
   A. Extradural hematoma
   B. Subdural hematoma
   C. Intracerebral hematoma
   D. None of the above

53. FNAC (Fine Needle Aspiration Cytology) can diagnose all the following EXCEPT
A. Papillary carcinoma of thyroid
B. Follicular carcinoma of thyroid
C. Anaplastic carcinoma of thyroid
D. Medullary carcinoma of thyroid

54. J. Cock's peculiar tumor is
A. Infected squamous cell carcinoma
B. Infected basal cell carcinoma
C. Infected, ulcerated sebaceous cyst
D. Infected, ulcerated dermoid cyst

55. All of the following are congenital cysts EXCEPT
A. External angular dermoid cyst
B. Sebaceous cyst
C. Branchial cyst
D. Thyroglossal cyst

56. Scan used preoperatively to localize parathyroid adenoma is
A. Thallium–Technetium scan
B. Radio–iodine scan
C. Technetium scan
D. Metal Iodo Benzyl Guanidine (MIBG) scan

DENTAL MATERIALS

57. In non zinc containing dental amalgam alloy the percentage of zinc present is
A. Less than 0.02%
B. Less than 0.1%
C. Less than 0.01%
D. None of the above

58. A uniform dispersion of minute droplets of one liquid within another liquid constitutes
A. Gels
B. Emulsions
C. Sols
D. Osmosis

59. When the two metals are completely miscible in the liquid state and they remain completely mixed on solidification, the alloy formed is called
A. Solid solution
B. Eutectic mixture
C. Peritectic mixture
D. Intermetallic compounds

60. The cleaning or etching solutions for acid etching are known as
A. Sealants
B. Bonding agents
C. Preconditioning solutions
D. Cleansing agents

61. The tin mercury phase formed during amalgamation is
A. Gamma phase
B. Gamma 1 phase
C. Gamma 2 phase
D. Alpha phase

62. The ability of the base to resist occlusal forces and to support the restoration is affected by
A. Compressive strength
B. Tensile strength
C. Young's modulus
D. Modulus of elasticity

63. The strength of the gypsum specimen when the water in excess of that required for the hydration of the hemihydrate is left in the specimen is called
A. Dry strength
B. Green strength
C. Water strength
D. Compressive strength

64. The plasticizer used in poly ether impression materials is
A. Poly ether polymer
B. Colloidal silica
C. Glycol ether
D. Di-vinyl polysiloxane (dimethyl siloxane)

65. Porosity formed due to simultaneous nucleations of solid grains and gas bubbles at the first moment that the metal freezes at the mold walls is called
A. Pinhole porosity
B. Gas inclusion porosity
C. Microporosity
D. Subsurface porosity

66. Strengthening of dental porcelain is done by
A. Increasing the compressive stress
B. Increasing the tensile stress
C. By introduction of residual compressive stresses into the surface of the material
D. By incorporating stress concentration

67. Austentite is an alloy of iron and carbon with the iron in
A. Alpha form
B. Beta form
C. Gamma form
D. None of the above

DENTAL ANATOMY AND HISTOLOGY

68. The transitory structure that is present in developing tooth germ
A. Enamel knot
B. Stratum intermedium
C. Cervical loop
D. All of the above

69. Secondary cementum is generally confined in
A. Cervical third of the root
B. Middle third of the root
C. Apical third of the root
D. No secondary cementum forms

70. The sequence of eruption of primary teeth is
A. ABCDE
B. ABDCE
C. ACBDE
D. ADBCE

71. The time taken for primary tooth root completion after eruption into oral cavity
A. 3 years
B. 1 year
C. 2 years
D. 1 month

72. The first sign of future deciduous teeth appears as a thickening of oral ectoderm of about
A. 25th day of intrauterine life
B. 34th day of intrauterine life
C. 56th day of intrauterine life
D. 20 weeks of intrauterine life

73. The stage of relatively rapid eruption from the time a tooth first penetrates the gingiva until it reaches the occlusal level is called
A. Pre emergent spurt
B. Post emergent spurt
C. Occlusal equilibrium
D. Dilaceration

ORAL PATHOLOGY AND ORAL MEDICINE

74. Complication of Vincent's angina is
A. Actinomycosis
B. Noma
C. Systemic candidiasis
D. Cellulitis

75. Teeth present at birth are called
A. Neonatal teeth
B. Primary teeth
C. Natal teeth
D. Accessory teeth

76. The most common teeth present at birth
A. Mandibular lateral incisor
B. Maxillary molars
C. Maxillary central incisors
D. Mandibular central incisors

77. Actinomycosis is a
A. Bacterial infection
B. Fungal infection
C. Viral infection
D. Parasitic infection

78. There may be multiple supernumerary teeth in one of the following conditions
A. Mongolism
B. Cleidocranial dysostosis
C. Hypothyroidism
D. Hypopituitarism

79. Bilateral symmetrical swelling of the mandible in a child is likely to be caused by
A. Acromegaly

B. Paget's disease
C. Cherubism
D. Dental cyst

80. Which of the following sugar present in the human diet is considered the most Caries promoting?
A. Sucrose
B. Fructose
C. Lactose
D. Glucose

81. Etiological factor for macro–glossia is
A. Atrophic glossitis
B. Oral submucous fibrosis
C. Syphilitic glossitis
D. Hurler's syndrome

82. NOT a type of lichen planus?
A. Atrophic
B. Reticular
C. Verrucous
D. Annular

83. Which clinical type of oral candidiasis has got the feature of white plaques that are scrapable?
A. Thrush
B. Erythematosus type
C. Hyperplastic type
D. None of the above

84. In which of the following type of tumor the HPV–6 can be detected?
A. Papilloma
B. CEOT
C. Sarcoma
D. Pyogenic granuloma

85. Naso Labial cyst is thought to arise from
A. Remnants of cell rests of Serre
B. Remnants of cell rests of Mallassez
C. Remnants of cell rests of embryonic lacrimal duct
D. Maxillary sinus lining epithelium

85. The circulating auto antibodies against the intercellular attachments of squamous epithelial cells are seen in
A. Scleroderma
B. Rheumatoid arthritis
C. Herpes zoster
D. Pemphigus vulgaris

87. The histiocytosis X is a spectrum of disorders which include the following condition
A. Eosinophilic granuloma
B. Hand Schuller–Christian disease
C. Letterer–Siwe disease
D. All of the above

88. Liesegang ring calcifications are seen in the following lesion
A. Amyloidosis
B. Pindborg tumor
C. Ossifying fibroma
D. Fibrous dysplasia

89. Hypodontia is a feature seen in
A. Gardener's syndrome
B. Ectodermal dysplasia
C. Paget's disease
D. Brown's tumor

90. Bell's palsy is triggered by
A. Exposure to cold
B. Tooth extraction
C. Local and systemic infection
D. Any of the above

91. Storiform pattern of fibrous tissue is seen in
A. Fibrosarcoma
B. Malignant fibrous histiocytoma
C. Neurofibroma
D. Ameloblastic fibroma

92. The following site is the common involvement in cases of myositis ossificans
A. Masseter
B. Hyoglossus
C. Stylohyoid
D. Lateral pterygoid

93. The risk of development of cancer is highest in the following lesions
A. Leukoplakia
B. Erythroplakia
C. Lichen planus
D. Leukoedema

94. **Lupus erythematosus is**
A. Reactive lesion
B. Degenerative condition
C. Auto immune disorder
D. Neoplastic condition

ORAL MEDICINE AND RADIOLOGY

95. **Nikolsky's sign is positive in**
A. Pemphigus
B. Recurrent Aphthous Stomatitis
C. Lichen planus
D. Erythema multiforme

96. **Normal serum alkaline phosphatase level is**
A. 100–400 Bodansky units
B. 1000–4000 Bodansky units
C. 0.1–0.4 Bodansky units
D. 1–4 Bodansky units

97. **Non–Neoplastic non–specific enlargement of the salivary gland**
A. Sialadenitis
B. Sialosis
C. Ptyalism
D. Sialorrhea

98. **Unusual extensibility of the tongue is a characteristic feature of**
A. Epidermolysis bullosa
B. Syphilis
C. Darier–White disease
D. Ehlers–Danlos syndrome

99. **Ectopic sebaceous glands in the mouth are called**
A. Linea alba buccalis
B. Heck's disease
C. Lingual varices
D. Fordyce spots

100. **Which is NOT a feature of Crest syndrome?**
A. Calcinosis
B. Endocrinopathies
C. Raynaud's phenomenon
D. Sclerodactyly

101. **Facial pain due to elongated Styloid process is called**
A. Cowden syndrome
B. Tic Dolorouex
C. Eagle's syndrome
D. Reiter's syndrome

102. **The term anamnesis is related to**
A. Diagnosis
B. Prognosis
C. Control
D. Prevention

ORAL RADIOLOGY

103. **Mathematical representation of inverse square law is**
A. $I_2/ I_1 = (D_2)^2/ (D_1)2$
B. $I_1/ I_2 = (D_2)^2/ (D_1)2$
C. $I_2/ I_1 = D_2/ D_1$
D. $I_1/ I_2 = D_2/ D_1$

104. **X–rays are produced at**
A. Anode
B. Cathode
C. Glass wall
D. Molybdenum focusing cup

105. **Quality of the X–ray beam is governed by**
A. KVp
B. mA
C. Filament current
D. Length of the X–ray tube

106. **Which is NOT a property of X–ray?**
A. Ionization
B. Action on photographic film
C. Excitation
D. Collimation

107. **Crimp marks in a radiograph are due to**
A. Droplets of fixing solution
B. Droplets of developing solution
C. Static electricity
D. Sharp bending of the film

ORTHODONTICS

108. Primate spaces present in primary dentition are

A. Inter dental space present in upper and lower anteriors
B. Spaces present mesial to lower canine and distal to upper canine
C. Space present distal to lower 1st molar and mesial to upper 1st molar
D. Space present distal to lower canine and mesial to upper canine

109. In primary dentition the anatomic structure used to determine the molar relationship

A. Mesio buccal cusp of primary 2nd molar
B. Distal plane of primary 1st molar
C. Mesial surface plane of primary 1st molar
D. Distal plane of primary 2nd molar

110. Midline diastema of maxillary central incisors at the age of 9 is indicative of

A. Mesiodens
B. Ugly duckling stage
C. Abnormal labial frenum
D. Any of the above

111. Cleft lip occurs due to non–union of

A. Maxillary and frontonasal process
B. Maxillary process and mandibular process
C. Maxillary process and palatine process
D. Frontonasal process and palatine process

112. The holding of teeth in an ideal aesthetic and functional positions is

A. Ideal occlusion
B. Normal occlusion
C. Retention
D. Functional occlusion

113. Apertognathia means

A. Anterior cross bite
B. Open bite
C. Posterior cross bite
D. Prognathism

114. Serial extraction is indicated in patients who have

A. Class II molar relation
B. Excessive overbite
C. Class I molar relation
D. Class III molar relation

115. Force maintained at some appreciable fraction of the original from one patient visit to the next is

A. Continuous force
B. Intermittent force
C. Interrupted force
D. None of the above

116. The Adam's clasp is made of 22 gauge wire or 0.7 mm or

A. 24 mil wire
B. 28 mil wire
C. 23 mil wire
D. 22 mil wire

117. Beta–titanium, an excellent choice for auxillary springs is nothing but

A. Nitinol
B. TMA
C. A–NiTi
D. Sentinol

118. Ectopic eruption is most likely to occur in

A. Eruption of maxillary first molars
B. Mandibular canines
C. Maxillary lateral incisors
D. Maxillary canines

119. The term Orthodontics was coined by

A. Hunter
B. Le foulon of France
C. Carabelli
D. Norman Kingsley

120. The relative mesial or distal angulations of the crown and the root along the line of force is called

A. Torque
B. Tip
C. Offset
D. Inclination of teeth

121. **Possible indicator of pubertal growth spurt on hand wrist films is sought as**
   A. Ossification of adductor sesamoid
   B. Appearance of hook of hamate
   C. Ossification of all the carpal bones
   D. Ossification of pisiform

122. **The point of intersection of dorsal contours of Mandibular processes and occipital bone is**
   A. Supramentale
   B. Articulare
   C. Condylion
   D. Pterygomaxillary

PEDODONTICS

123. **Some of the cause for recurrent salivary gland swelling is**
   A. Pleomorphic adenoma
   B. Abscess
   C. Punctuate sialectasis
   D. Frey's syndrome

124. **In a case of rampant caries the ideal procedure to perform in the first visit is**
   A. Diet control instructions
   B. Topical fluoride application
   C. Gross excavation and restoration of Teeth
   D. None of the above

P AND SD

125. **Which of the following level of fluorides in drinking water is associated with enamel Fluorosis?**
   A. 0.2 ppm
   B. 0.7 ppm
   C. 2.5 ppm
   D. 1.2 ppm

126. **A Gaussian distribution is**
   A. Normal distribution
   B. Log normal distribution
   C. Poisson distribution
   D. Variant distribution

127. **The type II error is the acceptance of a null hypothesis is true when it is**
   A. True
   B. Nonexistent
   C. Negative value
   D. False

128. **Sensitivity is usually expressed in**
   A. Units
   B. Alphabets
   C. Ascending order
   D. Percentage

129. **Secondary level of prevention includes**
   A. Health promotion
   B. Vaccination
   C. Early diagnosis and prompt treatment
   D. Rehabilitation

130. **If the ¼ is outside the 95% confidence limits with Normal deviation >2 then P will be**
   A. 0.05
   B. <0.05
   C. >0.05
   D. None of the above

131. **The tooth brushing method least likely to remove plaque in the gingival margin is the**
   A. Sulcular method
   B. Scrub method
   C. Modified still man
   D. Roll stroke

132. **Priority of five levels in relation to motivation was advocated by**
   A. Herzberg
   B. FW Taylor
   C. Douglas McGregor
   D. AH Winslow

133. **Hospital gives**
   A. Primary health care
   B. Comprehensive health care
   C. Specialized services
   D. Health education

134. Waste water from kitchen is

A. Sullage
B. Sewage
C. Garbage
D. Kitchen water

135. Residual chlorine of water should be

A. 1 mg/ltr after 1 hours
B. 1 mg/ltr after 2 hours
C. 0.5 mg/ltr after 1 hours
D. 0.5 mg/ltr after 2 hours

136. Removal of bacteria is

A. Better with slow sand filter
B. Better with rapid sand filter
C. Equal with both
D. Depends on hardness of water

137. A series may have all EXCEPT

A. No mode
B. One mode
C. Many modes
D. Negative mode

138. Correlation coefficient can range from

A. 0 to +1
B. 0 to 100
C. –1 to +1
D. –1 to 100

139. When sample size increases standard deviation

A. Decreases
B. Increases
C. Remains the same
D. May increase or decrease

140. In a 3 × 3 table, the number of degrees of freedom is

A. 4
B. 9
C. 3
D. 6

PROSTHODONTICS

141. Endosseous implants are examples of ridge

A. Preservation
B. Extension
C. Augmentation
D. Reconstruction

142. A simplified pantograph measures the following components

A. All the mandibular movements
B. Relationship of fossae in the temporo-mandibular joint
C. Hinge axis
D. Condylar inclination and mandibular side shift

143. Indicated finish margin with porcelain fused to metal restoration is

A. Shoulder
B. Labial shoulder with chamfer lingually
C. Heavy shoulder
D. Heavy chamfer

144. A device known as gothic arch tracer is used to record the mandibular movement in

A. Vertical plane
B. Horizontal plane
C. Sagittal plane
D. Transverse plane

145. The process of achieving limited removal of epithelial tissue in the sulcus while creating chamfer finish margin is called

A. Rotary curettage
B. Mechanic–surgical gingival retraction
C. Electro surgery
D. Periodontal curettage

146. The standard perforated tray for use with alginate impression materials may be brought to more customized contour by

A. Utility wax
B. Base plate wax
C. Beading wax
D. Boxing wax

147. The concept of lingualized occlusion was suggested by

A. Gysi
B. Mc Grane
C. Sears
D. Payne

148. The posterior speaking space was suggested by

A. Pound
B. Mc Grane
C. Niswonger
D. Silverman

149. Which of the following is an example of static method of recording centric relation?

A. Intra oral records
B. Needle house
C. Patterson
D. All of the above

150. The concept of occlusion that maintained the antero posterior plane of occlusion should be parallel with the denture foundation and not dictated by the horizontal condylar guidance is called

A. Lingualised concept
B. Balanced concept
C. Neutrocentric concept
D. Mutually protected concept

151. The use of selected initial roots in denture therapy is called

A. Overlay denture therapy
B. Biologic denture therapy
C. Submucosal vital root retention
D. Submerged denture therapy

152. Long span distal extension bases where rigidity is critical the major connector of choice is

A. Palatal strap
B. Antero posterior palatal bar
C. Closed horse shoe
D. Horse shoe

153. Ideally the depth of undercut on the proposed abutment teeth at the most desired location is

A. 0.010 inch
B. 0.015 inch
C. 0.020 inch
D. 0.030 inch

154. The abutment teeth that are to have cast inlays are classified as

A. Class I
B. Class II
C. Class III
D. Class IV

155. A ledge is created on the lingual surface of the full cast crown to accommodate the lingual clasp arm. The greatest advantage is that it provides

A. Appropriate contact
B. Appropriate under cut
C. Survey line
D. Guiding plane

156. The clasp most often used on the mandibular bicuspids when the most favorable retentive undercut is on the disto–buccal surface adjacent to edentulous area is

A. Ring clasp
B. Reverse loop clasp
C. Simple circlet clasp
D. Reverse approach circlet clasp

PERIODONTICS

157. Which of the following organisms predominant in early stage of plaque formation

A. Cocci
B. Filamentous colony
C. Actinomyces
D. Spirochete

158. Plaque lodged inter proximally is best removed by

A. Tooth brush
B. Mouth wash
C. Dental floss
D. Irrigation

159. The concept of oral prophylaxis and prevention in periodontal therapy was developed by

A. John W. Riggs
B. G. V. Black
C. Berhard Gottilieb
D. J. Leon Williams

160. The basal cells of the junctional epithelium show signs of proliferation and rete peg form in
- A. Stage I gingivitis
- B. Stage II gingivitis
- C. Stage III gingivitis
- D. Stage IV gingivitis

161. In periodontal disease, calculus is considered as
- A. Contributing factor
- B. Primary factor
- C. Etiological factor
- D. Governing factor

162. Povidine iodine is the choice of mouth rinse in cases associated with AIDS because
- A. It is a topical antimicrobial
- B. It is a topical anesthetic
- C. Its ability to aid in blood coagulation
- D. All of the above

163. Reactive ingredient present in tartar control tooth paste is
- A. Pyrophosphate
- B. Metaphosphate
- C. Carboxy methyl
- D. Bicarbonate

164. Computerized periodontal probe is
- A. CPITN probe
- B. Florida probe
- C. Michigan probe
- D. Jeffcoat probe

165. The pattern of bone destruction in periodontitis is determined by
- A. Depth of the pocket
- B. Suppuration
- C. Pathway of inflammation
- D. Composition of plaque

166. Instrumentation zone in periodontal therapy is
- A. The portion of the tooth where calculus (or) altered cementum is found
- B. CE Junction
- C. Exposed root surfaces
- D. Epithelial lining of periodontal pocket

167. Periochip is a commercially available local drug delivery system containing
- A. Doxycycline
- B. Chlorhexidine
- C. Minocycline
- D. Metronidazole

168. Lateral positioning of flap is done for
- A. Gingival recession
- B. High frenal attachment
- C. Increasing the width of attached gingiva
- D. Shallow vestibule

169. Bioglass is used in
- A. Root biomodification
- B. Resective osseous surgery
- C. Regenerative osseous surgery
- D. Mucogingival surgery

170. If an implant has lost some bone support, but bone loss is arrested, it is termed as
- A. Failed implant
- B. Failing implant
- C. Ailing implant
- D. Biointegration

171. Type of periodontitis which does not respond to therapy is
- A. Refractory periodontitis
- B. Juvenile periodontitis
- C. Rapidly progressive periodontitis
- D. Chronic adult periodontitis

172. Bio–brane is a commercially available as
- A. Root matrix protein
- B. Biodegradable membrane
- C. Bone graft material
- D. Non–bone graft material

CONS AND ENDO

173. The ratio of 1.618 to 1 constant which is used as a guide for dental esthetics is
- A. Golden proportion
- B. Geometric formula
- C. Fibonacci ratio
- D. Youthful ratio

174. When dental bur is sterilized by autoclaving, chemical used for protection of bur

A. Sodium nitrate
B. Sodium nitrite
C. Silver nitrate
D. Silver nitrite

175. In which of the condition "Piggy Back" wedging is indicated?

A. Proximal caries with gingival recession
B. Tooth with fluted surface
C. Class II with wide proximal box
D. Narrow class II cavity

176. Which of the following is a caries detector dye?

A. 1% basic fuschin in propylene glycol
B. 1% acid red in propylene glycol
C. 1% basic fuschin in ethylene glycol
D. 1% acid red in ethylene glycol

177. The limit of urinary mercury in microgram/g of creatinine attributed to extensive amalgam restoration is

A. 1 microgram/g of creatinine
B. 3 microgram/g of creatinine
C. 2 microgram/g of creatinine
D. 4 microgram/g of creatinine

178. Tick the odd one

A. Degassing
B. Desorbing
C. Annealing
D. Metalizing

179. Endo–extractor kit is a modification of

A. Endodontic plugger
B. Masserann kit
C. Endo box
D. Rubber dam kit

180. Tail file is also known as

A. Barbed broach
B. H file
C. R file
D. Rat file

181. The color code for No. 6 endodontic file is

A. White
B. Purple
C. Grey
D. Pink

182. Thymosin is a type of

A. Surgical curette
B. Miniature hand piece
C. Retrograde amalgam carrier
D. Retrograde amalgam condenser

183. Tick the odd one out

A. Abfraction
B. Crazing
C. Infraction
D. Infarction

184. Ruddle's solution is used as irrigating solution

A. In non vital bleaching
B. In vital bleaching
C. As Irrigation solution
D. For endo gram

185. For the balance of hand cutting instrument

A. Cutting edges of the working end should be centered over the long axis of the handle
B. The cutting edge centered on a line running at right angle to the long axis of the handle
C. It should have shorter, straighter shank
D. It should have solid handle

ORAL SURGERY

186. Leubke–Ochsenbein flap for periapical surgery is known as

A. Trapezoidal flap
B. Rectangular flap with sulcular incision
C. Submarginal flap
D. Triangular flap

187. Extra oral sutures should be removed around the .... day

A. Seventh
B. Third
C. Fourteenth
D. Tenth

188. Better healing of severely contused tissue occurs following

A. Extensive debridement
B. Thorough trimming of wound edges
C. Cleaning with strong antiseptics
D. Minimum debridement

189. An example of a synthetic absorptive suture is

A. Chronic catgut
B. Polyethylene
C. Polyglycolic acid
D. Polyamide

190. In cases of hypoglycemic coma induced by hypoglycemic drugs, which of the following may be tried if glucose for intravenous infusion is not available

A. Subcutaneous injection of 0.5 mg 1:1000 adrenaline
B. Subcutaneous injection of 1 mg of glucagon
C. Both of the above
D. None of the above

191. The drug of choice in the management of life threatening allergic reaction is

A. Corticosteroids
B. Antihistamines
C. Adrenaline
D. Diazepam

192. Walsham's forceps are used to

A. Remove teeth
B. Remove root
C. Clamp blood vessels
D. Reduce nasal bone fractures

193. Inferior alveolar nerve block is absolutely contra indicated in patients suffering from one of the following diseases

A. Thrombocytopenia
B. Hemophilia
C. Hypoprothrombinaemia
D. Von Willebrand's disease

194. The American Heart Association recommendation for infective endocarditis prophylaxis before minor surgeries is

A. 2 gms of amoxicillin
B. 3 gms of amoxicillin
C. 3 gms of amoxicillin followed by 500 mg after 6 hours
D. 2 gms of amoxicillin followed by 500 mg after 6 hours

195. The fascial space that is divided by the styloid process into an anterior and posterior compartment is

A. Pterygomandibular
B. Lateral pharyngeal
C. Retropharyngeal
D. Infratemporal

196. An absolute contraindication for extraction of teeth is

A. Hypertension
B. Myocardial infarction
C. Thyrotoxicosis
D. Central haemangioma

197. The cyst is 'deroofed' and the surrounding periosteum sutured to the margins of the cyst wall in

A. Decortication
B. Marsupialization
C. Saucerization
D. Enucleation

198. Bleeding from the ears is a sign in one of the following fractures

A. Condylar
B. Le Fort I
C. Le Fort II
D. Le Fort III

199. Saggital split osteotomy is a procedure done in the mandibular

A. Ramus
B. Body
C. Symphysis
D. Angle

200. After an extraction of teeth, ideally radiotherapy for oral cancer should be delayed for

A. Two weeks
B. Six weeks
C. One week
D. Three weeks

ANSWERS

HUMAN ANATOMY

1. **Ans: A**

   Ref: Di Fiore's Atlas of Histology, 11/E, p. 57

   Explanation
   - Histiocytes are fixed macrophages

2. **Ans: B**

   Ref: Osteology, RN Bajpai, 1/E, p. 4

3. **Ans: A**

   Ref: Sicher and DuBrul's Oral Anatomy, 8/E, p. 104

   Explanation
   - All the muscles of facial expression are supplied by the facial nerve which is the motor nerve of the face

4. **Ans: B**

   Ref: BD Chaurasia, 1/E, p. 328

   Explanation
   - Killian's dehiscense is the area in the posterior wall of pharynx the lower part of thyropharyngeus is a single sheet of muscle, not overlapped internally by upper and middle constrictors, it is limited inferiorly by the thick cricopharyngeal sphincter

5. **Ans: A**

   Ref: BD Chaurasia, 1/E, p. 280

6. **Ans: A**

   Ref: Sicher and DuBrul's Oral Anatomy, 8/E, p. 96

   Explanation
   - The mylohyoid muscle forms anatomically and functionally, the floor of oral cavity, hence it was termed as *oral diaphragm*

7. **Ans: D**

   Ref: BD Chaurasia, 1/E, p. 358

8. **Ans: C**

   Ref: BD Chaurasia, 1/E, p. 309

   Explanation
   - The first and second part of vertebral artery is related to stellate ganglion

PHYSIOLOGY

9. **Ans: B**

   Ref: Sembulingam, 4/E, p.47

   Explanation
   - Totally body water is 45–75% of body weight

10. **Ans: B**

    Ref: Ganong's, 23/E, p. 89

11. **Ans: C**

    Ref: Sembulingam, 4/E, p. 114

    Explanation
    - Vitamin K dependent clotting factors are II, VII, IX and X

12. **Ans: D**

    Ref: Guyton's, 11/E, p. 538–540

13. **Ans: D**

    Ref: Sembulingam, 4/E, p. 397

    Explanation

    Actions of Glucocorticoid
    - Carbohydrate metabolism
      - Promotes gluconeogenesis from amino acids
      - Inhibits glucose uptake (anti insulin action)
    - Protein metabolism
      - Decreases protein synthesis

- Accelerates protein catabolism
- Increases transport of amino acids

- Fat metabolism
  - Mobilization of fatty acids from adipose tissue
  - Increases concentration of fatty acids in blood
  - Increases utilization of fat from energy

14. Ans: A

Ref: Sembulingam, 4/E, p. 58

Explanation

- Plasma proteins are synthesized mainly from reticuloendothelial cells of liver

BIOCHEMISTRY

15. Ans: C

Ref: U. Sathyanarayana, U. Chakrapani, 3/E, p. 148

16. Ans: C

Ref: U. Sathyanarayana, U. Chakrapani, 3/E, p. 138

Explanation

- Niacin or Nicotinic acid is also known as Pellagra preventive factor of Goldberg
- The coenzyme of niacin (NAD^+ and NADP) can be synthesized by the essential amino acid tryptophan

17. Ans: D

Ref: U. Sathyanarayana, U. Chakrapani, 3/E, p. 216

Explanation

- In the liver, Bilirubin is conjugated with two molecules of glucuronate supplied by UDP glucuronate. This reaction is catalyzed by Bilirubin glucuronyl transferase (of smooth ER), that results in formation of a water soluble Bilirubin diglucuronide

GENERAL PATHOLOGY

18. Ans: B

Ref: Harsh Mohan, 3/E, p. 37

19. Ans: C

Ref: Harsh Mohan, 3/E, p. 238

20. Ans: A

Ref: Harsh Mohan, 3/E, p. 10

Explanation

- Cryostat or frozen section eliminates all the steps of tissue processing and paraffin embedding.
- The tissue is frozen to ice at about – 25°C which acts as embedding medium and then sectioned and stained.
- It used for the demonstration of fat, enzymes, etc.

21. Ans: C

Ref: Harsh Mohan, 3/E, p. 231

22. Ans: D

Ref: Robbin's Pathologic Basis of Disease, 7/E, p. 122

23. Ans: A

Ref: Harsh Mohan, 3/E, p. 231

MICROBIOLOGY

24. Ans: B

Ref: Ananthanarayan and Panicker's Text Book of Microbiology, 8/E, p. 31

25. Ans: A

Ref: Ananthanarayan and Panicker's Text Book of Microbiology, 8/E, p. 66

26. Ans: B

Ref: Ananthanarayan and Panicker's Text Book of Microbiology, 8/E, p. 444

Explanation

- During multiplication of virus in host cells, virus specified structures are produced and they are called Inclusion bodies
- They may be intracytoplasmic and intranuclear inclusions

Intracytoplasmic

1. Vaccinia – Gaurnier's bodies
2. Fowl pox – bollinger bodies
3. Molluscum contagiosum–molluscum bodies
4. Rabies – negri bodies

Intranuclear

1. Cowdry type A – herpes, yellow fever virus
2. Cowdry type B – adenovirus, poliovirus

Both

1. Measles virus
2. Basophilic inclusion bodies are found in adenovirus

27. Ans: C

Ref: Ananthanarayan and Panicker's Text Book of Microbiology, 8/E, p. 614

28. Ans: B

Ref: Ananthanarayan and Panicker's Text Book of Microbiology, 8/E, p. 40

29. Ans: B

Ref: Ananthanarayan and Panicker's Text Book of Microbiology, 8/E, p. 217

PHARMACOLOGY

30. Ans: D

Ref: KD Tripathi, 6/ E, p. 813

31. Ans: D

Ref: KD Tripathi, 6/ E, p. 681

32. Ans: D

Ref: KD Tripathi, 6/E, p. 205

Explanation

- It is a chimera monoclonal antibody which binds and neutralizes TM-±
- *Dosage:* 3–5 mg IV every 4 – 8 weeks

33. Ans: D

Ref: Stroke–Practical Management, C Warlow, 3/E, p. 830

Explanation:

- Triflusal is structurally related to aspirin and exerts its antiplatelet effect mainly through inhibition of platelet cyclo oxygenase. It is also involved in platelet aggregation to increase nitric oxide synthesis

34. Ans: A

Ref: KD Tripathi, 6/E, p. 450

35. Ans: B

Ref: KD Tripathi, 6/E, p. 729

36. Ans: D

Ref: KD Tripathi, 6/ E, p. 101

Explanation

- Neostigmine is a reversible anti-cholinesterase and prevents the breakdown of acetylcholine. Therefore it causes excessive salivation

GENERAL MEDICINE

37. Ans: B

Ref: Harrison, 17/E, Vol I, p. 1344

38. Ans: C

Ref: Davidson, 20/E, p. 616

Explanation

- The diagnosis of rheumatic fever, according to the revised Jones criteria is based upon two or more major criteria or one major and two or more minor criteria

39. Ans: C

Ref: Davidson, 20/E, p. 125

Explanation

- Defective formation of collagen impairs healing, that causes capillary haemorrhage and reduced platelet adhesiveness (normal platelets are rich in ascorbate)

40. Ans: B

Ref: Davidson, 20/E, p. 629

41. Ans: B

Ref: Harrison, 17/E,Vol. II, p. 1712

42. Ans: C

Ref: Davidson, 20/E, p. 384

43. Ans: B

Ref: Harrison, 17/E, Vol. I, p. 366

44. Ans: B

Ref: Davidson, 20/E, p. 1039

Explanation

- Leukemias are malignant disorders of the hematopoietic stem cell compartment associated with increased number of white cells in bone marrow and peripheral blood
- It is not transmitted through blood transfusions

45. Ans: B

Ref: Harrison, 17/E, Vol. II, p. 1976

46. Ans: D

Ref: Harrison, 17/E, Vol.II, p. 2382

47. Ans: C

Ref: Davidson, 20/E, p. 1127

GENERAL SURGERY

48. Ans: B

Ref: S. Das, 5/E, p. 613

Explanation

- *Rule of Two* followed while excising submandibular gland.

1. *Two common indications* – sialolith, radical neck dissection
2. *Protect two superficial nerves* – cervical and mandibular branches of facial nerve
3. *Protect two deep nerves* – lingual and Hypoglossal
4. *Divide two muscles* – platysma (superficial) and mylohyoid (deep)

49. Ans: C

Ref: S. Das, 5/E, p. 672

50. Ans: B

Ref: S. Das, 5/E, p. 598

Explanation

- It is generally advisable to perform at the age of 3 months when the baby is 5–6 kg

51. Ans: C

Ref: S. Das, 5/E, p. 601

52. Ans: A

Ref: S. Das, 5/E, p. 550

Explanation

- With advancing age, the duramater becomes more adherent to the scar and the hematoma takes sometimes to form, which is considered as *"lucid interval"*

53. Ans: B

Ref: S. Das, 5/E, p. 652

Explanation

- FNAC cannot distinguish between a benign follicular adenoma and follicular carcinoma as this distinction is mainly dependent on histology

54. Ans: C

Ref: S. Das, 5/E, p. 81

Explanation

- The formation of sebaceous cyst of the scalp and ulcerated excessive granulation tissue resembles fungating epithelioma. This is called as cock's peculiar tumour.

55. Ans: B

Ref: S. Das, 5/E, p. 76

56. Ans: A

Ref: S. Das, 5/E, p. 675

DENTAL MATERIALS

57. Ans: B

Ref: Phillips, 11/E, p. 496

58. Ans: B

Ref: Phillips, 11/E, p. 231

Explanation

- Emulsion: liquid in liquid

59. Ans: A

Ref: Phillips, 11/E, pp. 121 and 124

Explanation

- *Solid solution* – when the metals completely soluble in solid state. For example: Ag - Pd
- *Peritectic alloys* – when this limited solubility is accompanied by property of transformation at a particular temperature. For example: Ag - Sn
- *Hypoperitectic alloys* – Liquid $+\beta \rightarrow$ Liquid $+ \alpha$

60. Ans: C

Ref: Phillips, 11/E, pp – 383 and 384

Explanation

- Widely used surface conditioning agent is 37% phosphoric acid

61. Ans: C

Ref: Phillips, 11/E, p. 502

Explanation

1. γ - Ag_3Sn
2. γ_1 - Ag_2Hg_3
3. γ_2 - $Sn_{7-8}Hg$
4. η - Cu_6Sn_5
5. ε - Cu_3Sn

62. Ans: A

Ref: Phillips, 11/E, p. 460

Explanation

- Dental cements develop sufficient strength to resist condensation forces when they attain an initial set after 7 min

63. Ans: B

Ref: Phillips, 11/E, p. 271

Explanation

- *Wet strength or Green strength* is the strength obtained when the water in excess of that required for hydration of the hemihydrates is left
- *Dry strength* is when the excess water in the specimen may be two or more times as high as wet strength

64. Ans: C

Ref: Phillips, 11/E, p. 216

Explanation

- ***Polyether***
  - *First elastomer* to be used as an impression material
  - *Main chain* – copolymer of ethylene. oxide and tetrahydrofuron
  - *Initiator* – aromatic sulfonate ester
  - *Fillers* – colloidal silica
  - *Plasticizer* – glycol ether and phthalate

65. Ans: D

Ref: Phillips, 11/E, p. 346

Explanation

- Pin hole and gas inclusion porosities are due to the entrapment of gas during solidification
- Microporosity occurs from solidification shrinkage

66. Ans: C

Ref: Phillips, 11/E, p. 697

Explanation

Methods of strengthening dental porcelain

1. *Ion exchange* – introducing residual compressive strengths into the surface of a ceramic; also called as *Chemical tempering*
2. *Thermal tempering* – creates residual compressive stresses by rapidly cooling (quenching) the surface of object while it was in hot and softened (molten) state
3. *Dispersion strengthening* to reinforce them with a dispersed phase of a different material that is capable of hindering a crack from propagating through the material
4. *Transformation toughening* – when a small tough crystals are homogenously distributed in a glass, the ceramic structure is toughened because cracks cannot penetrate the fine particles easily

67. Ans: C

Ref: Phillips, 11/E, p. 639

DADH

68. Ans: A

Ref: Orban's, 12/E, p. 26

Explanation

- Cells in the centre of enamel organ are densely formed, called enamel knot
- Enamel knot and chord act as reservoir for the growing enamel organ

69. Ans: C

Ref: Orban's, 12/E, p. 142

Explanation

- Cellular cementum is also known as secondary cementum
- It is found in apical third of the root
- It is of 2 types
  - Cellular mixed fiber cementum
  - Cellular intrinsic fiber cementum

70. Ans: B

Ref: Wheeler's, 8/E, p. 38

71. Ans: B

Ref: Wheeler's, 8/E, p. 54

72. Ans: C

Ref: Orban's, 12/E, p. 22

Explanation

- At about 7th week, the primary epithelial band divides into an inner (lingual) process called dental lamina and outer (buccal) process called vestibular lamina
- The dental lamina serve as the primordium for the ectodermal portion of the deciduous teeth

73. Ans: B

Ref: Orban's, 12/E, p. 282

ORAL PATHOLOGY AND ORAL MEDICINE

74. Ans: B

Ref: Neville, 3/E, p. 205

75. Ans:

Ref: Neville, 3/E, p. 72

Explanation

- Natal teeth – present at birth
- Neonatal Teeth – within 30 days after birth

76. Ans: D

Ref: Neville, 3/E, p. 72

77. Ans: A

Ref: Shafer's, 6/E, p. 318

78. Ans: B

Ref: Shafer's, 6/E, p. 46

Explanation

- Multiple supernumerary teeth are seen in the following conditions
  1. Cleft lip and palate

2. Cleidocranial dysplasia
3. Gardener's syndrome

79. **Ans: C**

Ref: Shafer's, 6/E, p. 712

80. **Ans: A**

Ref: Shafer's, 6/E, p. 430

81. **Ans: D**

Ref: Shafer's, 6/E, p. 630

Explanation

Macroglossia is also seen in following aspects

1. Congenital or Developmental
   - Mongolism
   - Lingual thyroid
2. Inflammatory
   - Syphilis
   - Amoebic dysentery
   - Ludwig's angina
   - Pneumonia
   - Typhoid
   - Tuberculosis
   - Infected wound
   - Actinomycosis
3. Neoplasms
   - Hemangioma (diffuse)
   - Neurofibromatosis
   - Lymphangioma (diffuse)
4. Systemic
   - Pellagra
   - Down's syndrome
   - Myxedema
   - Acromegaly
   - Uremia
   - Gardener's syndrome
   - Diabetes
   - Scurvy
   - Dyskinesia chorea
   - Melkerson–Rosenthal syndrome
   - Sturge Weber syndrome
   - Hurler's syndrome
   - Beckwith's syndrome
   - Tuberous syndrome

82. **Ans: C**

Ref: Shafer's, 6/E, p. 601

83. **Ans: A**

Ref: Shafer's, 6/E, pp. 363 and 364

84. **Ans: A**

Ref: Shafer's, 6/E, p. 80

85. **Ans: C**

Ref: Shafer's, 6/E, p. 66

Explanation

- The nasolabial/nasoalveolar/ Kelstadt's cyst is not found within bone
- It arises at the junction of the globular process, lateral nasal process and the maxillary process as a result of proliferation of entrapped epithelium along the fusion line
- It may probably originate from the lower anterior part of the Nasolacrimal duct

86. **Ans: D**

Ref: Shafer's, 6/E, p. 817

87. **Ans: D**

Ref: Shafer's, 6/E, p. 743

Explanation

The clinical spectrum of histiocytosis X includes

- *Chronic and indolent* – Eosinophilic granuloma
- *Intermediate* – Hand Schuller Christian disease
- *Acute and fulminant* – Letterer Siwe disease

88. **Ans: B**

Ref: Shafer's, 6/E, p. 281

89. **Ans: B**

Ref: Shafer's, 6/E, p. 46

90. Ans: D

Ref: Neville, 3/E, p. 860

91. Ans: B

Ref: Shafer's, 6/E, p. 158

Explanation
- In malignant fibrous histiocytoma, the arrangement of spindle cells is seen as a storiform or criss cross pattern on low power magnification

92. Ans: A

Ref: Shafer's, 6/E, p. 860

Explanation
- The masseter muscle is often involved so that fixation of the jaw occurs
- The patient becomes transformed into a rigid organism sometimes encountered in circuses called "Petrified Man"
- Interestingly certain muscles tend to escape involvement, i.e. the larynx, diaphragm and perianal muscles

93. Ans: B

Ref: Shafer's, 6/E, p. 88

94. Ans: C

Ref: Shafer's, 6/E, p. 827

95. Ans: A

Ref: Shafer's, 6/E, p. 817

Explanation
- Nikolsky's sign is the loss of epithelium occasionally by rubbing apparently unaffected skin
- It is a characteristic feature of Pemphigus and is called by prevesicular edema which disrupts the dermal epidermal junction

96. Ans: D

Ref: Shafer's, 6/E, p. 938

97. Ans: B

Ref: Neville, 3/E, p. 470

Explanation
- Sialosis is also called as *'Sialadenosis'*.

98. Ans: D

Ref: Neville, 3/E, p. 757

Explanation
- 50% of patients with EDS can touch the tip of their nose with tongue (Gorlin's sign)

99. Ans: D

Ref: Neville, 3/E, p. 6

100. Ans: B

Ref: Shafer's, 6/E, p. 831

Explanation

CREST syndrome is a variant of systemic sclerosis

1. C - Calcinosis cutis
2. R - Reynaud's phenomenon
3. E - Esophageal dysfunction
4. S - Sclerodactyly
5. T - Telangiectasia

101. Ans: C

Ref: Shafer's, 6/E, p. 103

Explanation
- Eagle's syndrome consist of either elongation of the Styloid process or ossification of the stylohyoid ligament causing dysphagia, sore throat, otalgia, glossodynia, headache, vague orofacial pain or pain along the distribution of internal and external carotid arteries
- Probably the most consistent symptom is pharyngeal pain

102. Ans: A

Ref: Oral & Maxillofacial Medicine: The Basis of Diagnosis and Treatment, Crispian Scully, 2/E, p.3

Explanation
- History(Anamnesis) offers the diagnosis in about 80% of cases

ORAL RADIOLOGY

103. Ans: B

Ref: White and Pharaoh, 6/E, p. 12

104. Ans: A

Ref: White and Pharaoh, 6/E, p. 6

105. Ans: A

Ref: White and Pharaohs, 6/E, p. 7

Explanation

- Quality of X-ray depends upon KVP
- Quantity of X-ray depends upon MA

106. Ans: D

Ref: White and Pharoah, 6/E, p. 37

Explanation

- Collimation is a process to minimize radiation exposure to the patient

107. Ans: D

Ref: Robert P Langlais, 4/E, p. 326

Explanation

- Film crimping is seen as a crescent shaped radiolucency. It can be prevented by avoiding forceful pushing of film or bending of the film.

ORTHODONTICS

108. Ans: D

Ref: Bhalaji, 3/E, p. 41

Explanation

- These are physiological spaces
- Also called simian/anthropoid spaces
- Seen mesial to maxillary canines and distal to mandibular canines
- They help in placement of the canine cusps of the opposing areas

109. Ans: D

Ref: Bhalaji, 3/E, p. 42

Explanation

- *Flush terminal plane:* Distal surface of upper and lower second molars are in a vertical plane
- *Mesial step terminal plane:* The distal surface of lower second deciduous molar is more mesial than that of upper
- *Distal step terminal plane:* Distal surface of lower deciduous 2nd molar is more distal than upper

110. Ans: B

Ref: Bhalaji, 3/E, p. 48

Explanation

- It is a transient or self correcting malocclusion seen in maxillary incisor region between 8–9 years of age seen during eruption of the permanent canines

111. Ans: A

Ref: Bhalaji, 3/E, p. 440

112. Ans: C

Ref: Bhalaji, 3/E, p. 461

113. Ans: B

Ref: Orthodontics – Preperation Manual for Undergraduates , Sridhar Prem Kumar , 1/E, p. 529

Explanation

- *Laterognathia* is true skeletal cross bite
- *Deck Biss* means closed bite or 100% deep bite

114. Ans: C

Ref: Bhalaji, 3/E, p. 228

Explanation

- It is an interceptive orthodontic procedure
- Initiated in the early mixed dentition
- The term first used by Kjellgren (1929) later popularized by Nance

- Three methods
  - Dewel method – CD4
  - Tweed method – D 4 C
  - Nance – similar to Tweed

115. Ans: A

Ref: Bhalaji, 3/E, p. 201

Explanation

Types of forces

- *Continuous force* – active orthodontic force that decreases little in magnitude between appointment periods. For example: Light wire appliance
- *Intermittent force* – active orthodontic force that decays to zero magnitude prior to the next treatment of removable active plates
- *Interrupted force* – is an orthodontic or orthopedic force that is inactive for intervals of time between appointments. For example: Extra oral appliances worn only at night

116. Ans: B

Ref: Proffit, 4/E, p. 402

117. Ans: B

Ref: Gurkeerat Singh, 2/E, p. 334

118. Ans: D

Ref: Bhalaji, 3/E, p. 93

119. Ans: B

Ref: Gurkeerat Singh, 2/E, p. 5

120. Ans: B

Ref: Bhalaji, 3/E, p. 198

Explanation

Types of tooth movement

1. *Tipping* – movement of crown in one direction and root in opposite direction
   a. *Controlled* – occurs about a centre of rotation at its apex
   b. *Uncontrolled* – occurs about a centre of rotation apical to and very close to centre of resistance
2. *Bodily movement/translation* – line of action passes through centre of resistance of tooth
3. *Intrusion* – bodily displacement along its long axis in an apical direction
4. *Extrusion* – bodily displacement along its long axis in an occlusal direction
5. *Torquing* – reverse tipping characterized by lingual movement of root
6. *Uprighting* – tipping the roots back to get a parallel orientation

121. Ans: A

Ref: Bhalaji, 3/E, p. 168

Explanation

- The initial mineralization of seasmoid is usually attained during the accelerated period of the pubertal growth spurt. According to various skeletal maturity indicator methods
  1. Bjork, Grave, Brown – stage 4
  2. Singer – stage 3
  3. Hagg and taranger – stage 3
  4. Fishmann – stage 4

122. Ans: B

Ref: Bhalaji, 3/E, p. 148

PEDODONTICS

123. Ans: C

Ref: Shobha Tandon, 1/E, p. 684

124. Ans: C

Ref: Shobha Tandon, 1/E, p. 206

Explanation

First visit

- Gross excavation and restoration of lesion
- X–ray
- Application of topical fluoride

Second visit

- Analysis of diet chart
- Caries activity tests

Third visit

- Restoration of grossly decayed tooth and stainless steel crown
- Endodontic treatment

P AND SD

125. **Ans: D**

Ref: Soben Peter, 3/E, p. 327

126. **Ans: A**

Ref: Soben Peter, 3/E, p. 38

127. **Ans: D**

Ref: Soben Peter, 3/E, p. 42

128. **Ans: D**

Ref: Park, 20/E, p. 127

Explanation

- Sensitivity was introduced by Yerushalmy

129. **Ans: C**

Ref: Park, 20/E, p. 253

130. **Ans: B**

Ref: Park, 20/E, p. 753

131. **Ans: B**

Ref: Soben Peter, 3/E, p. 437

132. **Ans: A**

Ref: Primary Preventive Dentistry, Norman Q. Harris, 4/E, p. 396, 409

133. **Ans: B**

Ref: Park, 20/E, p. 45, 812

134. **Ans: A**

Ref: Park, 20/E, p. 667

135. **Ans: C**

Ref: Park, 20/E, p. 625

136. **Ans: A**

Ref: Park, 20/E, p. 623

Explanation

- When working ideally, slow sand filters have been shown to reduce total bacterial counts by 99.9 – 99.99% and *E.coli* by 99.9%

137. **Ans: D**

Ref: Park, 20/E, p. 750

138. **Ans: C**

Ref: Park, 20/E, p. 755

Explanation

- Correlation coefficient ranges from +1 to –1
- It is represent by r
  - If r is near +1, it indicates positive association
  - If r is near –1, it indicates negative association
  - If r is equal to 0, it indicates no association

139. **Ans: A**

Ref: Park, 20/E, p. 751

140. **Ans: A**

Ref: Park, 20/E, p. 756

Explanation

- d.f = (c – 1) × (r – 1)
  where c – number of columns rows
  r – number of rows

PROSTHODONTICS

141. **Ans: A**

Ref: Nallaswamy, 1/E, p. 775

142. **Ans: D**

Ref: Heartwell, 4/E, p. 246

Explanation

- The graphic tracings in a pantogram are recorded in three planes and are all the writings necessary to reproduce mandibular movements in order to develop a satisfactory occlusion

- The purpose of the mandibular recorder is to locate the centre of mandibular movement and at the same time records the paths of motion that these centers take in relation to a given plane in the face

143. Ans: B

Ref: Rosensteil, 4/E, p. 220

144. Ans: B

Ref: Nallaswamy, 1/E, p. 146

145. Ans: A

Ref: Nallaswamy, 1/E, p. 627

146. Ans: D

Ref: Zarb and Bolender, 12/E, p. 221

Explanation

- Alginate impression material will not support itself away from confines of the tray. So any areas of under extension need to be corrected with soft boxing wax before the impression is made

147. Ans: A

Ref: Winkler, 2/E, p. 228

148. Ans: D

Ref: Heartwell, 4/E, p. 281

Explanation

- It measures the vertical dimension when the mandible and muscles involved are in physiologic function of speech

149. Ans: A

Ref: Heartwell, 4/E, p. 290

Explanation

- The patterson technique and needle house technique are examples of the functional or chew in method

150. Ans: C

Ref: Heartwell, 4/E, p. 365

151. Ans: C

Ref: Heartwell, 4/E, p. 504

152. Ans: C

Ref: Nallaswamy, 1/E, p. 332

153. Ans: A

Ref: Mc Crackens, 20/E, p. 253

154. Ans: B

Ref: Rosensteil, 4/E, p. 308

155. Ans: C

Ref: Nallaswamy, 1/E, p. 103

156. Ans: D

Ref: Nallaswamy, 1/E, p. 360

PERIODONTICS

157. Ans: A

Ref: Carranza , 10/E, p. 141

158. Ans: C

Ref: Carranza, 10/E, p. 735

159. Ans: A

Ref: Ramjford, 20/E, p. 205

160. Ans: B

Ref: Carranza, 10/E, p. 358

161. Ans: A

Ref: Carranza, 10/E, p. 170

162. Ans: A

Ref: Carranza, 10/E, p. 529

163. Ans: A

Ref: Carranza, 10/E, p. 733

Explanation

- Calculus/tartar control tooth pastes contain pyrophosphates. They reduce the deposition of new calculus on tooth by interfering with crystal formation in calculus

164. Ans: B

Ref: Carranza, 10/E, p. 583

165. **Ans: C**

Ref: Carranza, 10/E, p. 453

166. **Ans: C**

Ref: Carranza, 10/E, p. 778

167. **Ans: B**

Ref: Carranza, 10/E, p. 809

Explanation

- Periochip is a small chip composed of a biodegradable hydrolysed gelatin matrix cross linked with gluteraldehyde into which 2.5 mg of chlorhexidine gluconate has been incorporated per chip

168. **Ans: A**

Ref: Carranza, 10/E, p. 1016

Explanation

- Described by Grupe and Warren in 1956
- Used to cover isolated denuded roots

169. **Ans: C**

Ref: Carranza, 10/E, p. 982

Explanation

- Bioactive glass consists of sodium and calcium salts, phosphates and silicone dioxide
- Particle size: 90–170 μm
- When it becomes coated with hydroxy-apatite
- Attracts osteoblasts that rapidly form bone

170. **Ans: C**

Ref: Carranza, 10/E, pp. 1186 – 1188

Explanation

- Ailing implants – arrested bone loss
- Failing implants – bone loss but no mobility
- Failed implants – bone loss + mobility

171. **Ans: A**

Ref: Carranza, 10/E, p. 104

172. **Ans: B**

Ref: Carranza, 10/E, p. 973

Explanation

- GTR is the method for the prevention of epithelial migration along the cemental-wall of the pocket
- It can be,
  - Non resorbable, For example: Expanded polytetrafluoroethylene
  - Resorbable – polylactic acid, vicryl (polyglactin 910) synthetic skin (biobrane); is freeze dried durameter

CONS AND ENDO

173. **Ans: A**

Ref: Sturdavent, 5/E, p. 628

Explanation

- According to the theory of golden proportions, a smile, when viewed from the front is considered to be esthetically pleasing, if each tooth in that smile (starting from midline) is approximately 60% of the size of the tooth immediately mesial to it. The exact proportion of the smaller tooth to the larger tooth is 0.618

174. **Ans: B**

Ref: Sturdavent, 5/E, p. 392

Explanation

- For autoclave sterilization burs can be protected by keeping them submerged in a small amount of 2% sodium nitrite crystals

175. **Ans: A**

Ref: Sturdavent, 5/E, p. 764

Explanation

- Piggy back wedging is indicated in ases where there is recession of the interproximal gingiva and gingival recession
- *Technique:* If the first wedge is placed significantly apical to the gingival margin, a second wedge usually smaller

than the first one may be piggy backed on the first wedge to adequately wedge the matrix band against tooth margins

176. Ans: A

Ref: Marzouk, 1/E, p. 33

177. Ans: D

Ref: Sturdavent, 5/E, p. 163

178. Ans: D

Ref: Sturdavent, 5/E, p. 920

179. Ans: B

Ref: Cohen, 9/E, p. 988

180. Ans: B

Ref: Clinical Endodontics, Leif Frontstad, 3/E, p. 158

Explanation

- The Root canal Rasps or Rat tail file are used to instrument and enlarge the root canals

181. Ans: D

Ref: Grossman, 12/E, p. 227

182. Ans: D

Explanation

- Answer is D, according to the key answers. But the question seems to be wrong. Hence no Reference is quoted

183. Ans: D

Ref: Sturdavent, 5/E, p. 425, 426

184. Ans: A

Ref: Cohen, 9/E, p. 962

185. Ans: A

Ref: Sturdavent, 5/E, p. 328

Explanation

- Balance is accomplished by designing the angles of the shank so that the cutting edge of the blade lies within the projected diameter of the handle and nearly coincides with the projected axis of the handle

ORAL SURGERY

186. Ans: D

Ref: Bhalaji, 1/E, p. 284

187. Ans: A

Ref: Kruger, Vol. 1, p. 342

188. Ans: D

Ref: Kruger, Vol. 1, p. 336

189. Ans: C

Ref: Neelima Malik, 2/E, p. 60

Explanation

- Gets absorbed within 60–90 days

190. Ans: C

Ref: Malamed Medical Emergencies in Dental Office, 6/E, p. 283

191. Ans: C

Ref: Malamed Local Anesthesia, 5/E, p. 328

Explanation

- Adrenaline/Epinephrine
  1. 0.3 ml of 1:1000 IM for adults
  2. 0.3 ml of 1:1000 IM for children
  3. 0.3 ml of 1:1000 IM for infants.

192. Ans: D

Ref: Neelima Malik, 2/E, p. 376

Explanation

Forceps	Use
Rowe's disimpaction forceps	Disimpaction of maxilla in Le-Fort fractures, To check for free movement of maxilla in Le-Fort osteotomy procedure
Hayton Williams Forceps	Used in conjunction with Rowe's disimpaction forceps
Asche's forceps	To reduce fractures of nasal bone and to align the nasal septum
Walsham's forcep	To manipulate the fractured nasal fragments

193. Ans: B

Ref: Malamed Local Anesthesia, 5/E, p. 145

194. Ans: A

Ref: Peterson, 4/E, p. 363

195. Ans: B

Ref: Neelima Malik, 2/E, p. 622

196. Ans: D

Ref: Peterson, 4/E, p. 118

197. Ans: B

Ref: Neelima Malik, 2/E, p. 463

Explanation

Indications

- Age–In young child with developing tooth buds
- In elderly, debilitated patients, marsupialisation is less stressful
- Proximity to vital structures
- To permit eruption of cysts
- Large cysts
- To maintain vitality of teeth

198. Ans: A

Ref: Neelima Malik, 2/E, p. 406

199. Ans: A

Ref: Neelima Malik, 2/E, p. 297

Explanation

- First described by Win Stanley in 1968

200. Ans: D

Ref: Peterson, 4/E, p. 409

2

KCET 2004

HUMAN ANATOMY

1. In a 15 year old type II collagen is present in

A. Skin
B. Bone
C. Cartilage
D. Basement membrane

2. The first branchial arch is called as

A. Maxillary arch
B. Mandibular arch
C. Hyoid arch
D. None

3. When a patient is asked to say "ah", if the uvula is drawn upwards to the left, the cranial nerve likely to be damaged is

A. Vagus
B. Right accessory
C. Left accessory
D. Hypoglossal

4. All of the following are examples of fibrous joints EXCEPT

A. Symphysis
B. Gomphosis
C. Sutural
D. Styloid process

5. First pharyngeal arch derivatives include which of the following structures?

A. Hyoid bone
B. Maxillary process
C. Stapes
D. Styloid process

6. Secretion of salivary gland is

A. Apocrine
B. Holocrine
C. Merocrine
D. Endocrine

PHYSIOLOGY

7. Following are the features of cretinism, EXCEPT

A. Pot–belly
B. Idiotic look
C. Normal intelligence
D. Stunted growth

8. The part of nephron "least permeable to water" is

A. Proximal tubule
B. Descending limb of loop of Henle
C. Ascending limb of loop of Henle
D. Collecting tubule

9. Hemophilia is due to deficiency of

A. Factor V
B. Factor VIII
C. Ca ions
D. Prothrombin

10. At neuromuscular junction following neurotransmitter is released

A. Nor–adrenaline
B. Glycine
C. Serotonin
D. Acetylcholine

BIOCHEMTRY

11. Following are extra pyramidal tracts EXCEPT
A. Reticulospinal
B. Corticospinal
C. Rubrospinal
D. Vestibulospinal

12. Liver cells cannot utilize ketone bodies as source of energy due to deficiency of?
A. Glucose 6 phosphatase
B. Thiophorase
C. Thiolase
D. Thiokinase

13. The hormone which exerts hypoglycemic effect is
A. Insulin
B. Glucagon
C. Growth hormone
D. Epinephrine

14. Scurvy is a deficiency disease of
A. Pyridoxine
B. Niacin
C. Riboflavin
D. Ascorbic acid

15. Urea synthesis takes place mainly in
A. Muscle
B. Liver
C. Kidney
D. Adipose tissue

16. Normal serum calcium level is
A. 5 to 7 mg%
B. 7 to 9 mg%
C. 9 to 11 mg%
D. 11 to 13 mg%

GENERAL PATHOLOGY

17. A lesion composed of microscopic vessels is called as
A. Hemangioma
B. Angioma
C. None
D. Hemangioma and Angioma

18. Which of the following tests will be abnormal in a patient with hemophilia?
A. Bleeding time
B. PTT (Partial thromboplastin time)
C. PT (Prothrombin time)
D. Platelet count

19. Kaposi's sarcoma is more commonly seen in patients with
A. AIDS
B. Amyloidosis
C. Leukemia
D. HSV infection

20. EBV is responsible for all EXCEPT
A. Nasopharyngeal carcinoma
B. Burkitt's lymphoma
C. Hepatoma
D. Infectious mononucleosis

21. Essential granulation tissue constituents include all EXCEPT
A. Fibroblasts
B. Macrophages
C. Polymorph giant cells
D. Budding blood vessels

22. Apoptosis is
A. Single cell necrosis
B. Intracytoplasmic accumulation
C. Neoplastic change in the cell
D. Degenerative change

23. Caisson disease refers to
A. Amniotic fluid embolism
B. Fat embolism
C. Arterial embolism
D. Gas embolism

24. All of the following malignancies metastasize EXCEPT
A. Basal cell carcinoma
B. Adenocarcinoma
C. Squamous cell carcinoma
D. Melanoma

MICROBIOLOGY

25. All of the following are biologic properties of IgG EXCEPT

A. Passes the placental barrier
B. Neutralizes bacterial toxins
C. Binds with organisms enhancing phagocytosis
D. Most efficient activator of complement system

26. Which of the following provides best guarantee for sterilization in the heat sterilizer?

A. Using chemical indicator strip or pouch
B. Recording a temperature/pressure readings from sterilizer gauge
C. Using a bacterial spore test
D. Determining the ability of a sterilizer to kill the hepatitis B virus

27. Borrelia vincenti is a

A. Mycoplasma
B. Mycobacteria
C. Spirochete
D. Chlamydia

28. Teichoic acid is present in

A. Cell wall of gram–positive organisms
B. Cytoplasm of gram–positive organisms
C. Cell wall of gram–negative organisms
D. Cytoplasm of gram–negative organisms

29. All of the following lab tests can be used to distinguish streptococcus mutans from other oral streptococci, EXCEPT

A. Gram staining
B. Fermentation of mannitol and sorbitol
C. Production of intracellular and extra cellular adherent polysaccharide
D. Colony morphology on saliva agar

30. Which of the following is NOT a characteristic of exotoxins?

A. Produced in minute amounts
B. Released from bacterial cell wall
C. Destroyed by proteolytic enzymes
D. Weakly antigenic

31. Which of the following are correctly matched?

A. Transfer of antibody from mother to child is through colostrum and acquired passive immunity naturally
B. Injection of antibodies (hepatitis) is artificially acquired passive immunity
C. Antigenic stimulus given by vaccine (polio) is artificial active immunity
D. All of the above

PHARMACOLOGY

32. Buprenorphine acts by following mechanism

A. Mu receptor antagonist
B. Kappa receptor antagonist
C. Mu receptor partial agonist
D. Kappa receptor partial agonist

33. Which of the following drugs undergoes "Hoffmann elimination"?

A. D–Tubocurarine
B. Acetylcholine
C. Atracurium
D. Acetazolamide

34. Mention the drug causing gynaecomastia, hirsutism, menstrual disturbance on long term use

A. Hydrochlorothiazide
B. Amiloride
C. Spironolactone
D. Acetazolamide

35. Magnesium tri–silicate should NOT be combined with

A. Aluminum hydroxide gel
B. Oxythiazine
C. Sucralfate
D. Ranitidine

36. INH induced neuropathy is treated with

A. Thiamine
B. Pyridoxine
C. Niacin
D. Riboflavin

37. Ibuprofen is contraindicated in
A. Patients having fever
B. Patients having asthma
C. Patients having amoebic dysentery
D. Patients having bronchitis

GENERAL MEDICINE

38. Confirmatory test for HIV infection is
A. ELISA
B. Western blot
C. RIA
D. None of the above

39. The most important investigation done in infective endocarditis is
A. 2–D echocardiography
B. ECG
C. Serial blood cultures
D. ASO titer

40. Which of the following is not correct about nephritic syndrome?
A. Proteinuria
B. Hypoalbuminemia
C. Hypolipidemia
D. Lipiduria

41. Which of the following represents the serologic evidence of recent Hepatitis B virus infection during "window" period?
A. HBs Ag
B. IgM anti HBC
C. Anti HBs
D. None of the above

42. Cryoprecipitate is a rich source of
A. Factor V
B. Factor VII
C. Factor VIII
D. Factor XII

43. All of the following conditions causes transudative pleural effusion EXCEPT
A. Cirrhosis of liver
B. Tuberculosis
C. Bronchogenic carcinoma
D. Rheumatoid arthritis

44. Hepatitis B infection spreads through all of the following routes EXCEPT
A. Blood transfusion
B. Sexual contact
C. Faeco oral route
D. Perinatal transmission

45. Treatment of choice for Pneumocystitis carinii pneumonia is
A. Trimethoprim/sulfamethoxazole
B. Erythromycin
C. Ofloxacin
D. Tetracycline

46. All of the following are bactericidal drugs against Mycobacterium tuberculosis EXCEPT
A. Rifampicin
B. Isoniazid
C. Pyrazinamide
D. Tetracycline

47. What are the symptoms of diabetes mellitus?
A. Polydypsia
B. Polyuria
C. Polyphagia
D. All of the above

GENERAL SURGERY

48. Punched out edge is a characteristic of which type of ulcer
A. Tuberculosis
B. Rodent ulcer
C. Syphilitic
D. Non specific

49. Cystic hygroma is
A. Lymphangiectasia
B. Cavernous haemangioma
C. Sebaceous cyst
D. All of the above

50. Early postoperative complication of tracheostomy are all EXCEPT
A. Apnoea
B. Haemorrhage

C. Pneumomediastenum
D. Tracheal Stenosis

51. Treatment strategy for Ludwig's angina includes
A. Amoxicillin plus metronidazole
B. Decompression of both submandibular triangles
C. Tracheostomy
D. All of the above

52. Symptoms of hyperthyroidism are the following EXCEPT
A. Emotional liability
B. Heat intolerance
C. Weight gain
D. Excessive appetite

53. Eighty percent of all salivary stones occur in
A. Parotid
B. Submandibular
C. Sublingual
D. Minor salivary glands

DENTAL MATERIALS

54. Mercury rich condition in a slow setting amalgam alloy system in a restoration results in
A. Accelerated corrosion
B. Fracture of the restoration
C. Marginal damage
D. All of the above

55. Ethoxy benzoic acid increases the strength and solubility of the cement
A. Zinc oxide eugenol
B. Polycarboxylate cement
C. Zinc phosphate cement
D. Silicate cement

56. If two elements form an intermetallic compound the mechanical properties of this compound
A. Are higher than those of either element
B. Are lower than those of either elements
C. Fall between those of the elements
D. Cannot be predicted

57. The term "Chroma aspect" in selection of artificial teeth refers to
A. Degree of saturation of hue
B. Intensity of value
C. Both value and hue
D. None of the above

58. Advantage of minimum mercury technique or Eames technique is all EXCEPT
A. High strength
B. Sets quickly
C. Need no squeezing of excess mercury
D. Greater plasticity and adapts well to cavity walls

59. Gold with highest strength and can be used in stress bearing areas
A. Gold foil
B. Mat gold
C. Spherical gold
D. Electralloy

60. When selecting a dental wire for its ability to withstand a certain stress without experiencing permanent deformation one should consult data tables for the property known as
A. Elastic limit
B. Fracture strength
C. Modulus of elasticity
D. Percent elongation

61. Inorganic phase of the composites aid in
A. Increasing the mechanical strength
B. Decreasing the coefficient of thermal expansion
C. Reducing the polymerization shrinkage
D. All of the above

62. The solder used for soldering two metal alloy parts should have fusion temperature
A. Below the fusion temperature of both the alloys
B. Above the fusion temperature of both of the alloys
C. Equal to either of the alloys
D. None of the above

63. The main advantage exhibited by the porcelain compared to the tooth colored restorations

A. Good marginal integrity
B. High tensile strength
C. Better color harmony
D. Highly insoluble

64. Knoop hardness number of the enamel is

A. 68
B. 110
C. 343
D. 450

65. Suck back porosity in the casting can be eliminated by

A. Increasing the mould metal temperature difference
B. Increasing the flow of molten metal
C. Flaring the point of the sprue attachment
D. None of the above

DADH

66. Congenital absence of teeth is most likely to affect the growth of

A. Palate
B. Maxillary sinus
C. Upper lip
D. Alveolus

67. Primary teeth begin to calcify at the age of

A. 4 to 5 weeks of fetal life
B. Between 4–6 months of fetal life
C. At birth
D. 2–4 months after birth

68. Deviation in which of the following stages of development of dentition result in supernumerary teeth

A. Apposition
B. Morpho differentiation
C. Initiation
D. Multiplication

69. When the jaw is opened

A. Condyles move upwards
B. Articular disc moves posteriorly
C. Lateral pterygoids contact
D. Condyles moves around vertical axis

70. Regarding teeth which statement is WRONG?

A. Enamel is harder than dentine
B. Enamel has no cells
C. Ameloblasts secrete enamel and dentine
D. Odontoblast produce dentine

71. The crown formation of all permanent teeth EXCEPT third molar is completed between

A. Birth to 6 years
B. Birth to 8 years
C. Birth to 12 years
D. 6 years to 12 years

72. The formation of which of the following does not represent normal physiological process of dentin formation

A. Primary and secondary dentin
B. Secondary dentin and circum pulpal dentin
C. Tertiary dentin and sclerotic dentin
D. All of the above

73. Which of the following has nonfunctional cusp?

A. Mandibular canine
B. Maxillary second premolar
C. Mandibular first premolar
D. Maxillary canine

ORAL PATHOLOGY AND ORAL MEDICINE

74. Internal resorption is characterized by

A. Pain on percussion
B. Slow dull continuous pain
C. No characteristic feature, symptom free
D. Increased pulpal pain when lying down

75. The most pronounced effect on the oral microflora by a reduction in rate of salivary flow is a

A. Significant increase in number of oral bacteria

B. Shift towards more acidogenic micro flora
C. Significant decrease in number of oral bacteria
D. Shift towards more aerobic micro flora

76. Actinomycosis is a
A. Bacterial infection
B. Viral infection
C. Fungal infection
D. Parasitic infection

77. The swollen degenerating epithelial cell due to acantholysis is
A. Antischkow cell
B. Tzank cell
C. Ghost cell
D. Prickle cell

78. The rate of malignant transformation is highest in
A. Leukoplakia
B. Oral submucous fibrosis
C. Oral lichen planus
D. Erythroplakia

79. Ackerman's tumor is an acronym for
A. Fibrous dysplasia
B. Epithelial dysplasia
C. Verrucous dysplasia
D. Basal Cell Carcinoma

80. Nikolsky's sign is positive in
A. Herpes labialis
B. Pemphigoid
C. Pemphigus
D. None of the above

81. Ghost cells are seen in
A. Ghost teeth
B. Pindborg's tumour
C. Odontogenic kerato cyst
D. Calcifying odontogenic cyst

82. Oral hairy leukoplakia is a feature of
A. White sponge nevus
B. Hairy cell leukemia
C. Speckled leukoplakia
D. None of the above

83. Liquefaction degeneration of basal cell layer is a histological feature of
A. Hairy leukoplakia
B. White sponge nevus
C. Oral lichen planus
D. Herpes zoster

84. Areca nut chewing is etiological factor in
A. Leukoedema
B. Oral submucous fibrosis
C. Erythema multiformae
D. Oral lichen planus

85. Oral co–carcinogenesis concept was suggested by
A. Thomas
B. Goldhaber
C. Shafer
D. Pindborg

86. Which of the following is NOT precancerous
A. Leukoplakia
B. Leukoedema
C. Verrucous hyperplasia
D. Erythroplakia

87. The inheritance pattern of dentinogenesis imperfecta is
A. Homozygous
B. Autosomal dominant
C. Recessive
D. X–linked recessive

88. Three stages in progression of acute odontogenic infection are
A. Periapical osteitis–cellulitis–abscess
B. Abscess–cellulitis–periapical osteitis
C. Cellulitis–Abscess–periapical osteitis
D. Periapical osteitis–abscess–cellulitis

89. The common site in oral cavity for lesion of lymphogranuloma venerum is
A. Gingiva
B. Tongue
C. Lips
D. Palate

90. Chronic sinus tract present at the angle of lower jaw, yellow purulent granular discharge, is due to

A. Tuberculosis
B. Staphylococcal infection
C. Actinomycosis
D. Histoplasmosis

91. A cyst can be differentiated from granuloma radiographically by injecting

A. Radiopaque dyes
B. Polyacrylamide gel
C. Sodium morrhuate
D. Corticosteroids

92. Grinspan syndrome is associated with

A. Leukoplakia
B. Lichen planus
C. Apthous ulcer
D. Oral submucous fibrosis

93. In hemophilia A there is deficiency of

A. Factor VIII
B. Factor V
C. Factor VI
D. Factor X

94. Peutz–Jegher syndrome is characterized by

A. Deafness
B. Multiple supernumerary teeth
C. Multiple intestinal polyps
D. Scleroderma

95. Cyst that has high recurrence rate is

A. Incisive canal cyst
B. Periapical cyst
C. Dentigerous cyst
D. Odontogenic Keratocyst

96. Routine assessment of jaw function does not consist of

A. Palpation of TM Joint
B. Determination of maximum opening
C. Observation of deviation
D. Arthrography

97. Which is best for diagnosis of primary herpes simplex infection?

A. Smear stained with Giemsa stain
B. Smear stained with Wrist's stain
C. Fluorescent staining of cytology smears
D. Routine cytology

98. Normal bleeding time is

A. 1 to 6 minutes
B. 8 to 10 minutes
C. 30–40 seconds
D. 40–50 seconds

99. Most common tumor associated with AIDS is

A. Carcinoma
B. Kaposi's sarcoma
C. Melanoma
D. Ewing's sarcoma

100. In sickle cell anemia there is

A. 75% to 100% hemoglobin S
B. 10% to 20% hemoglobin S
C. 20% to 30% hemoglobin S
D. 50% to 60% hemoglobin S

101. Patient's exaggerated concept that something is mechanically wrong in his/her occlusion or jaw is termed as

A. Bruxism
B. Skeletal malocclusion disharmony
C. Phantom bite
D. Juvenile occlusal disharmony

ORAL RADIOLOGY

102. Why an increased target–film distance is required in the paralleling techniques?

A. To avoid image magnification
B. To avoid distortion
C. To reduce scattered radiation
D. To improve film placement

103. Which of the following is not a type of particulate radiation?

A. Alpha particles
B. Beta particles
C. Protons
D. Nucleons

104. Thyroid dose from panoramic radiography is about

A. 0.022 mGy
B. 0.034 mGy
C. 0.051 mGy
D. 0.074 mGy

105. Of the following, which is the best projection to study the fracture of zygomatic arch

A. Lateral oblique view
B. PA Caldwell view
C. Submentovertex view
D. Lateral cephalometric view

106. Most commonly used color of the filter used in dark room safelight is

A. Blue
B. Red
C. Green
D. Yellow

ORTHODONTICS

107. Premature exfoliation of the primary mandibular canine is most often the sequale of which of the following

A. Caries
B. Trauma
C. Serial tooth extraction
D. Arch length inadequacy

108. Which of the following is a feature of Class I type 3 malocclusion

A. Posterior cross bite
B. Anterior crossbite
C. Mesial drifting of molars
D. Protrusion of mandibular incisors

109. In occlusion the teeth have

A. Cusp to cusp contact
B. Edge to edge contact
C. Marginal contact
D. Surface to surface contact

110. The condition in which the occlusal plane of the teeth lies nearer the Frankfort plane than it does in normal occlusion is termed

A. Distraction
B. Contraction
C. Attraction
D. Retraction

111. All of the following are dental characteristic of a skeletal class III malocclusion EXCEPT

A. Anterior cross bite
B. Distocclusion
C. Linguoversion of the mandibular molars
D. Posterior cross bite

112. In orthodontic treatment in order to avoid injuries to the tissues, the forces applied should not exceed the

A. Arterial blood pressure
B. Capillary blood pressure
C. Masticatory retrusion
D. Muscular forces of facial muscles

113. Orthodontic brackets attached directly to the tooth are retained by a

A. Compressive force
B. Hydrostatic force
C. Mechanical bond
D. Chemical bond

114. Eruption of the permanent maxillary second molar prior to the maxillary second premolar is

A. Normal and desirable
B. Abnormal and undesirable
C. Abnormal and desirable
D. Normal and undesirable

115. Frankfort horizontal plane is drawn from

A. Sella to nasion
B. Orbitale to nasion
C. Orbitale to porion
D. Sub nasion to nasion

116. Head gear applied to maxillary molars can improve antero-posterior skeletal dysplasia by

A. Maxillary growth redirection
B. Bilateral expansion of the palate
C. Anterior repositioning of the maxillary teeth
D. Stimulating growth of the mandible

117. The type of resorption seen when light continuous orthodontic forces are applied

A. Apical
B. Frontal or direct
C. Indirect or undermining
D. No resorption is seen

118. An early pre-pubertal growth spurt indicates

A. Metabolic disturbances
B. Fast maturing child
C. Endocrine dysfunction
D. Slow maturing child

119. "Growth spurt' refers to

A. Period of uniform growth
B. Period of sudden acceleration of growth
C. Axis of increased growth extending from head towards the feet
D. None of the above

120. Mechanism of bone growth is by

A. Bone deposition and resorption
B. Cortical drift
C. Displacement
D. All of the above

PEDODONTICS

121. What is the most common skeletal finding in cephalometric radiographs in a patient with a history of cleft palate and anterior cross bite

A. Maxillary retrusion
B. Mandibular protrusion
C. Mandibular retrusion
D. Maxillary protrusion

122. After 6 years of age, the lengthening of mandible occurs mainly

A. At the symphysis
B. Between the canines
C. Distal to first permanent molar
D. Along the lower border

123. "Fluoride syndrome" is a type of

A. Enamel hypoplasia
B. Dentin hypoplasia
C. Dental caries
D. Fluorosis

124. It is essential that restoration involving the proximal surfaces of deciduous teeth, restore the original mesio–distal dimensions of teeth primarily to

A. Maintain arch length
B. Maintain esthetics
C. Prevent food impaction
D. Prevent secondary caries

125. Familiarization can be solution of child's behavior problem, in the clinic, if the basis of problem is

A. Pain
B. Sibling rivalry
C. Fear
D. Parents

126. A mandibular lingual holding arch with the loops mesial to each molar band used in the children for

A. Correction of rotation
B. Regaining the space
C. Space maintenance only
D. Correction of distally tilted molar

127. When there is a large exposure of the pulp in a vital tooth with immature apex the treatment of choice is

A. Apexification
B. Apexogenesis
C. Pulpotomy
D. Pulpectomy

128. When natal teeth are present the most common preferable approach is to

A. Extract the teeth
B. Grind the sharp incisal edges
C. Take radiograph and determine the status of adjacent unerupted tooth
D. Retain the teeth if possible

129. Prolonged use of antibiotics in children can result in

A. Necrotizing ulcerative gingivitis
B. Candidiasis

C. Actinomycosis
D. Aphthous ulcer

130. During mixed dentition stage, which of the following appliance should be used as a space maintainer for missing primary molars in mandibular arch

A. Distal shoe
B. Nance holding arch
C. Passive lingual arch
D. Removable functional acrylic

131. When the cry of child is characterized by a siren like vocabulary it is called as

A. Compensatory
B. Frightened
C. Hurt
D. Obstinate

P AND SD

132. The Snyder test is designed to

A. Give a quantitative determination of acidogenic micro-organisms in the oral cavity
B. Predict the acidity of the saliva
C. Estimate the cariogenic potential of dental plaque
D. Identify the organisms involved in the carious process

133. Any principal/dean of recognized dental college can become a member of Dental Council of India. The maximum members in such category can be

A. Two
B. Three
C. Four
D. Six

134. The priority program of WHO is

A. Global eradication of small pox
B. Immunization against common disease of child hood
C. Surveillance of communicable disease
D. Child nutrition

135. The headquarters of UNICEF is situated at

A. Geneva
B. London
C. New York
D. Washington

136. The branch of biostatistics which deals with the birth, death and marriage is called as

A. Health
B. Medical
C. Demography
D. Vital

137. Awakening the fundamental desire to learn is known as

A. Motivation
B. Interest
C. Learning
D. Comprehension

138. "Nalgonda" technique of defluoridation was developed at

A. Chennai
B. Nagpur
C. Nalgonda
D. Bangalore

139. In a path finder survey, the examination carried out for various age groups in years are

A. 5, 10, 15, 35–44, 65–74
B. 5, 12, 15, 35–44, 65–74
C. 6, 12, 15, 35–44, 64–74
D. 5, 12, 15, 30–44, 65–74

140. When a circle is divided into different sectors corresponding to the frequencies of the variable in the distribution, the diagram is known as

A. Pie
B. Bar
C. Histogram
D. Pictogram

141. In lake water, the highest fluoride value ever recorded is 2800 ppm. In which country this lake is situated

A. Japan
B. Kenya
C. Libya
D. South Africa

142. According to WHO technical series published, CPITN probe is also known as

A. 611
B. 617
C. 621
D. 625

143. New Zealand type of school dental nurse can perform all of the following clinical duties EXCEPT

A. Prophylaxis
B. Pulp capping
C. Root canal treatment
D. Topical fluoride application

144. Sampling which involves grouping the population and then selecting the groups is known as

A. Cluster
B. quota
C. Systematic
D. Simple random

145. Dental auxillaries are not in existence in

A. America
B. India
C. Saudi-Arabia
D. New Zealand

146. "No Tobacco Day" is celebrated every year by the world on

A. 7th April
B. 31st May
C. 1st August
D. 5th December

PROSTHODONTICS

147. Which type of RPD can best resists the forces, to which it is subjected

A. Class I
B. Class II
C. Class III
D. Class IV

148. How far should be the border of maxillary major connector from the gingival crevices of the teeth

A. 1 mm
B. 4–6 mm
C. 1–2 mm
D. 0 mm

149. When a large inoperable palatal torus is present then the major connector of choice

A. Palatal strap
B. Antero-posterio palatal strap
C. Antero-posterior palatal bar
D. Complete palatal plate

150. Compared to resin base the main disadvantage of a metallic denture base in distal extension situation is that, metal bases

A. Are difficult to keep clean
B. Transfer thermal changes quickly to mucosa
C. Cannot be relined in event of ridge resorption
D. Are subjected to distortion and breakage

151. In distal extension base partial denture the impression is recorded in

A. Pressure impression technique
B. Mucostatic impression technique
C. Physiologic impression technique
D. Minimum pressure impression technique

152. Ante's law concerns with the

A. Degree of tipping allowable in the abutment tooth
B. Amount of increase in retentive factor with a full crown versus a 3/4th crown
C. Crown: Root ratio
D. Ratio of combined pericemental root surface area of the abutment teeth and pericemental root surface area of the teeth to be replaced

153. Extra retention in abutment teeth is obtained by

A. Dovetail
B. Screws, pins and grooves
C. Outline form
D. Increasing tooth reduction

154. Predictable compliment of optimum tooth preparation should satisfy

A. Biological requirement
B. Esthetic requirement
C. Combinations of compromises among the prevalence of biological and mechanical considerations
D. Biological, mechanical and esthetic requirement

155. Tissue displacement is commonly used to obtain

A. Adequate access to prepared tooth
B. To expose all necessary surfaces, both prepared and not prepared
C. Both of the above
D. None of the above

156. Post and core is indicated for

A. Vital tooth with primary caries
B. Badly damaged non-vital endodontically treated tooth
C. Badly damaged vital tooth
D. Tooth with fractured incisal third

157. When making complete denture the occlusal plane should be parallel to the

A. Frankfort horizontal plane only
B. Interpupillary line only
C. Camper's plane only
D. Campers plane and interpupillary line

158. The primary function of the compensatory curve, incorporated in complete denture is to provide

A. Stability in centric relation
B. Balanced occlusion, during lateral movement of mandible
C. An esthetically pleasing dentures
D. Balancing occlusal contacts, during protrusive movements

159. One of the major disadvantages to immediate denture treatment is

A. Pain associated with treatment
B. Difficulty in managing occlusion
C. Need for reline
D. No control over tooth placement and Shape

160. Over denture are indicated over retained roots instead of extracting them and making complete denture because

A. To preserve the alveolar bone
B. To allow proprioception from the periodontium of remaining teeth
C. Carrier for patient to adjust
D. All of the above

161. The gothic arch tracing device is used to record

A. The vertical dimension of occlusion
B. The centric relation
C. The centric occlusion
D. Vertical dimension at rest

PERIODONTICS

162. Basal lamina consists of

A. Type I collagen fibers
B. Type II collagen fibers
C. Type IV collagen fibers
D. Type III collagen fibers

163. Dendritic cells located among keratinocytes at all suprabasal levels and belonging to reticuloendothelial system derived from bone marrow are

A. Melanocytes
B. Langerhans cells
C. Lymphocytes
D. Merkel cell

164. One of the following systemic disease involving periodontal tissue is not a disorder of neutrophil functions

A. Agranulocytosis
B. Chediak–Higashi syndrome
C. Leukemia
D. Cyclic neutropenia

165. The predominant fiber groups affected in the early lesion of gingivitis are

A. Circular and dento gingival
B. Circular and horizontal
C. Circular and alveolar crest
D. Circular and trans septal

166. The distance between the bottom of calculus and alveolar crest in human periodontal pocket is constant having an approximate length of

A. 0.97 mm
B. 1.97 mm
C. 2.97 mm
D. 3.97 mm

167. Which of the following is not an instrument grasp during scaling procedure?

A. Pen grasp
B. Thumb grasp
C. Modified pen grasp
D. Palm and thumb grasp

168. Gracey curettes have an offset blade placed to the shank of the instrument at an angle of

A. 180 degrees
B. 100 degrees
C. 70 degrees
D. 50 degrees

169. The concept of calculus formation in which seeding agents induce small foci of calcification which enlarge and coalesce to form a calcified mass is termed as

A. Mineral precipitation
B. Calculus adaptation
C. Heterogeneous nucleation
D. None of the above

170. The inorganic component of sub gingival plaque is derived from

A. Saliva
B. Gingival crevicular fluid
C. Inorganic matter of tooth
D. Food debris

171. Gingival fluid from diabetics contain a reduced level of cyclic adenosine mono–phosphate which may lead to

A. Increased severity of gingival inflammation
B. Decreased severity of gingival inflammation
C. No response on gingiva
D. Epithelial desquamation

172. The overall effect of HIV is to gradually impair the immune system by interference with

A. Helper T lymphocytes
B. Natural killer cells
C. Plasma cells
D. Macrophages

173. The region in which cementum formation is most rapid is

A. Middle
B. Coronal
C. Apical
D. Inter–radicular

174. Alveolar bone proper is also known as

A. Lamina Lucida
B. Lamina densa
C. Lamina propria
D. Lamina dura

175. One of the following drugs can slow the loss of alveolar bone in periodontitis

A. Dexamethasone
B. Ibuprofen
C. Penicillin
D. Calcium channel blockers

CONS AND ENDO

176. In a pin retained amalgam restoration, use of pins

A. Does not reinforce the tooth
B. Weakens the tooth
C. Reinforces the amalgam structure
D. Improves retention of restoration

177. Which of the following restorative material is most biocompatible to the pulp

A. Silver amalgam
B. Composite resin
C. GIC II
D. Silicate cement

178. The rate of tarnish and corrosion of class II cast material having VHN 200 is

A. 0%
B. 2 to 3%

C. 5 to 10%
D. Less than 1%

179. Effective conditioning of the tooth enamel for retention purpose prior to insertion of tooth colored resin restoration using aqueous solution of phosphoric acid

A. 8 to 85%
B. As low as 15%
C. 35 to 50%
D. None of the above

180. A dental bur cuts the tooth structure more effectively when rake angle of bur is

A. Positive
B. Negative
C. Radial
D. None of the above

181. A 15% solution of EDTA has a pH of

A. 5.5
B. 7.3
C. 7.9
D. 7

182. Percussion is a dental diagnostic procedure used in determining whether

A. The tooth is vital
B. A pulp is hyperemic
C. A periodontitis exists
D. The pulp is metaplastic

183. Glass bead endodontics sterilizer is operated at temperature range

A. 425–475°F
B. 550–760°F
C. 285–330°F
D. 218–246°F

184. Average length of maxillary cuspid is

A. 26 mm
B. 33 mm
C. 21 mm
D. 18 mm

185. Urethane dimethacrylate based composite resin is cured by

A. Ultraviolet light
B. Visible light
C. Chemical means
D. None of the above

186. A giromatic hand piece for endodontic instrumentation operates by

A. Rotating motion
B. Oscillating motion
C. Zig zag motion
D. All

ORAL SURGERY

187. Toxic effect of local anesthetic include

A. Convulsions
B. Asystole
C. Methemoglobinemia
D. All of the above

188. The weakest part of the mandible where fracture occurs

A. Neck of the condyle
B. Angle of the mandible
C. Canine fossa
D. Symphysis

189. Foreign body aspirated during dental procedures can be retrieved by

A. Bronchoscopy
B. Gastroscopy
C. Arthroscopy
D. None of the above

190. Local reaction due to local anesthetic solution is

A. Pain
B. Local irritation
C. Haematoma
D. Dermatitis

191. In Jorgensen technique on IV sedation for dental procedure drugs used are

A. Pentobarbital
B. Mepiridine
C. Scopolamine
D. All of the above

192. Pick out odd drugs for anesthetic emergencies

A. Aminophylline
B. Epinephrine
C. Atropine sulphate
D. Amoxicillin

193. Nerves anaesthetized in incisive nerve block are

A. Incisive nerve only
B. Incisive and mental
C. Incisive and inferior alveolar
D. Mental and inferior alveolar

194. Masticator space infection usually results from

A. Infections of the last two lower molars
B. Non aseptic technique in local anesthesia
C. External or internal trauma to the mandibular angle region
D. All of the above

195. The horizontal fracture of maxilla is called as

A. Le fort I fracture
B. Floating jaw fracture of maxilla
C. Both of the above
D. None of the above

196. Pre auricular pain, grating sensation and partial trismus are the symptoms of

A. TM joint fibrous ankylosis
B. TM joint bony ankylosis
C. TM joint pain dysfunction syndrome
D. Ear infection

197. Which of the following is not a surgery for anterior open bite?

A. Thomas trapezoid osteotomy
B. Thomas' corticotomy
C. Thomas Y osteotomy
D. Limberg's osteotomy

198. Which of the following is NOT a sign of recovery of injured inferior alveolar nerve?

A. Pricking sensation
B. Hyperesthesia
C. Anesthesia
D. Partial return of sensation

199. Which of the following is/are known for recurrence?

A. Keratocyst
B. Ameloblastoma
C. Both of them
D. None of them

200. Spontaneous closure can be expected in

A. Chronic oroantral fistula
B. Acute oroantral fistula
C. Both chronic and acute oroantral fistula
D. None of the above

ANSWERS

HUMAN ANATOMY

1. Ans: C

Ref: Difiore's Atlas of Histology, 10/E, p. 56

Explanation

- It is also known as decompression sickness

2. Ans: B

Ref: Inderbir Singh, 8/E, p. 109

Explanation

Arch	*Nerve of arch*	*Muscles of arch*
First	Mandibular	Medial and Lateral Pterygoid, Masseter, Temporalis, Mylohyoid, Anterior belly of Digastric, Tensor tympani, Tensor palatini
Second	Facial	Muscles of face, Occipitofrontalis, Platysma, Stylohyoid, Posterior belly of Digastric, Stapedius, Auricular muscles
Third	Glosso pharyngeal	Stylopharyngeus
Fourth	Superior laryngeal	Muscles of Larynx
Fifth	Recurrent laryngeal	Muscles of Pharynx

3. Ans: B

Ref: BD Chaurasia, 1/E p. 320

Explanation

- All muscles of soft palate EXCEPT tensor veli palatini are supplied by pharyngeal plexus by accessory nerve through vagus

4. Ans: D

Ref: BD Chaurasia, 1/E p. 133

5. Ans: B

Ref: Inderbir Singh, 8/E, p. 107

6. Ans : C

Ref: Difiore's Atlas of Histology, 11/E, p. 43

PHYSIOLOGY

7. Ans: C

Ref: Sembulingam, 4/E, p. 367

Explanation

- A new born baby with thyroid deficiency may appear normal at the time of birth because thyroxin might have been supplied from mother. But a few weeks after birth, the baby starts developing the signs like sluggish movements and croaking sound while crying; unless treated immediately, the baby will be mentally retarded permanently

8. Ans: D

Ref: Sembulingam, 4/E, p. 295

9. Ans: B

Ref: Sembulingam, 4/E, p. 116

10. Ans: D

Ref: Sembulingam, 4/E, p. 175

11. Ans: B

Ref: Sembulingam, 4/E, p. 733

Explanation

Extrapyramidal tracts

- Medial longitudinal fasiculus
- Anterior and lateral vestibulospinal tracts
- Reticulospinal tract
- Rectospinal tract
- Rubrospinal tract
- Olivospinal tract

BIOCHEMISTRY

12. Ans: B

Ref: U. Sathyanarayana, U. Chakrapani, 3/E, p. 295

Explanation

- Acetoacetate is activated to aceto acetyl Co A by a mitochondrial enzyme thiophorase
- This enzyme is absent in liver

13. Ans: A

Ref: U. Sathyanarayana, U. Chakrapani, 3/E, p. 671

Explanation

- Insulin lowers blood glucose level (hypoglycemic effect) by promoting its utilization and storage and by inhibiting its production

14. Ans: D

Ref: SU. Sathyanarayana, U. Chakrapani, 3/E, p. 134

Explanation

- Pyridoxine–Neurological symptoms
- Niacin–Pellagra (3D's Dermatitis, Diarrhoea, Dementia and if not treated Death)
- Riboflavin–Cheilosis, glossitis, dermatitis

15. Ans: B

Ref: U. Sathyanarayana, U. Chakrapani, 3/E, p. 337

Explanation

- Urea is the end product of protein metabolism
- Urea is synthesized in liver (Krebs – Hensliet cycle)
- Urea synthesis is a 5 step cyclic process with 5 distinct enzymes of which first 2 enzymes are present in mitochondria while the rest are in cytosol.

16. Ans: C

Ref: U. Sathyanarayana, U. Chakrapani, 3/E, p. 406

Explanation

- Serum or plasma Ca: 9 – 11 mg/dl or 4.5–5.5 mEq/l

GENERAL PATHOLOGY

17. Ans: D

Ref: Robbin's Pathologic Basis of Disease, 7/E, p. 545

18. Ans: B

Ref: Robbin's Pathologic Basis of Disease, 7/E, p. 656

19. Ans:A

Ref: Robbin's Pathologic Basis of Disease, 7/E, p 256

20. Ans:C

Ref: Robbin's Pathologic Basis of Disease, 7/E, p 371

21. Ans: C

Ref: Harsh Mohan, 3/E, p. 136

Explanation

- Giant cells are characteristic of granuloma not granulation tissue

22. Ans: A

Ref: Harsh Mohan, 3/E, p. 38

Explanation

- Type III Collagen fibers are present in hyaline and elastic cartilage

23. Ans: D

Ref: Harsh Mohan 3/e p. 219

Explanation

- It is also known as decompression sickness

24. Ans: A

Ref: Robbin's Pathologic Basis of Disease, 7/E, p. 1242

MICROBIOLOGY

25. Ans: D

Ref: Ananthanarayan and Panicker's Text Book of Microbiology, 8/E, p. 97 to 98

26. Ans: C

Ref: Ananthanarayan and Panicker's Text Book of Microbiology, 8/E, p. 32

Explanation

- Dry heat – hot air oven – spores of non toxigenic strain of clostridium tetani
- Moist heat–autoclave – spores of Bacillus Stearothermophillus or Clostridium botulinum–below 100°C

27. Ans: C

Ref: Ananthanarayan and Panicker's Text Book of Microbiology, 8/E, p. 379

28. Ans: A

Ref: Ananthanarayan and Panicker's Text Book of Microbiology, 8/E, p. 17

Explanation

Feature	*Gram positive*	*Gram negative*
Thickness	Thicker	Thinner
Variety of aminoacids	Few	Several
Aromatic and sulphur containing aminoacids	Absent	Present
Lipids	Absent or scanty	Present
Teichoic acid	Present	Absent

29. Ans: A

Ref: Ananthanarayan and Panicker's Text Book of Microbiology, 8/E, p. 211

Explanation

- Presence of gram '+'ve cocci in chains is indicative of streptococcal infection. However smears are of no value in infections of throat or genitalia where streptococci may form part of the resident flora

30. Ans: D

Ref: Ananthanarayan and Panicker's Text Book of Microbiology, 8/E, p. 78

Explanation

Exotoxins	*Endotoxins*
Heat labile	Heat stable
Actively secreted by cells	Diffuse into surrounding medium
Readily separable from cultures by physical means such as filtration	Obtained only by cell lysis
Action often enzymatic	No enzymatic action
Specific pharmacological effect for each exotoxinaction	Non specific action common to all endotoxins
Specific tissue affinities	No specific tissue affinity
Active in very minute doses	Active only in very large doses
Highly antigenic	Weakly antigenic
Action specifically by antibody	Neutralization by antibody ineffective

31. Ans: D

Ref: Ananthanarayan and Panicker's Text Book of Microbiology, 8/E, pp. 86, 87

Explanation

Active Immunity	*Passive Immunity*
Produced actively by host's immune system	Received passively, no active host participation
Induced by infection or by immunogens	Readymade antibody transferred
Durable, effective protection	Transient, less effective
Immunological memory present	No memory
Negative phase may occur	No negative phase
Not applicable in the immunodeficient	Applicable in the immunodeficient
Immunity effective after lag period	Only immediate immunity

PHARMACOLOGY

32. **Ans: C**

Ref: KD Tripathi, 6/E, p. 465

33. **Ans: C**

Ref: KD Tripathi, 6/E, p. 27

Explanation

- Hoffman elimination refers to inactuva-tion of the drug in the body fluid by spontaneous molar rearrangement without the agency of any enzyme. For example: Atracurium

34. **Ans: C**

Ref: KD Tripathi, 6/E, p. 571

35. **Ans: C**

Ref: KD Tripathi, 6/E, p. 636

Explanation

- Antacids given concurrently reduce the efficacy of sucralfate

36. **Ans: B**

Ref: KD Tripathi, 6/E, p. 741

Explanation

- INH neurotoxicity is treated by pyridoxine – 100 mg/day
- Pyridoxine given prophylactically, 10 mg/day prevents neurotoxicity

37. **Ans: B**

Ref: KD Tripathi, 6/E, p. 192

GENERAL MEDICINE

38. **Ans: B**

Ref: Harrison, Vol. I, 17/E, p. 1165

39. **Ans: C**

Ref: Davidson, 20/E, p. 630

40. **Ans: C**

Ref: Davidson, 20/E, p. 480

Explanation

- Answer is C because in nephritic syndrome hypercholesterolemia is seen due to non –specific increase in lipoprotein synthesis by liver in response to low osmotic pressure

41. **Ans: B**

Ref: Davidson, 20/E, p. 965

Explanation

- HBsAg – Infection
- Anti HBsAg – Immunity
- HBC Ag – hidden component of viral core and is not detectable
- Anti HBCAg – latent phase
  IgM – acute
  IgG – chronic
- HBcAg – infectivity and viral replication
- Anti HBeAg – diminished viral replication and decreased infectivity

42. **Ans: C**

Ref: Davidson, 20/E, p. 1021

Explanation

- Each 10–20 ml cryoprecipitate contains fibrinogen factor VIII and Von Willebrand factor

43. **Ans: A**

Ref: Davidson, 20/E, p.664, 665

Causes of Pleural Effusion

Common Causes

- Pneumonia ('para-pneumonic effusion')
- Tuberculosis
- Pulmonary infarction
- Malignant disease
- Cardiac failure
- Subdiaphragmatic disorders (subphrenic abscess pancreatitis, etc.)

Uncommon Causes

- Hypoproteinemia (nephritic syndrome, liver failure, malnutrition)

- Connective tissue diseases (particularly systemic lupus erythematosus and rheumatoid arthritis)
- Acute rheumatic fever
- Post – myocardial infarction syndrome
- Meigs' syndrome (ovarian tumour plus pleural effusion)
- Myxoedema
- Uraemia
- Asbestos – related benign pleural effusion

44. Ans: C

Ref: Davidson, 20/E, p. 962

45. Ans: A

Ref: Davidson, 20/E, p. 390

Explanation

- Rx for Pneumo cystis carini pneumonia
  - Cotrimoxazole, Pentamidine or Clindamycin and Primaquime
  - Adjunctive corticosteroid therapy reduces mortality

46. Ans: D

Ref: Harrison, Vol. I, 17/E, p. 1032

47. Ans: A

Ref: Davidson, 20/E, p. 818

GENERAL SURGERY

48. Ans: C

Ref: S. Das, 5/E, p. 130

49. Ans: A

Ref: S. Das, 5/E, p. 625

Explanation

- It is a cystic swelling which contains multiple locules of clear lymph

50. Ans: D

Ref: Manipal Manual of Surgery, 2/E, p. 374

51. Ans: D

Ref: Manipal Manual of Surgery, 2/E, p. 35

52. Ans: C

Ref: S. Das, 5/E, p. 654

53. Ans: B

Ref: S. Das, 5/E, p. 616

Explanation

- Salivary calculi are more common in submandibular gland because the saliva of submandibular gland is more viscous and saturated in calcium salts

DENTAL MATERIALS

54. Ans: B

Ref: Phillip's, 11/E, 513

55. Ans: A

Ref: Phillip's, 11/E, 491

56. Ans: B

Ref: Phillip's, 11/E, p. 107

57. Ans: A

Ref: Phillip's, 11/E, p. 49, 50

Explanation

- Clark described color dimensions as
  1. Hue – dominant color of an object
  2. Chroma – degree of saturation of a particular hue
  3. Value – relative lightness or darkness of a color

58. Ans: D

Ref: Phillip's, 11/E, p. 521

59. Ans: D

Ref: Phillip's, 11/E, p. 550

60. Ans: A

Ref: Phillip's, 11/E, p. 87

61. Ans: D

Ref: Phillip's, 11/E, p. 403

Explanation

- The fillers which form the inorganic phase of the composites aid in
  1. Reinforcement of the matrix resin, resulting in hardness, strength and decreased wear
  2. Reduction in polymerization shrinkage
  3. Reduction in thermal expansion and contraction
  4. Improved workability by increasing viscosity
  5. Reduction in water sorption, softening and staining
  6. Increased radiopacity and diagnostic sensitivity through incorporation of heavy metals

62. Ans: A

Ref: Phillips, 11/E, p. 564

63. Ans: C

Ref: Phillips, 11/E, p. 711

64. Ans: C

Ref: Phillips, 11/E, p. 419

65. Ans: C

Ref: Phillip's, 11/E, p. 344

DADH

66. Ans: D

Ref: Orban's, 12/E, p. 2

Explanation

- Alveolar bone develops during the eruption of teeth and disappears after the tooth is extracted or lost

67. Ans: B

Ref: Wheeler's, 8/E, p. 35

Explanation

- Calcification of primary teeth begins in utero from 13 to 16 weeks / 4 – 6 months of fetal life
- By 18 – 20 weeks all the deciduous teeth start to calcify

68. Ans: C

Ref: Orban's, 12/E, p. 42

Explanation

- Lack of initiation–anodontia (complete/partial)
- Abnormal initiation–supernumerary teeth

69. Ans: C

Ref: Wheeler's, 8/E, p. 421

70. Ans: C

Ref: Orban's, 12/E, p. 65

Explanation

- The cells of inner enamel epithelium differentiate into ameloblasts and produce enamel matrix
- Enamel matrix is laid down only after the first layer of dentin is laid by the odontoblasts

71. Ans: B

Ref: Wheeler's, 8/E, p. 53

72. Ans: C

Ref: Berkovitz, 3/E, pp. 141 to 143

73. Ans: C

Ref: Wheeler's, 8/E, p. 247

ORAL PATHOLOGY AND ORAL MEDICINE

74. Ans: C

Ref: Shafer, 6/E, pp. 583, 584

75. Ans:B

Ref: Shafer 6/e pp. 426, 427

76. Ans: A

Ref: Shafer's 6/e p. 414

77. **Ans: B**

Ref: Shafer's, 6/E, p. 818

Explanation

- In Pemphigus vulgaris, prevesicular edema appears to be weakening this junction and the intercellular bridges between the epithelial cells disappear.
- This results in clumps of epithelial cells found lying free within the vesicular cells called Tzanck cells
- They show degenerative changes which include swelling of nucleus and hyper chromatic staining

78. **Ans: D**

Ref: Shafer's, 6/E, p. 93

79. **Ans: C**

Ref: Neville, 3/E, p. 422

Explanation

- Ackermans tumour is an synonym for verrucous carcinoma or snuff dipper's cancer as it was described by Ackerman in 1948

80. **Ans: C**

Ref: Shafer's, 6/E, p. 817

81. **Ans: D**

Ref: Shafer's, 6/E, p. 292

82. **Ans: D**

Ref: Shafer's, 6/E, p. 354

Explanation

- Oral hairy leukoplakia is caused by EBV frequently associated with HIV infection

83. **Ans: C**

Ref: Shafer's, 6/E, p. 802

Explanation

- As a result of the liquefaction degeneration which weakens the epithelial connective tissue interface, histologic clefts (i.e. Max – Joseph spaces) may form and on clinical examination blisters on the oral mucosa may be seen

84. **Ans: B**

Ref: Shafer's, 6/E, p. 98

85. **Ans: B**

Ref: Animal Models in Dental Research by Juam. M. Naria, p. 347

86. **Ans: B**

Ref: Shafer's, 6/E, p. 92

Explanation

- Leukoedema is a variant of normal mucosa

87. **Ans: B**

Ref: Shafer's, 6/E, p. 54

88. **Ans: D**

Ref: Shafer's, 6/E, p. 481

89. **Ans: B**

Ref: Shafer's, 6/E, p. 326

90. **Ans: C**

Ref: Shafer's, 6/E, p. 319

91. **Ans: B**

Ref: Clinical Outline of Oral Pathology, Diagnosis and Treatment, Lewis R Eversole, 3/E, p. 134

92. **Ans: B**

Ref: Shafer's, 6/E, p. 801

Explanation

- Grinspan syndrome is traid of lichen planus diabetes mellitus and vascular hypertension

93. **Ans: A**

Ref: Shafer's, 6/E, p. 785

94. **Ans: C**

Ref: Shafer's, 6/E, p. 22

Explanation

- Peutz -Jegher's syndrome is an autosomal dominantly inherited disorder characterized by intestinal hamartomatous polyps in association with mucocutaneous melanocytic macules

95. Ans: D

Ref: Shafer's, 6/E, p. 261

96. Ans: D

Ref: Shafer's, 6/E, p. 238

97. Ans: C

Ref: Shafer's, 6/E, p. 337

98. Ans: A

Ref: Shafer's, 6/E, p. 939

99. Ans: B

Ref: Shafer's, 6/E, p. 163

100. Ans: A

Ref: Shafer's, 6/E, p. 762

101. Ans: C

Ref: Silverman & Eversole, p. 344

ORAL RADIOLOGY

102. Ans: A

Ref: White and Pharoah, 6/E, p. 50

Explanation

Magnification = Object film distance/ Focal spot object distance

103. Ans: D

Ref: White and Pharoah, 6/E, p. 4

104. Ans: D

Ref: White and Pharoah, 6/E, p. 53

105. Ans: C

Ref: White and Pharoah, 6/E, p. 205

Explanation

Area of interest	*View*
Mandibular	Oblique body
Ramus	Lateral ramus and panoramic views
Coronoid	Water's view and lateral ramus
Condylar neck	Reverse towne and lateral ramus
Posterior maxilla	Panoramic view
Orbit	Water's view and PA cephalogram
Zygoma	Water's view
Zygomatic arch	SMV
Nasal bones	Lateral cephalogram
Nasal cavity	PA cephalogram

106. Ans: B

Ref: White and Pharoah, 6/E, p. 69

Explanation

- Safe lighting is low intensity illumination of relatively long wavelength (red) that does not rapidly affect open film but permits to see well enough to work in this area

ORTHODONTICS

107. Ans: D

Ref: Proffit, 4/E, p. 486

108. Ans: B

Ref: Bhalaji 3/E, p. 77

Explanation

- Class I modification of Dewey
  - Type 1 – crowded anteriors
  - Type 2 – protrusive maxillary incisors
  - Type 3 – Anterior cross bite
  - Type 4 – Posterior cross bite
  - Type 5 – Permanent molar has drifted mesially
- Class III modification of Dewey
  - *Type 1:* Each arch looks normal separately but on occlusion shows edge to edge relationship

- *Type 2:* Crowded mandibular incisors and lingual to maxillary incisors
- *Type 3:* Crowded maxillary incisors and in cross bite relation to mandibular incisors

109. Ans: D

Ref: Gurkeerat Singh, 2/E, pp. 56 and 57

110. Ans: C

Ref: Bhalaji, 3/E, p. 77

111. Ans: B

Ref: Bhalaji 3/E, pp. 75 and 77

Explanation

Feature of skeletal/true class III

- Excessive large mandible
- Forwardly placed
- Smaller than normal maxilla
- Retropositioned maxilla.

According to Lischer's classification

- Neutro occlusion – class I
- Distoocclusion – class II
- Mesioocclusion – class III

112. Ans: B

Ref: Bhalaji, 3/E, p. 186

113. Ans: C

Ref: Gurkeerat Singh, 2/E, pp. 340

114. Ans: B

Ref: Bhalaji 3/E, p. 92

Explanation

- Loss of a deciduous 2nd molar can cause a marked forward shift of the permanent first molar thereby blocking the eruption of the second premolar, which either gets impacted or is deflected to an abnormal position

115. Ans: C

Ref: Bhalaji 3/E, p. 148

116. Ans: A

Ref: Bhalaji 3/E, p. 371

Explanation

- Head gears are used for the purpose of reinforcement of anchorage or maxillary distallization
- Cervical head gear – increases facial height and causes distal movement of maxilla
- Occipital head gear – produces a distal and superior force on maxilla.

117. Ans: B

Ref: Bhalaji 3/E, p. 183

Explanation

- Light × continuous forces – direct or forward resorption
- Heavy × extreme forces hyalinization – Indirect or undermining resorption.

118. Ans: B

Ref: Bhalaji 3/E, Pg 9

Explanation

- Growth does not take place uniformly at all times. There seems to be periods when a sudden acceleration of growth occurs. This sudden increase in growth is termed growth spurt
- Any small deviations from the normal time of growth may not be always pathological. It may indicate a fast maturing child

119. Ans: B

Ref: Bhalaji 3/E, p. 9

120. Ans: D

Ref: Bhalaji 3/E, p. 15

PEDODONTICS

121. Ans: A

Ref: Shobha Tandon, 1/E, pp. 580

122. Ans: C

Ref: Shobha Tandon, 1/E, p. 73

123. Ans: B

Ref: Shobha Tandon, 2/E, p. 186

Explanation

- Increased fluoride exposure encourages remineralization and slows down progress of the caries in the pit and fissures of enamel while the cavitation continues in dentin and the lesion becomes masked by a relatively intact enamel surface. These hidden lesions are called as fluoride bombs or fluoride syndrome

124. Ans: A

Ref: Shobha Tandon, 1/E, pp. 382 and 385

Explanation

- Severe Caries results in a space loss of about 1 mm
- Retention of carious deciduous tooth by restoration is the best method of space maintenance

125. Ans: C

Ref: Shobha Tandon, 1/E, p. 148

126. Ans: B

Ref: Shobha Tandon, 1/E, p. 396

127. Ans: B

Ref: Shobha Tandon, 1/E, p. 357

Explanation

- Small pin point in a vital tooth – direct pulp capping
- Small exposure in a vital tooth – Pulpotomy
- Large exposure with immature apex in a vital tooth – apexogenesis
- Large exposure with immature apex in a non vital tooth – apexification
- Pulp exposure in a non vital tooth – RCT in permanent pulpectomy in primary teeth

128. Ans: D

Ref: Mc Donald's, 8/E, p. 183

129. Ans: B

Ref: Shobha Tandon, 1/E, p. 682

130. Ans: C

Ref: Shobha Tandon, 1/E, p. 394

131. Ans: D

Ref: Shobha Tandon, 1/E, p. 131

Explanation

Types of Cry

1. *Obstinate* – loud, high pitched, siren like wail, it is a temper tantrum to thwart dental treatment
2. *Frightened* – Convulsive breath catching sobs with torrent of tears
3. *Hurt* – may be loud accompanied by a small whimper – shows discomfort to the child
4. *Compensatory* – not a cry at all, slow monotone, to cope the unpleasant auditory stimuli

P AND SD

132. Ans: A

Ref: Soben Peter, 3/E, p. 361

133. Ans: C

Ref: Soben Peter, 3/E, p. 675

Explanation

Members of DCI consists of

1. One registered dentist
2. One member elected among themselves by DCI
3. Not more than 4 members elected from
    - Principals, vice principals, deans, director of dental college
    - Heads of dental wings of medical colleges
    - One member from each university established by law

4. One member to represent each state
5. 6 members nominated by central government of whom at least one should be a registered dental practitioner

134. Ans: B

Ref: Park, 20/E, p. 818

135. Ans: C

Ref: Park, 20/E, p. 820

Explanation

- UNICEF's regional office for South
- Central Asia region is in New Delhi

136. Ans: C

Ref: Park, 20/E, p. 411

137. Ans: A

Ref: Park 20/E, p. 588

Explanation

- Motivated person acts willingly and knowingly

138. Ans: C

Ref: Soben Peter, 3/E, p. 351

Explanation

- Developed by National Environmental Engineering Research Institute (NEERI) at Nagpur in 1961

139. Ans: B

Ref: Soben Peter, 3/E, p. 589

Explanation

Pathfinder survey

- The method used is a stratified cluster sampling technique
- Recommended ages – 5 years for primary teeth; 12, 15, 35, 44 and 65–74 for permanent teeth

140. Ans: A

Ref: Park, 20/E, p. 748

141. Ans: B

Ref: Soben Peter, 3/E, p. 276

142. Ans: C

Ref: Soben Peter, 3/E, p. 169

143. Ans: C

Ref: Soben Peter, 3/E, p. 630

144. Ans: A

Ref: Soben Peter, 3/E, p. 26

145. Ans: C

Ref: Soben Peter, 3/E, p. 631

146. Ans: B

Ref: Soben Peter, 3/E, p. 703

PROSTHODONTICS

147. Ans: C

Ref: Nallaswamy, 1/E, p. 381

148. Ans: B

Ref: Mc Crackens, 11/E, p. 38

149. Ans: C

Ref: Mc Crackens, 11/E, p. 63

Explanation

Indication of antero – posterior palatal bar

- Class I and II arches with excellent abutment and residual ridge support
- Long edentulous spans in Class II modification I arches
- Class IV arches with anterior RPD
- Inoperable palatal tori that do not extend to the junction of hard and soft palate

150. Ans: C

Ref: Zarb and Bolender, 5/E, p. 206

151. Ans: C

Ref: Nallaswamy, 1/E, p. 409

Explanation

Functional/physiological impressions:

- Mc Leans
- Hindle's
- Functional relining.

152. Ans: D

Ref: Rosensteil, 4/E, p. 95

153. Ans: B

Ref: Rosensteil, 4/E, p. 230

154. Ans: D

Ref: Rosensteil, 4/E, p. 209

Explanation

- The principles of tooth preparation may be divided into 3 broad categories
  1. Biologic considerations, which affects the health of the oral tissues
  2. Mechanical considerations which affects the integrity and durability of the restoration
  3. Esthetic considerations, which affect the appearance of the patient

155. Ans: C

Ref: Rosensteil, 4/E, p. 434

156. Ans: B

Ref: Nallaswamy, 1/E, p. 555

157. Ans: D

Ref: Nallaswamy, 1/E, p. 207

158. Ans: D

Ref: Nallaswamy, 1/E, p. 194

159. Ans: C

Ref: Zarb and Bolender, 5/E, p. 124

160. Ans: D

Ref: Zarb and Bolender, 5/E, p. 161

Explanation

Advantages of overdentures:

1. There is better maintenance of residual ridge integrity
2. Denture stability and retention
3. Better occlusal awareness, biting force and consequent neuromuscular control
4. Provides immense psychological support

161. Ans: B

Ref: Winkler, 2/E, p. 194

PERIODONTICS

162. Ans: C

Ref: Carranza, 10/E, p. 52

163. Ans: B

Ref: Carranza, 10/E, p. 51

Explanation

1. Keratinocytes – principal cells found in basal and suprabasal layers which differentiate to form the keratinized layer of epithelium
2. Non keratinocytes
   A. *Melanocytes:* Dendritic cells located in basal spinous layer of epithelium. They synthesize melanin
   B. *Langerhans cells:* Dendritic cells located among keratinocytes at all suprabasal layers; they are antigen presenting cells and belong to the reticulo-endothelial system
   C. *Merkel cells:* Are non dendritic cells that function as tactile receptors

164. Ans: C

Ref: Carranza, 10/E, p. 297

Explanation

- Leukocyte (Neutrophil) disorders are those that affect production or function of leukocytes resulting in severe periodontal destruction
- They are:
  1. Neutropenia
  2. Agranulocytosis
  3. Chediak – Higashi syndrome
  4. Lazy Leukocyte syndrome
  5. Leukocyte adhesion deficiency
  6. Papillon Lefevre syndrome
  7. Down syndrome

165. **Ans: A**

Ref: Carranza, 10/E, p. 358

166. **Ans: B**

Ref: Carranza 10/E, p. 445

Explanation

- The distance between apical end of junctional epithelium and alveolar bone is relatively constant
- The distance between apical extent of calculus and alveolar crest in human periodontal pockets is most constant, i.e. 1.97 mm
- The distance from attached plaque to bone is never less than 0.5 mm and never more than 2.7 mm

167. **Ans: B**

Ref: Carranza, 10/E, p. 766

Explanation

The instrument grasps are:

1. Standard pen grasp
2. Modified pen grasp – ensures greatest control in performing intraoral procedures
3. Palm and thumb grasp – used for stabilizing instruments during sharpening and for manipulating air and water syringes

168. **Ans: C**

Ref: Carranza, 10/E, p. 755

Explanation

- Ideal offset angle – 60° but it may range from 60 – 70°

169. **Ans: C**

Ref: Carranza, 10/E, p. 175

Explanation

Theories on mineralization of calculus

1. *Booster mechanism theory:*
   - Increase in pH of saliva causes precipitation of calcium phosphate salts by lowering the precipitation constant
   - Colloidal proteins bind calcium and Phosphate ions and maintain a super-saturated solution with respect to calcium phosphate salts
2. *Epitactic concept/Heterogenous nucleation:*
   - Seeding agents induce small foci of calcification that enlarge and coalesce to form a calcified mass

170. **Ans: B**

Ref: Carranza, 10/E, p. 140

171. **Ans: A**

Ref: Gururaja Rao, 2/E, p. 174

172. **Ans: A**

Ref: Carranza, 10/E, p. 513

173. **Ans: C**

Ref: Carranza, 10/E, p. 77

Explanation

- Cementum formation is most rapid in apical region where it compensates for tooth eruption, which itself compensates for attrition

174. **Ans: D**

Ref: Carranza, 10/E, p. 79

175. **Ans: B**

Ref: Carranza, 10/E, p. 814

Explanation

- The ability of NSAIDs to block PGE_2 production thereby reducing inflammation and inhibiting osteoclastic activity in the periodontal tissue

CONS AND ENDO

176. **Ans: D**

Ref: Sturdavent, 5/E, p. 817

177. **Ans: B**

Ref: Sturdevant's, 6/E, 547

178. Ans: C

Ref: Sturdavent, 5/E, p. 219

Explanation

Of the given options

1. Amalgam – if placed directly causes galvanic action
2. Composite – should not be applied directly on the tooth
3. Silicate – has very low pH causes damage

179. Ans: A

Ref: Sturdavent, 6/E, p. 848

180. Ans: C

Ref: Sturdavent, 5/E, p. 248

181. Ans: A

Ref: Sturdavent, 6/E, p. 356

182. Ans: B

Ref: Ingle, 5/E, p.505

Explanation

- The recommended regime for irrigation is to employ 17% EDTA for 1 minute followed by a final rinse with NaOCl

183. Ans: C

Ref: Grossman, 12/E, p. 60

184. Ans: A

Ref: Grossman, 12/E, p. 174

Explanation

- Temperature ranges between 425°F– 475° F or 218°C–246°C.

185. Ans: A

Ref: Grossman, 12/E, p. 185

186. Ans: C

Ref: Grossman, 12/E, p. 230

Explanation

- The giromatic hand piece activates a stainless steel, barbed broach, K I file or K–reamer in the root canal through a 90° reciprocating arc at a speed up to 3000 cycles/min

ORAL SURGERY

187. Ans: D

Ref: Malamed Local Anesthesia, 5/E, p. 313

188. Ans: A

Ref: Killey's, 4/E, p. 10

Explanation

- Forces of range 425 lbs produces fractures of the condylar neck which is the weakest part of the mandible

189. Ans: A

Ref: Peterson, 4/E, p. 31

190. Ans: B

Ref: Malamed Local Anesthesia, 5/E, p. 296

191. Ans: D

Ref: Neelima Malik, 2/E, p. 172

192. Ans: D

Ref: Peterson, 4/E, p. 26

193. Ans: B

Ref: Malamed Local Anesthesia, 5/E, p. 250

194. Ans: D

Ref: Neelima Malik, 2/E, p. 618

195. Ans: C

Ref: Neelima Malik, 2/E, p. 354

Explanation

1. Le Fort I–horizontal/Guerin's/fracture
2. Le Fort II–pyramidal/subzygomatic
3. Le Fort III–transverse/suprazygomatic

196. Ans: D

Ref: Neelima Malik, 2/E, p. 242

Explanation

- Various symptoms of MPDS

Table 2.1: Associated symptoms in MPDS

Neurologic	*Gastro –intestinal tract*	*Musculo skeletal*	*Otologic*
Tingling	Nausea	Fatigue	Tinnitus
Numbness	Vomiting	Tension	Ear pain
Blurred vision	Diarrhoea	Shift joint pains	Dizziness
Twitches	Constipation	Tiredness	Vertigo
Trembling	Indigestion	Weakness	Diminished hearing
Lacrimation	Dry mouth		

- Cardinal symptoms of MPDS
  - I. pain or discomfort (unexplained nature), anywhere about the head or neck
  - II. limitation of motion of the jaw
  - III. Joint noises – grating, clicking, snapping, etc
  - IV. Tenderness to palpation of the muscles of mastication (Negative recent history of trauma, infection, ear or joint or maxillary sinus pathosis)

Ref to Table 2.1

197. Ans: D

Ref: Text Book of Oral Surgery, Gustav O Kruger, 6/E, p. 612

198. Ans: C

Ref: Malamed, 5/E, p. 289

199. Ans: C

Ref: Neelima Malik, 2/E, p. 442

200. Ans: B

Ref: *Neelima Malik, 2/E, p. 576*

3

KCET 2005

HUMAN ANATOMY

1. **Nerve passing through the center of cavernous sinus is**
   A. Oculomotor nerve
   B. Trochlear nerve
   C. Abducent nerve
   D. Maxillary nerve

2. **Structures passing through superior constrictor muscle and base of skull are**
   A. Stylopharyngeus and glossopharyngeal nerve
   B. Auditory tube and levator palatine muscle
   C. Internal laryngeal nerve and superior laryngeal vessels
   D. Recurrent laryngeal nerve and inferior laryngeal vessels

3. **Inferior salivatory nucleus supplies**
   A. Lacrimal gland
   B. Parotid gland
   C. Submandibular salivary gland
   D. Sub lingual salivary gland

4. **Hassall's corpuscles are seen in**
   A. Prostate
   B. Spleen
   C. Thymus
   D. Liver

5. **Which of the following paranasal sinuses is formed before birth?**
   A. Maxillary sinus
   B. Frontal sinus
   C. Ethmoid sinus
   D. Mastoid air sinus

PHYSIOLOGY

6. **Sharp momentary pain elicited by pulp is caused by**
   A. A delta fibers
   B. C fibres
   C. A alpha fibers
   D. None of the above

7. **Renin is secreted by**
   A. Cells in proximal tubules
   B. Cells in distal tubules
   C. Macula Densa
   D. Juxtaglomerular Cells

8. **Calcium absorption is increased by**
   A. Increased Na^+ absorption
   B. Hypercalcemia
   C. Iron over load
   D. 1, 25 dihydroxycholecalciferol

9. **When the radius of the resistance vessels is increased, which of the following is increased?**
   A. Capillary blood flow
   B. Systolic blood pressure
   C. Diastolic blood pressure
   D. Hematocrit

10. **Which of the following has the greatest effect on the ability of blood to transport oxygen?**
   A. CO2 content of red blood cells
   B. pH of plasma
   C. Amount of hemoglobin in the blood
   D. Capacity of the blood to dissolve Oxygen

11. In infants, defecation often follows a meal. The cause of colonic contraction in this situation is

A. The gastroileac reflex
B. The enterogastric reflex
C. Gastrocolic reflex
D. Increased circulatory levels of CCK

12. Principle cation that requires for absorption of D–Glucose is

A. K^+
B. Na^+
C. Ca^{++}
D. Mg^+

BIOCHEMISTRY

13. Mucopolysaccharide which function as a lubricant and shock absorber in synovial fluid is

A. Heparin
B. Hyaluronic acid
C. Keratin sulphate
D. Chondroitin–4–sulphate

14. Figlu excretion test is used to detect

A. Folic acid deficiency
B. Biotin deficiency
C. Pantothenic acid deficiency
D. Vitamin B_{12} deficiency

15. Biological value (fuel value) of fat is

A. 4.0 KC/g
B. 5.4 KC/g
C. 7.0 KC/g
D. 9.0 KC/g

16. Electron transport chain and ATP synthesizing structures are located in

A. Outer membrane of mitochondria
B. Mitochondrial matrix
C. Inner membrane of mitochondria
D. Microsomes

GENERAL PATHOLOGY

17. Serum alkaline phosphatase is raised in all of the following EXCEPT

A. Paget's disease
B. Fibrous dysplasia
C. Osteomyelitis
D. Hyperparathyroidism

18. Enzymatic digestion is the predominant event in the following type of necrosis

A. Coagulative necrosis
B. Caseous necrosis
C. Liquefactive necrosis
D. Fibrinoid necrosis

19. Sago spleen is found in

A. Chronic inflammation
B. Amyloidosis
C. Tuberculosis
D. Syphilis

20. Langhan's type of giant cell is found in

A. Fat necrosis
B. Malignancy
C. Tuberculosis
D. Acute inflammation

21. Transudate differs from exudates in having the following EXCEPT

A. Few inflammatory cells
B. Glucose content
C. Low protein content
D. Low specific gravity

22. Nutmeg liver is seen in

A. Thrombosis
B. Embolism
C. CVC liver
D. Alcoholism

23. Hydatid cysts are due to infection with

A. Hymenilepis nana
B. Diphyllobothrium latum
C. Echinococcus granulosus
D. Ascaris Lumbricoides

24. Chloromas are a feature of

A. Lymphomas
B. Leukemia
C. Leukoedema
D. Leukoplakia

MICROBIOLOGY

25. Which of the following viruses are NOT implicated in human malignancies?

A. Epstein–Barr virus
B. Herpes simplex virus type I
C. HTLV 1
D. Papilloma virus

26. Secretory immunoglobulin is

A. IgA
B. IgE
C. IgG
D. IgM

27. The temperature and pressure at which spores are killed during sterilization by autoclave are

A. 102°C temp and pressure is 8 lb/sq. inch for 10min
B. 105°C temp and pressure is 8 lb/sq. inch for 10min
C. 110°C temp and pressure is 8 lb/sq. inch for 10min
D. 121°C temp and pressure is 8 lb/sq. inch for 10min

28. Rice water stools are seen in infections with

A. Proteus
B. Shigella
C. Vibrio cholera
D. Salmonella

29. Donavan bodies are seen in bone marrow and splenic aspiration smears in infection with

A. Leishmania donovani
B. Lymphogranuloma venereum
C. Klebsiella pneumonia
D. Haemophilus ducreyi

30. The commonly done screening test for HIV infection is

A. Radio immuno assay
B. ELISA
C. Fluorescent antibody technique
D. Electrophoresis

PHARMACOLOGY

31. Therapeutic Index is a measure of

A. Safety of a drug
B. Toxicity of a drug
C. Efficacy of a drug
D. All of the above

32. Dissociative anesthesia is produced by

A. Lignocaine
B. Nitrous oxide
C. Diazepam
D. Ketamine

33. Contra indications for the use of corticosteroids are all the following EXCEPT

A. Peptic ulcer
B. Herpes simplex Infection
C. Diabetes Mellitus
D. Severe acute bronchial asthma

34. Obtundents are

A. Abrasives
B. Mummifying agents
C. Sweetening agents
D. Dentine desensitizers

35. Malignant hyperthermia is caused by

A. Atropine
B. Aspirin
C. Succinyl choline
D. None of the above

GENERAL MEDICINE

36. The term poikilokaryosis refer to

A. Alteration of nuclear–cytoplasmic ratio
B. Division of nuclei without division of cytoplasm
C. Large, prominent nuclei
D. Loss of polarity and disorientation of Cells

37. The invasion of living tissues by larvae of certain species of flies is called

A. Helminthiasis
B. Myiasis
C. Myelofibrosis
D. Moniliasis

38. Which of the following is indicative of left ventricular failure?

A. Neck vein distension
B. Ascitis
C. Anorexia
D. orthopnoea

39. Lobar pneumonia is usually caused by

A. Klebsiella pneumoniae
B. Streptococcus pyogenes
C. Pneumococci
D. Staphylococcus aureus

40. All of the following contribute to hepatic encephalopathy EXCEPT

A. Antibiotic therapy
B. Hypokalemia
C. Gastro–intestinal bleeding
D. Cirrhosis

41. Intravenous drug abusers have following disease EXCEPT

A. Hepatitis B
B. Polyneuritis
C. Endocarditis
D. None

42. Blood borne hepatitis are all EXCEPT

A. Hepatitis B
B. Hepatitis C
C. Hepatitis D
D. Hepatitis E

43. Massive splenomegaly is seen in

A. Typhoid
B. Infective endocarditis
C. Acute leukemia
D. Portal hypertension

44. Drug of choice for dermatitis herpetiformis

A. Rifampicin
B. Corticosteroid
C. Acyclovir
D. Dapsone

45. All of the following are clinical features of Infective endocarditis EXCEPT

A. Anemia
B. Pyrexia
C. Hepatomegaly
D. Splenomegaly

46. The commonest cause of jaundice in India is

A. Anti–tubercular drugs
B. Viral hepatitis
C. Liver cancer
D. Stone in common bile duct

47. Commonest mode of death in patients of Hypertension is

A. Epistaxis
B. Gastro–intestinal bleeding
C. Heart failure
D. Kidney failure

48. Vasovagal shock is precipitated due to activation of

A. Parasympathetic system
B. Sympathetic system
C. Dilation of all vessels
D. None of the above

49. Mannitol is given in head injury patients to

A. Decrease hematoma formation
B. Decrease intracranial pressure
C. To differentiate cerebral edema and hematoma formation
D. To decrease osmolarity of blood

50. Paresis means

A. Total loss of sensory function
B. Total loss of motor function
C. Incomplete paralysis
D. None of above

GENERAL SURGERY

51. In cerebral concussion the pupils are

A. Constricted and reacting to light
B. Dilated and not reacting to light
C. Dilated and reacting to light
D. Constricted and not reacting to light

52. Primary closure of wounds fail if there is

A. Tight closure
B. Haematoma formation
C. When no drainage is present
D. All of the above

53. Cystic hygroma is a

A. Haemangioma
B. Lymphangioma
C. Lung abscess
D. Liver cirrhosis manifestation

54. Marjolin's ulcer is a

A. Malignant ulcer found on skin of face
B. Malignant ulcer found on the scar of burn
C. Trophic ulcer
D. Tropical ulcer characterized by absence of pain

55. Positive Murphy's sign is indicative of

A. Peritonitis
B. Perforation of peptic ulcer
C. Acute appendicitis
D. Tender gall bladder

56. Pyelography is a method by which dye is injected to visualize

A. Parotid gland
B. Liver
C. Kidney
D. Spleen

57. Coles' fracture is associated with

A. Mandible
B. Knee
C. Ankle
D. Wrist

58. Cold abscess formation is due to

A. Presence of acute inflammation
B. Formation of caseous pus with signs of acute inflammation
C. Formation of caseous pus without signs of acute inflammation
D. Infected cyst

DENTAL MATERIALS

59. The blue light used to polymerize composite resin is harmful to eye if one looks at it, which portion of the eye is affected

A. Cornea
B. Retina
C. Lens
D. None of the above

60. Once triturated the dental amalgam should be condensed with in

A. 5 minutes
B. 6 minutes
C. 3 minutes
D. 15 minutes

61. Which of the following impression materials is more biocompatible?

A. Polysulphide
B. Condensation silicone
C. Addition silicone
D. Polyether

62. According to ADA specification No. 3, TypeI impression compound, at 45°C, should have a minimum flow

A. More than 65%
B. More than 75%
C. More than 85%
D. More than 95%

63. Which of the following impression material is most biocompatible?

A. Polysulphide
B. Condensation Silicone
C. Addition Silicone
D. Polyether

64. Which of the following is NOT a direct restorative material?

A. Dentin bonding agent
B. Composite resin
C. Dental amalgam
D. Dental ceramic

65. Loss of gloss test in gypsum product is an indication for

A. Adequate mixing time
B. Adequate working time
C. Initial set
D. Final set

66. Rouge, used as dental abrasive, is chemically known as

A. Tin oxide
B. Iron oxide
C. Ethyl silicate
D. Zirconium silicate

67. Casting porosity, which is caused by the inability of air to escape through the pores in the investment

A. Localized shrinkage porosity
B. Suck–back porosity
C. Back pressure porosity
D. Micro porosity

68. Particle size of micro filled composite restorative resin is in the following range

A. 0.04–0.4 micrometer
B. 0.4–1 micro meter
C. 0.5–3 micrometer
D. 8–12 micrometer

69. Which of the following is a castable dental ceramic?

A. Aluminous porcelain
B. IPS–empress 2
C. In–ceram
D. Dicor

70. In visible light cured denture base resin, Camphoroquinone serves as the

A. Activator
B. Initiator
C. Retarder
D. Filler

DADH

71. In the absence of a second premolar the roots of the primary second molar will most likely

A. Resorb at normal site
B. Resorb more slowly than normal
C. Resorb more rapidly than normal
D. Show no resorption as the initiator force is absent

72. Abnormality in morphodifferentiation stage of tooth development results in

A. Mottled enamel
B. Mesiodens
C. Dens in dente
D. Dentinogenesis imperfecta

73. The oblique ridge runs from the disto-buccal cusp to

A. Mesiobuccal
B. Mesiolingual
C. Distolingual cusp
D. None of the above

74. The human teeth are

A. Haplodont
B. Triconodont
C. Bunodont
D. All of the above

75. The formation of hard tissues initiates in the

A. Bud stage
B. Cap stage
C. Advanced bell stage
D. Early bell stage

76. The most accepted dentine sensitivity theory is

A. Transduction theory
B. Hydrodynamic theory
C. Direct neuronal theory
D. None of the above

ORAL PATHOLOGY AND ORAL MEDICINE

77. Presence of ammonia in the saliva will

A. Increase plaque formation
B. Decrease plaque formation
C. Have no effect on plaque
D. Increase calculus formation

78. **Phlegmon is a**
   A. Sexually transmitted disease
   B. Type of cellulitis
   C. Type of osteomyelitis
   D. Venereal disease

79. **Which type of odontogenic keratocyst is more aggressive, more common and more likely to reccur**
   A. Orthokeratinised
   B. Parakeratinised
   C. Nonkeratinised
   D. Dekeratinised

80. **The epithelium of a dentigerous cyst is**
   A. 15–20 cell thick
   B. 6–10 cell thick
   C. 2–4 cell thick
   D. 1–2 cell thick

81. **The Swiss cheese appearance is seen in microscopic picture of**
   A. Lichen planus
   B. Adenoid cystic carcinoma
   C. Ameloblastoma
   D. Pleomorphic adenoma

82. **Candidiasis associated with dentures is**
   A. Acute pseudo membranous
   B. Acute atrophic
   C. Chronic hyperplastic
   D. Chronic atrophic

83. **Monroe's abscess is seen in**
   A. Leukoplakia
   B. White spongy nevus
   C. Psoriasis
   D. Lichen planus

84. **Mask–like appearance of face with narrowing of oral aperture and rigidity of the mucosa is characteristic of**
   A. Progressive systemic sclerosis
   B. Tetanus
   C. Multiple sclerosis
   D. Osteomalacia

85. **Intraepithelial vesicle is the feature found in**
   A. Lichen planus
   B. Pemphigus
   C. Bullous pemphigoid
   D. All of the above

86. **Double lip is one of the features of**
   A. Albright's syndrome
   B. Frey's syndrome
   C. Aldrich syndrome
   D. Ascher's syndrome

87. **The capacity to reproduce skin lesion at sites of injury in psoriasis is called**
   A. Koebner's phenomenon
   B. Nikolsky's sign
   C. Chvostek's sign
   D. Raynaud's phenomenon

88. **Swelling of the nasolabial fold with no radiographic findings is suggestive of**
   A. Median palatine cyst
   B. Periapical cyst
   C. Nasopalatine cyst
   D. Nasoalveolar cyst

89. **Gustatory sweating is seen in**
   A. Auriculotemporal syndrome
   B. Facial palsy
   C. Myofacial pain dysfunction syndrome
   D. Mikulicz's disease

90. **Complete obliteration of pulp is seen in all the following EXCEPT**
   A. Type I dentinogenesis imperfecta
   B. Type II dentinogenesis imperfecta
   C. Type III dentinogenesis imperfecta
   D. Dentinal dysplasia

91. **Epstein pearls are cysts that arise from**
   A. Squamous tissue of the mucosa
   B. Herpes simplex virus type I
   C. Rests of Malassez
   D. Dental Lamina

92. **Paul–Bunnel test is positive in**
   A. Infectious mononucleosis

B. Multiple myeloma
C. Malignant melanoma
D. Rubella

93. The cell body seen in microscopic picture of Lichen planus is
A. Lipschutz bodies
B. Barr bodies
C. Civatte bodies
D. Koilocyte body

94. A disease that only affects formation and eruption of tooth but DOES NOT cause hypoplasia is
A. Hypoparathyrodisim
B. Hyperparathyroidism
C. Rickets
D. Syphilis

95. Juvenile rheumatoid arthritis is called
A. Still's disease
B. Cushing's syndrome
C. Addison's disease
D. Von Recklinghausen's syndrome

RADIOLOGY

96. Target lesions are seen in
A. Erythroplakia
B. Pemphigus
C. Erythema multiforme
D. Lichen planus

97. The overall degree of darkening of exposed film is known as
A. Contrast
B. Density
C. Sharpness
D. Fog

98. The Filter in an X–ray apparatus is made up of
A. Aluminium
B. Lead
C. Molybdenum
D. Tungsten

99. Choose the false statement among the four
A. X–rays are ionizing rays
B. X–rays can be focused
C. X–rays cannot be seen or touched
D. X–rays can cause mutation

100. Injecting radio–opaque dye into the joint space to visualize the joint is referred to as
A. Arthroscopy
B. Arthrography
C. Orthopantomography
D. Arthroplasty

101. The compton effect is seen when
A. X–rays strike on Film
B. X–rays strike on skin
C. X–rays interact with matter
D. X–rays interact with emulsion coating on film

ORTHODONTICS

102. The best age for giving a functional appliance for correcting skeletal dysplasia in girls is
A. 6–8 years
B. 10–11 years
C. 13–14 yeas
D. After 18 years

103. The optimal time to employ an orthodontic appliance that takes advantage of growth is during
A. Late primary dentition
B. Early mixed dentition
C. Late mixed dentition
D. Early permanent dentition

104. A retained lower deciduous incisor will usually
A. Deflect the permanent tooth labially
B. Deflect the permanent tooth lingually
C. Causes ankylosis of the underlying permanent tooth
D. Causes impaction of underlying permanent tooth

105. The difference between the amount of space needed for the permanent incisors to erupt and the space available for them is called

A. Primate space
B. Leeway space
C. Interdental space
D. Incisor liability

106. Rotation of the teeth around its long axis is known as

A. Axioversion
B. Transversion
C. Perversion
D. Torsiversion

107. The most common tooth to get impacted (excluding the third molars) is

A. Maxillary canine
B. Mandibular canine
C. Maxillary II premolar
D. Mandibular II premolar

108. The face that is long and narrow is said to be

A. Mesoprosopic
B. Leptoprosopic
C. Euryprosopic
D. Brachyprosopic

109. Lisping is associated commonly with which of the following malocclusions

A. Anterior deep bite
B. Anterior crowding
C. Anterior open bite
D. Anterior retroclination

110. The average angle of convexity as in Down's Cephalometric analysis is

A. 0 degree
B. 25 degree
C. 82 degree
D. 84 degrees

111. Fishman's SMI is a method of evaluation of

A. Symmetry of the dental arch
B. Skeletal maturity
C. Arch length discrepancy
D. Prognathism of maxilla

112. Which of the following analysis is used to assess the tooth size discrepancy between the upper and lower teeth?

A. Wits analysis
B. Korkhaus analysis
C. Bolton analysis
D. Moyers analysis

113. The type of tooth movement most notorious for relapse is

A. Tipping
B. Translation
C. Torquing
D. Rotation

114. Rapid palatal expansion using a Hyrax screw is an example for

A. Extra–oral anchorage
B. Intermaxillary anchorage
C. Muscular anchorage
D. Reciprocal anchorage

115. The most important disadvantage of removable appliance is

A. They are dependent on patient co–operation
B. They are NOT hygienic
C. They are ineffective in treating deep bite
D. Fabrication is cumbersome

116. Shape memory is a characteristic of which of the following wires?

A. Beta–titanium
B. Alpha–titanium
C. Nickel–titanium
D. Chrome–cobalt

117. The force exerted by wire is

A. Directly proportional to the cube of the length of the wire
B. Inversely proportional to the cube of the length of the wire
C. Directly proportional to the fourth power of the length of the wire
D. Inversely proportional to the fourth power of the length of the wire

118. Delaire's Facemask is used in the treatment of

A. Mandibular retrognathism
B. Maxillary retrognathism
C. Mandibular ankylosis
D. Maxillary prognathism

119. Which of the following is a fixed functional appliance?

A. Bionator
B. Bow activator
C. Herbst appliance
D. Kinetor

120. In classical Begg Mechano therapy, bite opening is primarily effected in

A. Stage I
B. Stage II
C. Stage III
D. Stage IV

PEDODONTICS

121. The ugly duckling stage of dentition in a child is corrected by the eruption of which tooth?

A. Central incisor
B. Lateral incisor
C. Canine
D. First molar

122. Which of the following procedure is replaced by the use of occlusal sealants?

A. Occlusal amalgam restoration
B. Topical fluoride restoration
C. Prophylactic odontomy
D. All

123. The Green stains frequently seen in children's teeth are caused by

A. Chromogenic bacteria
B. Acute necrotizing gingivitis
C. Enamel defects
D. Vitamin B deficiency

124. Most common cause of acute generalized gingival inflammation in a preschool child

A. Acute herpetic gingivostomatitis
B. Acute necrotizing gingivitis
C. Aphthous stomatitis
D. Vitamin B deficiency

125. On the first dental visit, basic fear of a child under the age of 2 is related to

A. Fear of injection
B. Anxiety over being separated from parent
C. Anxiety regarding instruments used to perform dental treatment
D. NOT understanding the reason for dental treatment

126. The success of calcium hydroxide pulpotomy is determined by the

A. Formation of calcified bridge
B. Formation of hard base to support the restoration
C. Continuation of root formation and apexogenesis
D. All of the above

127. Teeth usually emerge when

A. ¼ of their roots are complete
B. ½ of roots are complete
C. ¾ of roots are complete
D. After completion of root formation

128. In primary molars when proximal portion of Class II cavity preparation extends deep gingivally, a satisfactory gingival seat is NOT obtained because

A. Enamel rods extend occlusally in gingival third
B. Buccal and lingual surface converge occlusally
C. Primary teeth have marked cervical constriction
D. All of the above

P AND SD

129. Bias is any systematic error in determination of association between

A. Relative risk and attributable risk
B. Incidence and prevalence
C. Exposure and disease
D. Disease and environmental factors

130. Salt fluoridation was pioneered by

A. US public health commission
B. Switzerland
C. New Zealand
D. Singapore

131. "Loss of head" in water purification is related to

A. Filtration capacity
B. Disinfection of water
C. Fluoridation of water
D. Chlorination of water

132. Stipulated lethal dose of fluoride in adults

A. 1–2 gm/kg of body weight
B. 2.5–3.5 gm/kg of body weight
C. 3.5–4 gm/kg of body weight
D. 5–10 gm/kg of body weight

133. DMF score for any one individual can range from

A. 0–28
B. 0–32
C. 0–48
D. 0–64

134. Revised Dean's fluorosis index has

A. Five point scale
B. Six point scale
C. Seven point scale
D. Nine point scale

135. Which of the following is NOT an indicator for nutritional status?

A. Vital signs
B. Weight and height
C. Mid arm circumference
D. Prevalence of low birth weight

136. Primordial prevention, a new concept receiving special attention in the prevention of

A. Acute disease
B. Chronic disease
C. Epidemics
D. Pandemics

137. Repeated topical application of a fluoride agent will NOT produce tooth mottling because

A. The concentration in topical agent is NOT as high as required for mottling
B. The saliva neutralizes the excess fluoride delivered by topical agent
C. It is NOT fluoride that produces the mottling seen in Fluorosis
D. The tooth is already calcified and cannot be altered in this fashion

138. Select the FALSE principle for DMF Score

A. Last permanent molars are included in scoring
B. Naturally exfoliated teeth should not be taken into consideration
C. Teeth extracted due to orthodontic treatment or periodontal disease or impaction should not be considered
D. Endodontically treated tooth should be considered

139. Which of the following is the WRONG statement?

A. 2% NaF solution is recommended as caries preventive agent
B. 2% NaF solution can be prepared by dissolving 0.2 gm of NaF powder in 10 ml of distilled water in plastic bottle
C. If NaF aqueous solution is stored in glass bottle, then the fluoride ions of solution can react with silica of glass forming Si F2, thus reducing the availability of free active fluorides to anticaries activity
D. 2% NaF application should be carried out at the age 3, 7, 12, 18

140. Prevention of disease has.........levels

A. One
B. Two
C. Three
D. Four

141. Teeth selected for scoring of PHP–M (Personal Hygiene Performance Modified) are

A. Six

B. Twelve
C. Eighteen
D. Twenty four

142. DMFT and DMFS indices represent

A. Decayed teeth index
B. Missing/surface teeth index
C. Filled teeth index
D. Caries index

143. Which of the following sugars contribute least to dental caries?

A. Fructose
B. Galactose
C. Sucrose
D. Xylitol

PROSTHODONTICS

144. Fovea palatini are formed

A. Behind the vibrating line
B. In front of vibrating line
C. On the vibrating line
D. Has no relation to the vibrating line

145. The stability of denture refers to

A. Resistance against vertical forces
B. Resistance against horizontal forces
C. Resistance to removal in the opposite direction
D. Mobility of dentures

146. The Gothic arch tracing device is used to record

A. The vertical dimension of occlusion
B. The centric relation
C. Centric occlusion
D. Orientation relation

147. Reduced interocclusal distance in complete denture

A. Reduces biting forces
B. Increases biting force
C. Is NOT related to biting force
D. Causes increased soreness

148. Difficulty in use of metallic denture bases is

A. Less margin of error in posterior palatal seal
B. Lack of tissue tolerance
C. Increased weight of dentures
D. Difficulty in getting accuracy of fit

149. Antes law states that

A. Combined periodontal ligament area of the abutment tooth should equal or exceed that of tooth or teeth to be replaced
B. Combined periodontal ligament area of the abutment tooth should be less than that of tooth or teeth to be replaced
C. Combined periodontal ligament area of the abutment tooth should be at least double that of tooth or teeth to be replaced
D. Ante's law has now been proved to be Obsolete

150. The Pontic of maxillary posterior region should be

A. Sanitary
B. Point contact
C. Bullet nose
D. Saddle

151. A full veneer crown is one that

A. Fully veneers one surface of a tooth
B. Covers whole of the clinical crown of a tooth
C. Is basically a porcelain veneer
D. Covers more than 7/8th of the tooth

152. Margin for all ceramic crowns should be

A. Feather edge
B. Shoulder
C. Shoulder with bevel
D. Chamfer

153. The ideal occlusal clearance for a complete cast crown is

A. 0.5 mm
B. 1.5 mm
C. 2 mm
D. 2.5 mm

154. Indirect retainers in bilateral distal extension base removable partial dentures are based on

A. Class I lever principle
B. Class II lever principle
C. Class III lever principle
D. Combination of more than one of the Above

155. Least preferred maxillary major connector is

A. Single palatal strap
B. Anterior-posterior palatal bar
C. Horse shoe shaped major connector
D. Complete palatal coverage

156. Back action clasp is a modification of

A. Embrasure clasp
B. Half and half clasp
C. Reverse action clasp
D. Ring clasp

PERIODONTICS

157. Gingival fluid is a

A. Transudate
B. Exudate
C. Can be either of the two (transudate or exudate)
D. Neither of the two (transudate and exudate)

158. Burtonian line is a linear pigmentation of gingival margin due to overexposure to

A. Bismuth
B. Silver
C. Lead
D. Arsenic

159. The flap technique for pocket elimination which also increase the width of attached gingiva is

A. Coronally repositioned flap
B. Apically repositioned flap
C. Laterally displaced flap
D. Modified widman flap

160. In modified widman flap

A. Internal bevel incision is the last incision
B. Interdental papilla is eliminated
C. Posterior areas are difficult to access the bone
D. Crevicular incision is made from the base of the pocket

161. For root planing and sub gingival scaling of mesial surface in posterior teeth, Gracey curettes

A. No. 7–8 are used
B. No. 9–10 are used
C. No. 11–12 are used
D. No. 13–14 are used

162. Coronoplasty should be carried out in patients with

A. Occlusal prematurities
B. Parafunctional habits
C. Signs of trauma from occlusion
D. All of the above features

163. The periodontal fibers which are more resistant to forces along the long axis are

A. Apical
B. Oblique
C. Alveolar crest
D. Horizontal

164. Electro–surgery or surgical diathermy uses controlled high frequency electrical current in the range of

A. 1.5–7.5 million cycles/second
B. 7.5–10.0 million cycles/second
C. 15–20 million cycles/second
D. 25–30 million cycles/second

165. A glycoprotein that promotes new attachment and increased cell proliferation is

A. Fibronectin
B. Fibropectin
C. Glycogen
D. Glycosaminoglycan

166. Healing of a graft of intermediate thickness is completed by

A. 3 weeks

B. 5 weeks
C. 10 weeks
D. 16 weeks

167. The offset angle of Gracey curette between the blade and shank is
A. 70 degrees
B. 60 degrees
C. 80 degrees
D. 90 degrees

168. CADIA is used to assess
A. Occlusal trauma
B. Furcation involvement
C. Gingival enlargement
D. Periodontal disease progression

169. DNA probe
A. Measures periodontal pocket depth
B. Identifies a particular micro–organism
C. Calculate the length of gingival epithelium attachment
D. Is NOT useful in all the above three

170. The graft with maximum osteogenic potential is
A. Allograft
B. Xenograft
C. Auto–cortical
D. Auto–cancellous

CONS AND ENDO

171. Apicoectomy is
A. Periapical curettage
B. Retrograde restoration
C. Surgical removal of root
D. Surgical removal of root tip of endodontically treated tooth

172. Most of the routinely used burs in conservative dentistry have
A. Positive rake
B. Negative rake
C. Neutral rake
D. None of the above

173. In a class V preparation, during application of rubber dam the punch of the tooth to be restored should be made
A. According to the template supplied
B. According to the existing arch form
C. Labial to the position of the tooth to be operated
D. Lingual to the position of the tooth to be operated

174. Lentulospirals are used for
A. Locating canal orifice
B. Pulp extirpation
C. Enlarging coronal third root canal
D. Application of root canal sealer

175. Penetrating corrosion in an amalgam restoration is caused by
A. Ag–Hg phase
B. Sn–Hg phase
C. Cu–Sn phase
D. All the above

176. Which among the following statements is TRUE?
A. Files have more flutes than reamers
B. Reamers have more flutes than files
C. Both have the same number of flutes
D. Files and reamers have no flutes

177. According to ISO standardization, root canal files and reamers should have a taper of
A. 0.02 mm per cm
B. 0.02 mm per mm
C. 0.03 mm per cm
D. 0.03 mm per mm

178. One of the purpose of etching beveled enamel surface is to
A. Increase surface energy
B. Produce macro under cut
C. To increase convenience
D. To prevent caries

179. The Masserann Kit technique for removing solid objects

A. Is very short procedure
B. Is more successful in posterior teeth than in anterior ones
C. Requires frequent radiographic monitoring
D. Is better than the ultrasonic technique

180. The angle of the beveled resected root

A. Should be sufficient to provide access to perform the retro preparation
B. Should be at 45 degrees of the facial surface
C. Shall enable the removal of 1 to 2 mm of apex to ensure that apical ramifications are NOT present
D. Should be at 60 degrees to the facial Surfaces

181. A pulp is inflamed as a result of deep caries and cavity preparation, which of the following helps the best to resolve the inflammation

A. Calcium hydroxide
B. No medication/material available presently which can promote pulp healing
C. Mineral trioxide aggregate
D. Poly antibiotic preparation

182. Which of the following Principles of the cavity preparation is NOT considered much in modern methods of restorative dentistry?

A. Extension for prevention
B. Convenient form
C. Removal of the undermined enamel
D. Removal of the carious enamel

183. Rounding of the axio–pulpal line angle in a proximo–occlusal preparation is considered as a part of

A. Refining the line form
B. Retention form
C. Resistance form
D. Convenient form

184. As per the raise of frictional heat in using various rotary cutting instruments is concerned which one of the following is the most kind to the pulp

A. Stainless steel bur
B. Diamond bur
C. Carbide bur
D. Carbon steel bur

185. Which of the following is least likely to be used as a pit and fissure sealant?

A. Cyanoacrylates
B. Urethane dimethacrylate
C. Gold alloy
D. BIS–GMA

ORAL SURGERY

186. Time taken for osseointegration of implants in the maxilla is

A. 4 months
B. 2 months
C. 6 months
D. 8 months

187. The recommended time interval between surgery and placing load in the posterior mandible is

A. 2 months
B. 3 months
C. 4 months
D. 5 months

188. The proximal segment of horizontally unfavorable mandibular angle fracture is displaced

A. Inferiorly
B. Posteriorly and medially
C. Anteriorly and superiorly
D. Anteriorly and laterally

189. Surgical management of Ludwig's Angina includes

A. Application of heat
B. Incision and decompression
C. Drainage through closed dwelling catheter
D. Both B and C

190. Gunning splints are used when the patient is

A. Dentulous
B. Edentulous
C. Children
D. Young Adults

191. Ecchymosis in the mastoid region seen after a fracture bone is known as

A. Chvostek's sign
B. Battle sign
C. Guerin's sign
D. Tinel's sign

192. Direct interdental wiring is also known as

A. Risdon's wiring
B. Gilmer's wiring
C. Stout's wiring
D. Eyelet wiring

193. The following structures are divided when the angle of the mandible is exposed through the submandibular incision

A. Skin, superficial fascia, platysma, deep cervical fascia and medial pterygoid muscles
B. Skin, superficial fascia, deep cervical fascia and masseter muscle
C. Skin, platysma, deep cervical fascia and masseter muscle
D. Skin, superficial fascia, platysma, deep cervical fascia and masseter muscle

194. The "Red Line" in Winter's classification of impacted teeth represents

A. The depth at which the impacted tooth is located
B. The angulations of the second molar
C. The summit of the alveolar bone covering the impacted tooth
D. The level of occlusal plane

195. Hyperbaric oxygen therapy is indicated in

A. Pulmonary hypertension
B. Myocardial infarction
C. Syncope
D. Osteoradionecrosis

196. "Kelsey Fry technique" refers to the removal in

A. Impacted maxillary 3rd molars
B. Impacted mandibular 3rd molars
C. Impacted mandibular canine
D. Impacted maxillary canines

197. "Dumb–bell" shaped swelling is characteristic of which type of odontogenic space infections

A. Submandibular space
B. Buccal space infection
C. Submasseteric space infection
D. Temporal space infection

198. Infection from the dangerous area of the face spreads to the cavernous sinus via the

A. Neural sheath
B. Emissary veins
C. Orbital fissure
D. Ethmoidal air sinuses

199. BP blade used for the "Hilton method" is

A. No. 10
B. No. 11
C. No. 12
D. No. 15

200. Visor osteotomy is

A. An orthognathic surgical procedure
B. A cancer resection procedure
C. A fracture reduction and fixation procedure
D. A preprosthetic procedure

ANSWERS

HUMAN ANATOMY

1. **Ans: C**

   Ref: BD Chaurasia, 1/E, p. 205

   Explanation

   Structures passing through the centre of sinus
   - Internal carotid artery
   - Abducent nerve

   Structures in the lateral wall of the sinus
   - M - Maxillary nerve
   - O - Oculomotor nerve
   - T - Trochlear nerve
   - T - Trigeminal ganglion
   - O - Ophthalmic nerve

2. **Ans: B**

   Ref: BD Chaurasia, 1/E, p. 328

   Explanation
   - The large gap between the upper concave border of the superior constrictor and the base of the skull is semilunar and is known as the sinus of Morgagni
   - Structures passing through this gap are
     1. Auditory tube
     2. Levator veli palatini muscle
     3. Ascending palatine artery
   - Option A is through the gap between superior and middle constrictors
   - Option C is between middle and inferior constrictors
   - Option D is between lower border of inferior constrictor and esophagus

3. **Ans: B**

   Ref: BD Chaurasia, 1/E, p. 245

   Explanation
   - Parotid gland–inferior salivatory nucleus – otic ganglion
   - Submandibular gland–superior salivatory nucleus–submandibular ganglion
   - Lacrimal gland–lacrimatory nucleus–geniculate ganglion and pterygopalatine ganglion

4. **Ans: C**

   Ref: Di Fiore's Atlas of Histology, 11/E, p. 202

   Explanation
   - They contains whorls of flattened epithelial cells

5. **Ans: A**

   Ref: BD Chaurasia, 1/E, p. 338

PHYSIOLOGY

6. **Ans: A**

   Ref: Ganong, 23/E, p.167

7. **Ans: D**

   Ref: Sembulingam, 4/E, p. 284

   Explanation
   - It is a hormone that plays an important role in maintenance of blood pressure

8. **Ans: D**

   Ref: Sembulingam, 4/E, p. 372

   Explanation
   - It is a steroid hormone synthesized from vitamin D. Its main action is to increase the blood calcium level by increasing the calcium absorption from small intestine

9. **Ans: A**

   Ref: Ganong, 23/E, p. 543

10. **Ans: C**

    Ref: Sembulingam, 4/E, p. 640

Explanation

- Oxygen combines with Hb in blood and is transported as oxyhaemoglobin. Maximum amount (95%) of O_2 is transported in this form

11. Ans: C

Ref: Sembulingam, 4/E, p. 252

12. Ans: B

Ref: Sembulingam. 4/E. p. 261

BIOCHEMISTRY

13. Ans: B

Ref: U.Sathyanarayana and U.Chakrapani, 3/E, p. 23

14. Ans: A

Ref: U.Sathyanarayana and U.Chakrapani, 3/E, p. 152

Explanation

- Folic acid is associated with histidine metabolism in which formimino-glutamate is formed and is excreted in urine. Excretion of FiGLU in urine is used to assess folic acid deficiency

15. Ans: D

Ref: U.Sathyanarayana and U.Chakrapani, 3/E, p. 503

Explanation

Biologic/calorific/fuel values are as follows:

1. Carbohydrates–4
2. Fats–9
3. Proteins–4

16. Ans: C

Ref: U.Sathyanarayana and U.Chakrapani, 3/E, p. 226

Explanation

- The mitochondrial matrix is rich in enzymes responsible for citric acid cycle, β oxidation of fatty acids and oxidation of amino acids

GENERAL PATHOLOGY

17. Ans: C

Ref: Harshmohan, 36/E, p. 415

Explanation

- Serum Alkaline phosphatase levels is a marker of osteoblastic activity. Its levels are raised in active bone growth or pathologic conditions associated with high osteoblastic activity

18. Ans: C

Ref: Harsh Mohan, 3/E, p. 37

19. Ans: B

Ref: Harsh Mohan, 3/E, p. 60

20. Ans: C

Ref: Harsh Mohan, 3/E, p. 110

Explanation

Giant cells	*Condition*
Foreign body giant cells	Chronic infective granuloma, leprosy, tuberculosis
Langhans giant cells	Tuberculosis, sarcoidosis
Touton giant cells	Xanthoma
Aschoff giant cells	Rheumatic nodules

21. Ans: B

Ref: Harsh Mohan, 3/E, p. 189

Explanation

Ref to Table 3.1

22. Ans: C

Ref: Harsh Mohan, 3/E, p. 199

23. Ans: C

Ref: Harsh Mohan, 3/E, p. 181

24. Ans: B

Ref: Text Book of Pathology, Datta, 2/E, p. 820

Table 3.1

Feature	*Transudate*	*Exudate*
Definition	Filtrate of blood plasma without changes in endothelial permeability	Oedema of inflamed tissue associated with increased vascular permeability
Character	Non – inflammatory oedema	Inflammatory oedema
Protein content	Low (less than 1 g/dl); hence no tendency to coagulate	High (2.5 – 3.5 g/dl), readily coagulates due to high content of fibrinogen and other coagulation factors
Glucose content	Same as in plasma	Low (less than 60 mg/dl)
Specific gravity	Low (less than 1.015)	High (more than 1.018)
pH	> 7.3	< 7.3
LDH	Low	High
Effusion LDH/Serum LDH ratio	> 0.6	> 0.6
Cells	Few cells, mainly mesothelial cells and cellular debris	Many cells, inflammatory as well as parenchymal
Examples	Oedema in congestive cardiac failure	Purulent exudate such as pus

Explanation

- A peculiar localized tumour is known to develop in AML, on the skin and in bones specially over the eyebrow. This tumour has a greenish colour when freshly incised and is known as chloroma or granulocyte tumour

MICROBIOLOGY

25. Ans: B

Ref: Ananthnarayan,, 8/E, p. 564

26. Ans: A

Ref: Ananthanarayan and Panicker's Text Book of Microbiology, 8/E, p. 99

27. Ans: D

Ref: Ananthanarayan and Panicker's Text Book of Microbiology, 8/E, p. 32

28. Ans: C

Ref: Ananthanarayan and Panicker's Text Book of Microbiology, 8/E, p. 306

Explanation

- The cholera stool is a colorless watery fluid with flecks of mucus said to resemble water in which rice has been washed. Hence it is called as rice water stools. It has a characteristic sweet offensive odor

29. Ans: A

Ref: Satish Gupte, 9/E, p. 396

Explanation

- The infection with L.donovan's reticular cells of Billroth cord are increased and packed with amastigote form of parasite (L.D bodies of Leishmania donovani bodies)

30. Ans: B

Ref: Ananthanarayan and Panicker's Text Book of Microbiology, 8/E, p. 578

Explanation

- Screening test–ELISA
- Confirmatory test–western blot test

PHARMACOLOGY

31. Ans: A

Ref: K.D Tripathi Medical Pharmacology, 6/ E, p. 55

Explanation

- Therapeutic index = median lethal dose/ median effective dose or LD^{50}/ED^{50}

32. Ans: D

Ref: K.D Tripathi Medical Pharmacology, 6/ E, p. 376

33. Ans: D

Ref: K.D Tripathi Medical Pharmacology, 6/E, p. 287

34. Ans: D

Ref: Padmaja, 1/E, p. 322

35. Ans: C

Ref: K.D Tripathi Medical Pharmacology, 6/E, p. 372

Explanation

- Patients with a genetically determined reaction malignant hyperthermia have an abnormal RYR (Ryanodine receptor) calcium channel at the sarcoplasmic reticulum of the skeletal muscles which is triggered by halothane isoflurane to release massive amounts of Ca^{2+} intracellularly causing persistent muscle contraction and increased heat production succinyl choline accentuates the condition.

GENERAL MEDICINE

36. Ans: B

Ref: Harrison, 17/E, Vol. 1, p. 357

37. Ans: B

Ref: Davidson, 20/E, p. 299

38. Ans: D

Ref: Harrison, 17/E, Vol. 2, p. 1446

39. Ans: A

Ref: Davidson, 20/E, p. 690

40. Ans: D

Ref: Davidson, 20/E, p. 950

41. Ans: B

Ref: Davidson, 20/E, p. 292

Explanation

- Disease seen in IV drug abusers
  1. HIV, hepatitis infection
  2. Skin-deep infections or abscess formation
  3. Joints-pain and redness with associated osteomyelitis
  4. Breathlessness and endocarditis
  5. New murmurs or cardiac decompensation
  6. Myalgia and muscle pain
  7. Abdominal pain
  8. Hepatitis encephalopathy

42. Ans: D

Ref: Davidson 20/E p. 962

43. Ans: D

Ref: Davidson, 20/E, p. 957

44. Ans: D

Ref: Davidson, 20/E, p. 896

Explanation

- In dermatitis herpetiformis, the rash usually responds to a gluten free diet but some patients require additional treatment with dapsone (100–150 mg daily)

45. Ans: C

Ref: Davidson, 20/E, p. 631

Explanation

Clinical features of infective endocarditis

- Sub conjunctival haemorrhage
- Varying murmurs, conduction disorders cardiac failure

- Haematuria
- Osler's nodes
- Petechial rash
- Cerebral embolic
- Roths spots in fundi
- Poor dentition
- Splenomegaly
- Systemic emboli
- Digital clubbing and sphincter haemorrhages
- Loss of pulses

46. Ans: B

Ref: Davidson, 20/E, p. 962

47. Ans: C

Ref: Davidson, 20/E, p. 611

48. Ans: A

Ref: Davidson, 20/E, p. 553

Explanation

- Vasovagal syncope is usually triggered by a reduction in venous return due to prolonged standing excessive heat or a large meal
- It is mediated by the Bezold-Jarisch reflex, which is characterized by initial sympathetic activation that then leads to vigorous contraction of the relatively under filled ventricles
- This stimulates ventricular mechanoreceptors and in turn produces parasympathetic vagal activation and sympathetic withdrawal causing bradycardia, vasodilation, i.e. Syncope

49. Ans: B

Ref: Davidson, 20/E, p. 198

Explanation

- To control intracranial pressure osmotic diuretic mannitol 20% 100–200 ml (0.25–0.5 g/kg) coupled with volume replacement

50. Ans: C

Ref: Harrison's, 13/E,Vol 1, p. 117

GENERAL SURGERY

51. Ans: C

Ref: S. Das, 5/E, p. 545

52. Ans: D

Ref: S. Das, 5/E, p. 7

Explanation

Factors affecting wound healing

General	Local
Age	Position of wound
Nutrition	Blood supply
Hormones	Tension movement
Others–anaemia, infection, jaundice, Diabetes	Exposure to ionizing radiation Necrosis Impaired lymph drainage UV light Faulty technique of closure Foreign bodies

53. Ans: B

Ref: S. Das, 5/E, p. 625

54. Ans: B

Ref: S. Das, 5/E, p. 108

Explanation

- It is a squamous carcinoma which arises in a chronic benign ulcer or scar

55. Ans: D

Ref: S. Das, 5/E, p. 918

Explanation

- During deep palpation of the right upper quadrant the patient is asked to take deep breath in and out, patient complains of acute pain during deep inspiration with inspiratory arrest when tender inflammable gall bladder comes down and touches the palpating finger. This is Murphy's Sign.

56. Ans: C

Ref: S. Das, 5/E, p. 1160

Explanation
- Also called as intravenous *urography/ pyelogram*
- Is a radiological procedure used to visualize disturbances of the urinary system

57. Ans: D

Ref: S. Das, 5/E, p. 352

Explanation
- A cole's fracture is a fracture of the radius within 2.5cm of the wrist with or without avulsion of the ulnar styloid process and with a characteristic deformity. The lower fragment is usually shifted backwards with a tilt radially

58. Ans: C

Ref: S. Das, 5/E, p. 66

DENTAL MATERIALS

59. Ans: C

Ref: Phillips, 11/E, p. 47

60. Ans: C

Ref: Phillips, 11/E, p. 527

Explanation
- The working time of amalgam is short so condensation should be as rapid as possible and a fresh mix of amalgam should be made if condensation takes longer than 3 or 4 minutes

61. Ans: A

Ref: Phillip's, 11/E, p. 229

Explanation
- Comparison of different impression materials reveals that polysulfide results in the lowest cell death count and set polyether impression material produces the highest cell cytotoxicity scores

62. Ans: C

Ref: Skinner's, 9/E, p. 97

63. Ans: A

Ref: Phillip's, 11/E, p. 229

64. Ans: D

Ref: Phillip's, 11/E, p. 659

65. Ans: D

Ref: Phillip's, 11/E, p. 261

66. Ans: B

Ref: Phillip's, 11/E, p. 370

67. Ans: C

Ref: Phillip's, 11/E, p. 346

68. Ans: A

Ref: Phillip's, 11/E, p. 419

69. Ans: D

Ref: Phillip's, 11/E, p. 681

Explanation
- Dicor – castable ceramic
- Dicor MGC – Machinable glass ceramic
- Empress and IPS empress 2 – pressable glass ceramic

70. Ans: B

Ref: Phillip's, 11/E, p. 737

Explanation
- Light cure – denture base resins
- Visible light – activator
- Initiator – camphoroquinone

DADH

71. Ans: B

Ref: Orban's, 12/E, p. 301

72. Ans: A

Ref: Orban's, 12/E, p. 42

73. **Ans: B**

Ref: Wheeler's, 8/E, p. 277

74. **Ans: C**

Ref: Wheeler's, 8/E, p.107

Explanation
- Bunodont – teeth bearing conical cusps
- Triconodont – teeth bearing 3 cups in line
- Haplodont – tooth bearing single cone

75. **Ans: D**

Ref: Orban's, 12/E, p. 28

76. **Ans: B**

Ref: Orban's, 12/E, p. 96

ORAL PATHOLOGY AND ORAL MEDICINE

77. **Ans: B**

Ref: Shafer's, 6/E, p. 426

78. **Ans: B**

Ref: Shafer's, 6/E, p. 501

79. **Ans: B**

Ref: Shafer's, 6/E, p. 261

80. **Ans: B**

Ref: Shafer's, 6/E, p. 256

81. **Ans: B**

Ref: Shafer's, 6/E, p. 234

Explanation
- The cribiform pattern in adenoid cystic carcinoma shows basaloid epithelial cell rests that form multiple cylindrical cysts like patterns resembling swiss cheese or honey comb pattern

82. **Ans: D**

Ref: Shafer's, 6/E, p. 365

83. **Ans: C**

Ref: Shafer's, 6/E, p. 804

Explanation
- Monro's abscesses are intraepithelial microabscesses seen in psoriasis

84. **Ans: A**

Ref: Shafer's, 6/E, p. 831, 832

85. **Ans: B**

Ref: Shafer's, 6/E, p. 818

Explanation

Intraepithelial vesicle	Pemphigus Herpes Erythema multiformae
Sub epithelial vesicle	Pemphigoid Bullous pemphigoid Dermatitis herpetiformis Skin lesion of Erythema Multiformae

86. **Ans: D**

Ref: Neville, 3/E, p.6

87. **Ans: A**

Ref: Anil Ghom Text book of Oral Pathology, 1/E, p. 187

88. **Ans: D**

Ref: Shafer's, 6/E, p. 66

Explanation
- Superficial erosion of the outer surface of the maxilla may be produced by pressure of the nasoalveolar cyst, but it should be noted that they are not primarily central lesions and therefore may not be visible on the radiograph

89. **Ans: A**

Ref: Shafer's, 6/E, p. 848

Explanation
- The auriculotemporal syndrome(Frey's syndrome,Gustatory sweating) is an unusual phenomenon. This arises as a result of damage to the auriculo-temporal nerve and subsequent reinnervation of sweat glands by parasympathetic salivary fibers

90. Ans: C

Ref: Shafer's, 6/E, p. 54, 56

91. Ans: D

Ref: Shafer's, 6/E, p. 262

Explanation

- Epstein's pearls – Mid palatine raphe
- Bohn's nodules – function of hard and soft palate

92. Ans: A

Ref: Shafer's, 6/E, p. 774

93. Ans: C

Ref: Shafer's, 6/E, p. 802

Explanation

- *Civatte/Hyaline/Cytoid bodies:* They are degenerating basal keratinocytes which appears as homogenous eosinophillic globules
- *Other options:*
  - Lipschutz bodies–Herpes simplex virus
  - Barr body – X - chromosomes of female
  - Koilocytes – squamous papilloma

94. Ans: B

Ref: Anil Ghom's Text book of Oral Pathology, 1/E, p. 674

95. Ans: A

Ref: Shafer's, 6/E, p. 740

Explanation

- Rheumatoid arthritis in children when it involves the TMJ, may cause a malocclusion of the class II division I with protrusion of maxillary incisors and an anterior open bite

96. Ans: C

Ref: Shafer's, 6/E, p. 806

Explanation

- A concentric ring like appearance of the lesions, resulting from the varying shades of erythema termed as target, iris or bull's eye
- It is most commonly seen on hands, wrists and ankles

ORAL RADIOLOGY

97. Ans: B

Ref: White and Pharoah, 6/E, p. 58

Explanation

Other options:

- Contrast – difference between light and dark regions of an X-ray film
- Sharpness – ability of radiograph to define an edge precisely

98. Ans: A

Ref: White and Pharoah, 6/E, p. 11

99. Ans: B

Ref: White and Pharoah, 6/E, p. 5

100. Ans: B

Ref: White and Pharoah 6/E p. 478

101. Ans: C

Ref: White and Pharoah, 6/E, p. 14

Explanation

- Three types of beam attenuations
  1. Coherent scattering/thompson scattering
  2. Photoelectric absorption – critical in diagnostic imaging
  3. Compton – scattering

ORTHODONTICS

102. Ans: A

Ref: Bhalaji, 3/E, p. 9, 10

Explanation

- Growth modification by means of functional and orthodontic appliances elicit better response during growth spurts, i.e.
  - Boys: 8–11 years

- Girls: 7 – 9 years
- Therefore A is the nearest answer

103. Ans: C

Ref: Bhalaji, 3/E, p.10, 333

104. Ans: B

Ref: Bhalaji, 3/E, p. 92

Explanation

- *Prolonged retention of deciduous anteriors*– lingual or palatal eruption of their permanent successors
- *Prolonged retention of buccal teeth*– permanent teeth erupt buccally or lingually or may be impacted

105. Ans: D

Ref: Bhalaji, 3/E, p. 44

106. Ans: D

Ref: Bhalaji, 3/E, p. 77

Explanation

- Lischer's modification of angle's classification includes:
  1. Mesioverison–Mesial to normal position
  2. Distoversion–distal to normal position
  3. Transversion–transposition of two teeth
  4. Axiversion–Abnormal axial inclination of a tooth.
  5. Torsiversion–Rotation of tooth around its long axis

107. Ans: A

Ref: Bhalaji, 3/E, p. 450

Explanation

- Frequency of impaction commonly seen in descending order
- Mandibular 3rd molar–maxillary 3rd molar–maxillary canine–mandibular premolars–maxillary premolar–mandibular canine–maxillary incisors

108. Ans: B

Ref: Bhalaji, 3/E, p. 121

Explanation

- Facial form is classified into:
  1. Mesoprosopic – average or normal face
  2. Euryprosopic – broad an short face
  3. Leptoprosopic – broad and narrow face

109. Ans: C

Ref: M. S Rani, 3/E, p. 41

110. Ans: A

Ref: Bhalaji, 3/E, p. 151

Explanation

- Angle of convexity – angle formed by intersection of a line form nasion to point A and a line from point and to pogonion
  - It reveals the convexity or concavity of the skeletal profile
  - Average value – ranges between 2.5 to 10
  - Increased angle of convexity–prominent maxilla
  - Decreased angle of convexity–retrognathic mandible

111. Ans: B

Ref: Bhalaji, 3/E, p. 168

Explanation

- System for evaluation of skeletal maturation was proposed by Leonard. S. Fishman in 1982
- System discrete adolescent skeletal maturity indicators (SMIs)

112. Ans: C

Ref: Bhalaji, 3/E, p. 178

Explanation

- According to Bolton, there exists a ratio between mesiodistal widths of maxillary and mandibular teeth
- Over all ratio: sum of mandibular 12 × 100 = 77.2 %
  - If ratio is <77.2%-maxillary anterior excess
  - If ratio is >77.2%-mandibular anterior excess

113. Ans: D

Ref: Bhalaji, 3/E, p. 396

Explanation

- Rotation has a very high risk of relapse due to stretching of supra alveolar and transseptal gingival fibres which readapt very slowly to new position
- Pericision or circumferential supracrestal fibrotomy is an adjunctive surgical procedure where the gingival fibres are incised to prevent relapse

114. Ans: D

Ref: M. S. Rani, 3/E, p. 227

115. Ans: A

Ref: Bhalaji, 3/E, p. 272

116. Ans: C

Ref: Bhalaji, 3/E, p. 315

117. Ans: B

Ref: Bhalaji, 3/E, p. 289

Explanation

$F = D^4/L^3$

Where F – force

D – Diameter of wire

L – Length of wire

Hence $F \alpha D^4$ and $F \alpha 1/L^3$.

118. Ans: B

Ref: Bhalaji, 3/E, p. 374

Explanation

- Delaire facemask used the chin and forehead for support

119. Ans: C

Ref: Bhalaji, 3/E, p. 358

Explanation

- Given by Emil Herbst
- Fixed functional appliance

Indications:

- Connection of class II malocclusion due to retrognathic mandible
- Anterior repositioning splint in patients having TMJ
- Specific post adolescent patients
- Mouth breathers
- Uncooperative patients

120. Ans: A

Ref: Bhalaji, 3/E, p. 322

Explanation

- Three stages of Begg appliance therapy;
  1. Stage I – alignment, correction of crowding rotation, correction, closure of anterior spaces and achieving edge to edge anterior bite
  2. Stage II – alignment of remaining extraction space while maintaining previous corrections
  3. Stage III – Up righting and torquing to achieve normal axial inclination of the teeth

PEDODONTICS

121. Ans: C

Ref: Shoba Tandon, 1/E, p. 116

Explanation

- This is known as broadbent phenomenon

122. Ans: C

Ref: Shoba Tandon, 1/E, p. 233

Explanation

- Hyatt (1923)–Prophylactic odontomy
- Bodecker (1955)–Fissure eradication
- Buonocore (1955)–P and F sealant with bonded resin
- Bowen (1965)–BIS-GMA as P and F sealants

123. Ans: A

Ref: Shoba Tandon, 1/E, p. 719

124. Ans: A

Ref: Shoba Tandon, 1/E, p. 661

125. Ans: B

Ref: Shoba Tandon, 1/E, p. 132

126. Ans: A

Ref: Shoba Tandon, 1/E, p. 340

127. Ans: C

Ref: Shoba Tandon, 1/E, p. 111

Explanation

- Tooth crowns pierce the bony alveolar crest – 2/3rd root development is complete
- ¾ root development complete – tooth emerges into oral cavity
- 2–3 years after eruption – root development is completed

128. Ans: C

Ref: Shoba Tandon, 1/E, p. 289

P AND SD

129. Ans: C

Ref: Joseph John, 1/E, p. 76

130. Ans: B

Ref: Joseph John, 1/E, p. 210

Explanation

- First introduced in Switzerland in 1995, with 5 mg of potassium iodide and 90 mg of sodium fluoride per kg

131. Ans: A

Ref: Joseph John, 1/E, p. 26

132. Ans: B

Ref: Soben Peter, 3/E, p. 326

133. Ans: A

Ref: Joseph John, 1/E, Pg. 124

134. Ans: B

Ref: Park and Park, 20/E, p. 565

135. Ans: A

Ref: Soben Peter, 3/E, p. 204

136. Ans: B

Ref: Park and Park, 20/E, p. 39

137. Ans: D

Ref: Soben Peter, 3/E, p. 292

Explanation

- Enamel surface of newly erupted teeth undergoes rapid maturation and immature and porous enamel acquires fluoride rapidly

138. Ans: D

Ref: Soben Peter, 3/E, p. 292

Explanation

- Teeth NOT included in DMF score are
  - Third molars
  - Unerupted teeth
  - Congenitally missing and supernumerary teeth
  - Teeth removed for reasons other than dental caries such as for orthodontic treatment or impaction or cosmetic purpose
  - Endodontically treated teeth
  - Retained primary teeth

139. Ans: D

Ref: Soben Peter, 3/E, p. 299

Explanation

- The four visit procedure of application of NaF is at the age of 3, 7, 11, 13 years

140. Ans: D

Ref: Park and Park, 20/E, p. 39

Explanation

- Levels of prevention
  1. *Primordial prevention:* Prevention of diseases in countries or population groups in which they have NOT appeared

2. *Primary prevention:* Action taken prior to the onset of disease
3. *Secondary prevention:* Action which halts the progress of a disease as its incipient stage and prevents complications
4. *Tertiary prevention:* Rehabilitation when the disease process has advanced beyond its early stages

141. Ans: A

Ref: Soben Peter, 3/E, p. 136

Explanation
- Patient's hygiene performance index
- Introduced by Podshadley AG and Haley J.V in 1968
- Teeth and surfaces to be examined

Tooth	*Surface*
16	Buccal
11	Labial
26	Buccal
36	Lingual
31	Labial
46	Lingual

142. Ans: D

Ref: Soben Peter, 3/E, p. 177

143. Ans: D

Ref: Soben Peter, 3/E, p. 246

Explanation
- Sucrose is the most cariogenic followed by fructose
- Xylitol, mannitol and sorbitol have-no ability to initiate caries or support caries

PROSTHODONTICS

144. Ans: A

Ref: Zarb and Bolender, 5/E, p. 217

Explanation
- The vibrating line passes about 2 mm in front of the fovea palatini
- These are indentations near the midline of the palate formed by a coalescence of several mucous glands ducts

145. Ans: B

Ref: Heartwell, 4/E, p. 195

Explanation
- Stability is the resistance to horizontal movement
- It decreases with the loss of vertical height of the ridges or with the increase in flabby movable tissue

146. Ans: B

Ref: Winkler, 2/E, p. 194

147. Ans: A

Ref: Heartwell, 4/E, p. 230

148. Ans: C

Ref: Zarb and Bolender, 12/E, p. 206

149. Ans: A

Ref: Rosensteil, 4/E, p. 95

150. Ans: B

Ref: Rosensteil, 4/E, p. 628

151. Ans: B

Ref: Nallaswamy, 1/E, p. 503

152. Ans: B

Ref: Nallaswamy, 1/E, p. 572

Explanation
- Metal crown preparation – chamfer
- All ceramic preparation – shoulder
- Metal ceramic/PTM – lingual chamfer and labially shoulder

153. Ans: B

Ref: Rosensteil, 4/E, p. 263

Explanation
- Complete cast metal crown – 1.5 mm on functional cusps; 1 mm on nonfunctional cusps
- All ceramic crown – 1.5 mm

154. **Ans: B**

Ref: Nallaswamy, 1/E, p. 382

155. **Ans: C**

Ref: Nallaswamy, 1/E, p. 332

Explanation
- Under stress the horse shoe shaped major connector may tend to straighten out

156. **Ans: D**

Ref: Nallaswamy, 1/E, p. 362

PERIODONTICS

157. **Ans: B**

Ref: Carranza, 10/E, p. 344

158. **Ans: C**

Ref: Carranza, 10/E, p. 306

Explanation
- Bismuth – bluish black discoloration of gingiva
- Lead – linear steel gray pigmentation (burtonian line)

159. **Ans: B**

Ref: Carranza, 10/E, p. 943

160. **Ans: D**

Ref: Carranza, 10/E, p. 929

Explanation
- Internal bevel incision – is the first incision, and flap is reflected to expose the underlying bone and root
- Crevicular incision – made from the base of the pocket to the crest of the bone
- Interdental incision separates the collar of gingiva that surround the tooth

161. **Ans: C**

Ref: Carranza, 10/E, p. 772

Explanation
- 1 – 2 and 3 – 4 anterior teeth
- 5 – 6 Anterior and premolar
- 7 – 8 and 9 – 10 Facial and lingual surfaces of posterior
- 11 – 12 Mesial surface of posterior teeth
- 13 – 14 Distal surface of posterior teeth

162. **Ans: C**

Ref: Carranza, 10/E, p. 853

Explanation
- Coronoplasty/occlusal adjustment/occlusal equilibrium is the selective reshaping of occlusal surfaces with the goal of establishing a stable, non traumatic occlusion

163. **Ans: B**

Ref: Carranza, 10/E, p. 70

164. **Ans: A**

Ref: Carranza, 10/E, p. 899

165. **Ans: A**

Ref: Carranza, 10/E, p. 974

166. **Ans: C**

Ref: Carranza, 10/E, p. 1010

Explanation

Graft (thickness)	*Time taken for healing*
Intermediate thickness (0.75 mm)	10.5 weeks
Thicker grafts (1.75 mm)	16 weeks

167. **Ans: B**

Ref: Carranza, 10/E, p. 755

168. **Ans: D**

Ref: Carranza, 10/E, p. 587

Explanation
- CADIA – Computer assisted densitometric image analysis
- It is an objective method that follows alveolar bone density changes quantitatively over time thereby demonstrating the prevalence of progressing lesions in periodontitis

169. **Ans: B**

Ref: Carranza, 10/E, p. 593

Explanation

- A probe is a known nucleic acid molecule (DNA or RNA) from a specific microorganism artificially synthesized and labelled for its detection when placed with a plaque samples
- DNA probes are available for multiple bacteria including A. Actinomycetemcomitans, P. gingivalis, B. intermedius

170. **Ans: D**

Ref: Carranza, 10/E, p. 977

CONS AND ENDO

171. **Ans: D**

Ref: Ingle's, 6/E, p.1252

172. **Ans: B**

Ref: Sturdavent, 5/E, p. 356

173. **Ans: C**

Ref: Sturdavent, 5/E, p. 469

Explanation

- This is done to compensate for the extension of the dam to the cervical area

174. **Ans: D**

Ref: Cohen, 9/E, p. 257

175. **Ans: B**

Ref: Sturdavent, 5/E, p. 157

176. **Ans: A**

Ref: Grossman, 12/E, p. 228

177. **Ans: B**

Ref: Grossman, 12/E, p. 226

178. **Ans: A**

Ref: Sturdavent, 5/E, p. 246

Explanation

- Acid etching transforms the smooth enamel into an irregular surface and increases its surface free energy

179. **Ans: C**

Ref: Cohen, 9/E, p. 988

180. **Ans: A**

Ref: Grossman, 12/E, p. 406

181. **Ans: B**

Ref: Sturdavent, 5/E, p. 102

182. **Ans: A**

Ref: Sturdavent, 5/E, p. 290

Explanation

- Black noted that in tooth preparation for smooth surface caries, the restoration should be extended to areas that are normally self cleansing to prevent recurrence of caries. This principle was known as extension for prevention. However this practice has been virtually eliminated now because of modern preventive and conservative measures.

183. **Ans: C**

Ref: Sturdavent, 5/E, p. 305

Explanation

- Rounding external angles, e.g. axiopulpal line angles, reduces the stress on the tooth and increasing the resistance to fracture of the restorative material

184. **Ans: C**

Ref: Sturdavent, 5/E, pp. 350, 362

185. **Ans: C**

Ref: Sturdavent, 5/E, p. 571

ORAL SURGERY

186. **Ans: B**

Ref: Peterson, 4/E, p. 322

Explanation

Region of Implant Placement	*Minimum Integration Time*
Anterior mandible	3 months
Posterior mandible	4 months
Anterior maxilla	6 months
Posterior maxilla	6 months
Into bone graft	6 to 9 months

187. Ans: B

Ref: Peterson, 4/E, p. 322

Explanation

Region of Implant Placement	*Minimum integration Time*
Anterior mandible	3 months
Posterior mandible	4 months
Anterior maxilla	6 months
Posterior maxilla	6 months
Into bone graft	*6 to 9 months*

188. Ans: C

Ref: Killey's, 4/E, p. 12

Explanation

- The fractures of mandible are under the influence of medial pterygoid
  1. Horizontally unfavourable – upward displacement of posterior fragment
  2. Vertically unfavourable – lingual displacement of posterior fragment

189. Ans: D

Ref: Neelima Malik, 2/E, p. 60

190. Ans: B

Ref: Killey's, 4/E, p. 87

Explanation

- It was described by gunning in 1866

191. Ans: B

Ref: Killey's, 4/E, p. 26

192. Ans: B

Ref: Neelima Malik, 2/E, p. 331

193. Ans: D

Ref: Neelima Malik, 2/E, p. 389

194. Ans: A

Ref: Neelima Malik, 2/E, pg 127

Explanation

Winter's WAR lines

- *White line* – corresponds to the occlusal plane. It indicates the difference in occlusal level of 2nd and 3rd molars
- *Amber line* – represents the bone level. This line denotes the alveolar bone covering the impacted tooth and the portion of tooth not covered by the bone
- *Red line* – is drawn perpendicular form the amber line to an imaginary point of application of the elevator. It indicates the amount of bone that will have to be removed before elevation

195. Ans: D

Ref: Neelima Malik, 2/E, p. 667

Explanation

Hyperbaric O_2 therapy is used in treatment of various conditions

- Osteoradionecrosis
- Decompression sickness and air embolism
- Chronic refractory osteomyelitis
- Co poisoning
- Gas gangrene

196. Ans: B

Ref: Neelima Malik, 2/E, p. 132

Explanation

- It was described originally by sir William Kelsey Fry and later popularized by Steward

197. Ans: D

Ref: Laskin, Vol. 2, p. 223

198. Ans: B

Ref: Neelima Malik, 2/E, p. 634

199. Ans: B

Ref: Peterson, 4/E, p. 354

200. Ans: D

Ref: Neelima Malik 2/E, p. 434

Explanation

- The goal of visor osteotomy is to increase the height of the mandibular ridge for denture support

4

KCET 2006

HUMAN ANATOMY

1. The nerve which lies in association to Wharton duct is

A. Facial
B. Spinal accessory
C. Hypoglossal
D. Lingual

2. Inferior meatus of nasal cavity contains the opening of

A. Maxillary sinus
B. Middle ethmoidal sinus
C. Nasolacrimal duct
D. Frontal sinus

3. The artery that passes forwards through cavernous sinus is

A. Supra trochlear artery
B. Supra orbital artery
C. Internal carotid artery
D. Anterior ethmoidal artery

4. Accessory meningeal artery enters cranial cavity through

A. Foramen lacerum
B. Foramen rotundum
C. Foramen spinosum
D. Foramen ovale

5. Basic metabolic unit of bone is

A. Osteon
B. Osteoblast
C. Osteocyte
D. Osteoclast

6. The following muscles are supplied by mandibular nerve EXCEPT

A. Tensor tympani
B. Tensor veli palatini
C. Levator veli palatini
D. Mylohyoid

7. Mastoid air sinus is posteriorly related to

A. Cavernous sinus
B. Sigmoid sinus
C. Straight sinus
D. Spheno parietal sinus

8. The medial surface of the neck of the mandible is related to the

A. Inferior alveolar nerve
B. Lingual nerve
C. Auriculo temporal nerve
D. Chorda tympani nerve

PHYSIOLOGY

9. The chief cation in extra cellular fluid

A. Sodium
B. Potassium
C. Calcium
D. Magnesium

10. The feature of slow pain is

A. No projection to reticular nucleus
B. Carried by Aδ fibers
C. Poor localization
D. Glutamate is the neuro transmitter

11. Cyanosis is bluish discoloration of skin due to more than ….. gms/100 ml in blood of deoxygenated hemoglobin

A. 2
B. 5
C. 8
D. 10

12. Normal blood flow pattern is
- A. Predominantly stream line
- B. Predominantly turbulent
- C. Streamline and turbulent in equal ratio
- D. None of the above

13. Coronary blood flow to the left ventricle is predominantly from
- A. Right coronary artery and during diastole
- B. Right coronal artery and during systole
- C. Left coronal artery and during systole
- D. Left coronal artery and during diastole

14. Secretions of the parafollicular cells of the thyroid gland are stimulated by
- A. Increase in serum calcium
- B. Increase in serum thyroxin
- C. Decrease in serum calcium
- D. Decrease in serum thyroxin

15. Platelets adhere to the subendothelial collagen through one of the following
- A. Platelet factor 4
- B. Fibronectin
- C. Von Willebrand factor
- D. None of the above

BIOCHEMISTRY

16. The following carbohydrate is called animal starch
- A. Glucose
- B. Fructose
- C. Sucrose
- D. Glycogen

17. Lesch nyhan syndrome is due to deficiency of
- A. HGPRTase (total)
- B. PRPP glutamine amino transferase
- C. CTP synthetase
- D. OMP decarboxylase

18. Thyroxine is derived from
- A. Tyrosine
- B. Tyramine
- C. Taurine
- D. Tryptophan

19. The storage form of carbohydrates in our body is
- A. Starch
- B. Glycogen
- C. Sucrose
- D. Cellulose

GENERAL PATHOLOGY

20. One of the following is NOT capable of replication
- A. Neuron
- B. Liver
- C. Kidney
- D. None of the above

MICROBIOLOGY

21. On an average in the saliva of an adult man the lactobacilli count is
- A. 50,000/ml
- B. 75,000/ml
- C. 70,000/ml
- D. 30,000/ml

22. Gas gangrene is NOT caused by
- A. Clostridium welchii
- B. Clostridium septicum
- C. Clostridium emotines
- D. Clostridium tetani

23. Lophotrichous flagella are seen in
- A. Spirilla
- B. Vibrio
- C. Pseudomonas
- D. Klebsiella

24. The efficacy of moist heat sterilization is tested by using spores of
- A. Bacillus anthracis
- B. Bacillus cereus
- C. Bacillus subtilis
- D. Bacillius stearothermophilus

25. Microscope was invented by
- A. Louis Pasteur

B. Hippocrates
C. Robert Koch
D. Leeuwen Hock

26. Plasmid is transmitted to other bacteria in

A. Transformation
B. Transduction
C. Conjugation
D. All of the above

27. The immunoglobulin which crosses placenta is

A. IgG
B. IgM
C. IgA
D. IgD

28. Diphtheria toxin acts by

A. Increasing levels of cramps
B. Inhibiting protein synthesis
C. Inhibiting acetyl choline release
D. Inhibiting glucose transport

PHARMACOLOGY

29. Optic neuritis is the side effect of

A. Rifampicin
B. Isoniazid
C. Ethambutol
D. Pyrazinamide

30. Following are the prodrugs EXCEPT one

A. Levodopa
B. Enalapril
C. Epinephrine
D. Proguanil

31. Which one of the following drugs is NOT a cardio selective (β1) beta blocker?

A. Metaprolol
B. Alprenolol
C. Atenolol
D. Esmolol

32. Which one of the following drugs is NOT an aminoglycoside?

A. Kanamycin
B. Tobramycin
C. Erythromycin
D. Streptomycin

33. 'Second gas effect' is exerted by the following gas when co–administered with halothane

A. Nitrogen
B. Cyclopropane
C. Nitrous oxide
D. Helium

34. Amphotericin B is NOT effective in the following fungal disease

A. Cryptococcosis
B. Histoplasmosis
C. Blastomycosis
D. Dermatophytosis

35. Antispastic drug used in treating trigeminal neuralgia is

A. Gabapentin
B. Nortriptyline
C. Clonazepam
D. Baclofen

36. Among the following drugs which is not an immunosuppressive agent

A. Levamisole
B. Azathioprine
C. Cyclosporin
D. Corticosteroid

GENERAL MEDICINE

37. Exudative pleural effusion is seen in all EXCEPT

A. Tuberculosis
B. Rheumatoid disease
C. SLE
D. Cardiac failure

38. Acromegaly is due to increased

A. Growth hormone
B. Thyroid hormone
C. Adrenaline
D. Parathyroid hormone

39. Serum amylase is elevated in

A. Pancreatitis
B. Intestinal ischemia
C. Ruptured ovarian cyst
D. All of the above

40. Asterixis is caused by all EXCEPT

A. Hepatic failure
B. Renal failure
C. Hypo capnia
D. Phenytoin toxicity

41. The most common cause of mitral regurgitation in a patient who has no evidence of mitral stenosis is

A. Congenital
B. Mitral valve prolapse
C. Rheumatic heart disease
D. Secondary to aortic valve disease

42. A patient with hypertension

A. Will always have symptoms
B. Will not be able to reduce blood pressure without drug treatment
C. Will usually not have an underlying identifiable cause or condition
D. Can always have the blood pressure controlled by single drug

43. If a patient presents with generalized pruritis the following condition should be considered as possibility

A. Cholestatic jaundice
B. Addison's disease
C. Acromegaly
D. Myxedema

44. Diseases typically acquired by man from animals include

A. Hepatitis A
B. Cholera
C. Tuberculosis
D. Leptospirosis

45. Flask shaped ulcer is a feature of

A. Cholera
B. Amoebiasis
C. Sarcoidosis
D. Bacillary dysentery

46. Antibiotic recommended for prophylaxis of bacterial endocarditis in patients who are allergic to penicillin

A. Clindamycin
B. Azithromycin
C. Clarithromycin
D. All the above

47. Disease of the liver can produce bleeding tendencies because

A. Synthesis of Vitamin K is decreased
B. Production of prothrombin is low
C. Plasma protein levels are low
D. All of the above

48. In which of the following condition, immune mediated damage is implicated

A. Hemophilia
B. Congenital heart disease
C. Rheumatic fever
D. All the above

49. Presence of Bence–Jones proteins is a characteristic feature of

A. Infectious mononucleosis
B. Multiple myeloma
C. Malignant melanoma
D. Paget's disease

GENERAL SURGERY

50. The following thyroid disease are diagnosed by FNAC EXCEPT

A. Follicular carcinoma
B. Papillary carcinoma
C. Medullary carcinoma
D. Malignant lymphoma

51. Cause of persistence of a sinus and fistulas

A. Foreign body
B. Unrelieved distal obstruction
C. Presence of malignancy
D. All of the above

52. Carcinoma lip commonly occur in

A. Upper lip skin surface

B. Vermillion border of lower lip
C. Commisures
D. Mucosal surface of upper lip

53. The most common thyroid cancer is

A. Anaplastic
B. Medullary
C. Papillary
D. Follicular

54. Which statement is FALSE regarding thyroglossal cyst?

A. Almost always arises in the midline
B. Vestigeal remnant of second branchial cleft
C. Sistrunk's operation is indicated
D. Moves upward on protrusion of the Tongue

55. Branchial cyst is located at

A. The junction of middle third and lower third of sternomastoid at anterior border
B. The junction of upper third and middle third of sternomastoid at its posterior border
C. The junction of middle third and lower third of sternomastoid at its posterior border
D. The junction of upper third and middle third of sternomastoid at its anterior border

DADH

56. The epithelial lining of the maxillary air sinus is

A. Simple squamous
B. simple cuboidal
C. ciliated columnar
D. stratified squamous non keratinized

57. Band of fibrous tissue which slings the tooth between the walls of the crypt according to Sicher is

A. Hammock ligament
B. Gomphosis
C. Dento alveolar ligament
D. Fibrosis

58. To protrude the mandible the following muscles will contract in conjunction with stabilizing of the opening muscles

A. Outer and inner layers of temporalis
B. Contraction of posterior fibers of temporalis and geniohyoid
C. Lateral and medial pterygoid muscles
D. Mylohyoid and temporalis

59. Mesial developmental depression is the characteristic feature of

A. Maxillary first premolar
B. Maxillary second premolar
C. Mandibular first premolar
D. Mandibular second premolar

DENTAL MATERIALS

60. The process of heating a cast alloy to eliminate composition difference is

A. Hardening heat treatment
B. Softening heat treatment
C. Homogenization
D. Crystallization

61. Type IV gold alloy contains

A. 2% gold
B. 13% gold
C. 75% gold
D. 80% gold

62. Galvanism is

A. Tarnishing
B. Electrolytic corrosion
C. Chemical corrosion
D. Annealing

63. Shape memory exhibited by

A. Beta titanium
B. Nickel titanium
C. Cobalt chromium
D. Nickel chromium

64. Non gamma 2 alloy is

A. Resistant to marginal leakage
B. Resistant to discoloration
C. Resistant to sensitization
D. Resistant to corrosion

65. The irreversible hydrocolloid impression material used in removable partial denture prosthesis construction is

A. Agar agar
B. Alginate
C. Silicone
D. Thiokol

66. How much minimum amount of alloy percentage by weight of noble elements is present in high noble metals?

A. 60% by weight of noble elements
B. 30% gold
C. 40% by weight of noble elements
D. Less than 40% by weight of noble elements

67. How much fraction of methyl mercury is absorbed from the gut?

A. 20%
B. 50%
C. 80%
D. 100%

68. The average particle size of powdered gold is

A. 10 μm
B. 15 μm
C. 30 μm
D. 0.1 μm

69. Loss of gloss test in gypsum product is an indication for

A. Adequate mixing time
B. Adequate working time
C. Initial set
D. Final set

70. Stabilization of stainless steel is achieved by addition of

A. Carbon
B. Chromium
C. Nickel
D. Titanium

71. The best method to control gelation time while mixing alginate material is

A. Alter the temperature of water
B. Alter the water/powder ratio
C. Increase the mixing time
D. Reduce the percentage of retarder

72. The modulus of elasticity of an alloy refers to

A. Flexibility
B. Ductility
C. Stiffness
D. Malleability

ORAL PATHOLOGY AND ORAL MEDICINE

73. Sjogrens syndrome refers to disease of

A. Thyroid gland
B. Parotid gland
C. Parathyroid gland
D. Multiple endocrine glands

74. Abtropfung (or) dropping off effect is seen in

A. Intradermal nevus
B. Junctional nevus
C. Compound nevus
D. Blue nevus

75. Physiologic wearing of a tooth as a result of tooth to tooth contact is

A. Attrition
B. Abrasion
C. Erosion
D. All the above

76. "Triangular frontal defect" occurs in

A. Crouzon disease
B. Crouzon syndrome
C. Cranio facial dysostosis
D. All the above

77. Difference between ranula and mucous cyst is presence of

A. Epithelial lining in ranula
B. Mucous glands in mucocele
C. Extravasation of mucous in mucocele
D. Transparency of ranula

78. In hypoplastic amelogenesis imperfecta

A. Shape normal, enamel soft
B. Shape abnormal, enamel brown
C. Shape abnormal, enamel normal
D. Shape abnormal, enamel soft

79. On inspection of mouths of patients with malabsorption following may be observed

A. Leukoplakia
B. Aphthous ulcers
C. Black tongue
D. Macroglossia

80. Hutchinson triad–notched central incisors, blindness and deafness are seen in

A. Primary syphilis
B. Secondary syphilis
C. Tertiary syphilis
D. Congenital syphilis

81. Squamous cell carcinoma most common in mouth is in

A. Upper lip
B. Lower lip
C. Tongue
D. Floor of mouth

82. The fundamental defect in Down syndrome is the presence of an extra chromosome in the affected individual karyotype; this was proven by

A. Le Jeune
B. Turpin
C. Gautier
D. All of the above

83. Usually the natal teeth are

A. Supernumerary primary incisors
B. Prematurely erupted primary teeth
C. Variations of Epstein pearls
D. Variations of Bohn's nodules

84. Condition like Treacher Collin syndrome and hemifacial microsomia, the defect is primarily in

A. Origin and migration of neural crest cells
B. Germ layer formation
C. Differentiation of tissues
D. Neural tube formation

85. Radiographic image of Botryoid odontogenic cyst has a

A. Multilocular radiolucent appearance
B. Unilocular radiolucent appearance
C. Solitary radio–opaque appearance
D. Salt and pepper appearance

86. In hemolytic anemia the radiographic appearance of lamina dura is

A. Normal
B. Lost
C. Less Radio opaque
D. More radio opaque

87. Dilaceration of a permanent incisor is resulted due to

A. Extrusion of deciduous predecessor
B. Intrusion of deciduous predecessor
C. Avulsion of deciduous predecessor
D. None of the above

88. Leukodema has a characteristic sign that it

A. Disappears on stretching
B. Remains fluctuant throughout
C. Is not fluctuant
D. Has a malignant potential

89. Sialosis is

A. Non–inflammatory non–neoplastic swelling of major salivary glands
B. Disease associated with sailors
C. Stone in salivary gland
D. Sialorrhea

90. Oral pathognomonic sign of measles

A. Fordyce's spots
B. Koplick's spots
C. Café–Au–lait spots
D. Purpuric spots

91. Osteomyelitis is defined as an inflammation of

A. Periosteum of the bone
B. Haversian system of the bone
C. Medullary portion of the bone
D. Cortical bone

92. Ludwig's angina begins usually in

A. Sub–lingual space
B. Sub–mental space
C. Sub–maxillary space
D. Sub–masseteric space

93. Acute lymphonodular pharyngitis is caused by

A. Coxsackie virus A–16
B. Coxsackie virus A–10
C. Coxsackie virus A–6
D. Coxsackie virus A–22

94. Pathognomonic feature of cervicofacial actinomycosis is

A. Involvement of submandibular region
B. Presence of multiple discharging sinuses
C. Presence of sulphur granules in the pus
D. Presence of non healing tooth socket

95. Salivary calculi are most commonly discovered in

A. Parotid gland duct
B. Stenson's duct
C. Maxillary sinus
D. Submandibular duct

96. In AIDS, Hairy leukoplakia is found most commonly in which location

A. Hard palate
B. Buccal mucosa
C. Lateral border of tongue
D. Soft palate

97. Malignancy in pleomorphic adenoma is indicated by

A. Rapid enlargement
B. Pain
C. Facial nerve paralysis
D. All of the above

98. Patients with Sjogren's syndrome have higher incidence of

A. Papillary carcinoma thyroid
B. Pleomorphic adenoma
C. Malignant lymphoma
D. None of the above

99. Boggy gums are seen in

A. Scurvy
B. Leukemia
C. Polycythemia
D. Only A and B

100. Which type of ameloblastoma appears to be aggressive with a marked activity for recurrence

A. Follicular ameloblastoma
B. Plexiform ameloblastoma
C. Granular cell ameloblastoma
D. Acanthomatous–ameloblastoma

ORAL RADIOLOGY

101. Radiation causes the following biological effects in younger tissues and organs

A. Carcinogenesis
B. Teratogenesis
C. Mutagenesis
D. All the above

102. The X–ray tube is evacuated to facilitate

A. The movement of electrons
B. The oxidation of filament
C. The production of electrons
D. The collision of electrons

103. The energy of resultant photon is numerically

A. Double the energy of electron that hits the nucleus of target atom
B. More than the energy of electron that hits the nucleus target atom
C. Less than the energy of electron that hits the nucleus of a target atom
D. Equal to the energy of electron that hits the nucleus of a target atom

104. The use of intensifying screens results in

A. Greater clarity in a radiograph
B. Recording of minute details
C. Reduction of dose to the patient
D. Reduction of the speed of the film

ORTHODONTICS

105. A Time period usually required for erupting premolar tooth to move through one mm of bone is

A. 1–2 months
B. 4–5 months
C. 6–9 months
D. 10–12 months

106. Severe crowding is

A. Crowding of more than 2 mm
B. Crowding of more than 5 mm
C. Crowding of more than 8 mm
D. Crowding of more than 10 mm

107. South end clasp by Stephens is more effective on

A. Upper central incisors
B. Canines
C. First molars
D. On any tooth

108. RESPOND is a

A. Invisible retainer
B. Braided wire used in pea for alignment
C. Adhesive-pre coated (APC) bracket system
D. Clear bracket

109. Myofunctional exercises were first advocated by

A. Robin, 1902
B. Moyers, 1925
C. Rogers, 1918
D. Kingsley, 1930

110. The main aim of Frankel appliance is to influence

A. Function of tongue
B. Temporomandibular joint
C. Outer neuro muscular envelop
D. Control of vertical dimension

111. Implant studies on jaw rotations were conducted by

A. Moss
B. Belchier
C. Bjork
D. Sicher

112. Child has a flush terminal plane early in mixed dentition, movement of the lower molar forward relative to the upper molar by

A. 1 mm
B. 1.5 mm
C. 2 mm
D. 3.5 mm

113. When the twin block appliance is enlarged in full closure the upper and lower bite blocks interlock at

A. 45° angle
B. 60° angle
C. 70° angle
D. 90° angle

114. The sequence in which growth of jaw occurs is

A. Width–length–height
B. Height–width–length
C. Length–height–width
D. Width–height–length

115. Patient friendly functional appliance

A. Bionator
B. Activator
C. Twin block
D. Frankel

116. In Catalan's appliance (inclined plane) the plane should be at approximately 45 degrees to

A. Occlusal plane
B. Long axis of the tooth
C. Curve of Spee
D. Facial plane

117. Imbrication denotes

A. Teeth which are irregularly arranged within the arch due to lack of space for them
B. Lack of space due to extra teeth
C. Spacing of teeth
D. Crowding in the posterior segment of arch

118. The combined width of deciduous canines and first and second molar is greater than that of the permanent canine and premolars in the lower is by

A. 3 mm
B. 1.7 mm
C. 1 mm
D. Equal

PEDODONTICS

119. Distal shoe appliance is contra indicated in

A. Hemophilia
B. Congenital heart disease
C. Rheumatic fever
D. All of the above

120. Technique considered as the 'Corner stone of behavior management' is

A. Voice control
B. Tell–show–do
C. Hand over mouth exercise
D. Reinforcement

121. 'Window of Infectivity' in children is possibly seen in age group of

A. 6–18 months
B. 19–33 months
C. 34–48 months
D. 36–60 months

122. Most of the cerebral palsy children are

A. Spastic
B. Dyskinetic
C. Ataxic
D. Mixed

123. Prophylactic restoration (odontotomy) was introduced by

A. Hyatt
B. Bodecker
C. Buonocore
D. Hermann

124. Place of the child in the pedodontic treatment triangle is

A. At the base
B. In the centre
C. At the apex
D. None of the above

125. Complete pulpectomy technique for primary molars is developed by

A. Garcia–Godoy
B. Buckley
C. Starkey
D. Sweet

126. The deciduous molar relation indicative of a developing Angles class II malocclusion

A. Flush terminal plane
B. Mesial step
C. Distal step
D. None of the above

P AND SD

127. "The Cigarette Act of 1975' was introduced by the Government of India on

A. 1st April 1976
B. 15th May 1975
C. 1st June 1976
D. 18th January 1975

128. April 7th is observed as

A. World Anti–AIDS day
B. Doctors day
C. World health day
D. Anti–Tobacco day

129. The "Swish and Swallow' technique is

A. Water fluoridation program
B. Salt fluoridation program
C. Milk fluoridation program
D. Class–room based fluoride tablet program

130. Case control study is

A. Prospective study
B. Retrospective study
C. Longitudinal study
D. None of the above

131. The prevention of emergence of development of risk factors in countries where they have not appeared is what type of prevention?

A. Primary

B. Secondary
C. Tertiary
D. Primordial

132. The earliest phase in public health is
A. Disease control
B. Health promotion
C. Social engineering
D. Health for all

133. The dental auxillary who fabricate dentures directly to patients is called
A. Dental lab technician
B. Expanded function dental auxillary
C. Denturist
D. Dental assistant

134. Beneficience is
A. To do no harm
B. To do good
C. Justice
D. Respect for persons

135. The ideal physical quality of life index score for any country should be
A. 0
B. 50
C. 100
D. Infinity

136. The Consumer Protection Act was passed by the Parliament in the year
A. 1996
B. 1976
C. 1986
D. 2000

137. The test used to evaluate the caries activity in very young children is
A. Calorimetric Snyder test
B. The swab test
C. Susceptibility test
D. Alban test

138. The study that attempts to do no more than describe the pattern of occurrence of disease or a condition relative to other characteristics of the population is
A. Descriptive epidemiology
B. Specific epidemiology
C. Clinical epidemiology
D. General epidemiology

139. Duraphat is a
A. Fluoride mouth wash
B. Fluoride varnish
C. Fluoride tooth paste
D. Fluoride gum paint

140. Fluorspar used in water fluoridation is
A. Sodium fluoride
B. Calcium fluoride
C. Sodium silico fluoride
D. Silico fluorides

141. Histogram is
A. Areas of segments in circle compound
B. Pictorial representation
C. Series of blocks
D. Bars separated by appropriate spaces

PROSTHODONTICS

142. Gingival retraction cord impregnated with epinephrine is contraindicated in
A. Cardiovascular disease
B. Diabetes
C. Hyperthyrodisim
D. All of the above

143. Trubyte tooth indicator is
A. Reinforced tooth for posterior segment
B. Determine the size of the maxillary lateral incisor
C. To measure the length of the lip
D. To determine the size of maxillary central incisor

144. The maximum bite force for person wearing complete denture when compared to person with natural teeth appears to be less by how many times
A. 5–6 times
B. 4–5 times
C. 3–4 times
D. 2–3 times

145. Which of the following is NOT a mouth temperature wax

A. Adaptol
B. Korecta type I
C. HL physiologic paste
D. Lowa wax

146. Posterior palatal seal is recorded when the head is bent at

A. 150°
B. 30°
C. 60°
D. 45°

147. Size of the bur for preparing lingual rest seat for an RPD is

A. 1/4th of an inch
B. 3/4th of an inch
C. ½ an inch
D. 1 inch

148. When the ceramic crown is contra-indicated

A. More conservative restoration
B. Less conservative restoration
C. Three–quarter crown
D. Laminate veneer

149. Conservative alternative to full coverage for improving the appearance of an anterior tooth is

A. Full veneer metal crown
B. Porcelain jacket
C. Three–quarter crown
D. Root canal treated tooth

150. The angle between occlusal rest and the vertical minor connector from which it originates is

A. 90°
B. 100°
C. 120°
D. Less than 90°

151. "Fishbelly' design refers to which type of pontic in fixed partial denture?

A. Saddle
B. Hygienic
C. Ovate
D. Modified ridge lap

152. Continuous clasp is a type of

A. Kennedy's multiple circumferential clasps
B. Embrasure clasp
C. Combination clasp
D. None of the above

PERIODONTICS

153. During scaling and root planing procedures optional angulation is between

A. 35 and 45 degrees
B. 45 and 90 degrees
C. 10 and 20 degrees
D. More than 90 degrees

154. The operator position to perform scaling in mandibular right posterior sextant on lingual aspect is

A. Front position
B. Left side of the patient
C. Right side of the patient
D. Back position

155. Langer technique is used in

A. Sub epithelial connective tissue grafts
B. Free soft tissue autografts
C. Fenestration operation
D. Vestibular extension operation

156. For interproximal areas of diastema or for wide proximal space to properly adapt the proximal papilla against the bone, the recommended technique of suturing method is

A. Interdental ligation
B. Horizontal mattress suture
C. Continuous, independent slight suture
D. Closed anchor suture

157. When osseous defects amenable to regeneration are present, the technique of choice in order of first preference is

A. Modified Wildman flap
B. Apically displaced flap

C. Scaling and root planning
D. Papilla preservation flap

158. Specific and non specific hypothesis was delineated by

A. Walter Loesche
B. William Hunter
C. Socransky
D. Slot

159. Electronic transducer used to measure gingival crevicular fluid is

A. Periotron
B. Perio Test
C. Perio Scan
D. Perio Scope

160. Furcation defects are often diagnosed by

A. Naber's probe
B. DNA probe
C. William probe
D. Michigan probe

161. Frenectomy is a surgical procedure where in

A. Gingiva is removed
B. Bone is removed
C. Frenum is only incised
D. Frenum is completely removed

162. Transfer of the patient from active treatment status to a maintenance program for total patient care is a

A. Step forward
B. Step backward
C. Definitive step
D. Premature step

163. The pH at which citric acid should be applied for root biomodification

A. 1
B. 2
C. 2.5
D. 3

164. The brushing technique that can be recommended for the routine patient with or without periodontal involvement

A. Bass method
B. Modified Stillman method
C. Charter's method
D. Leonard technique

165. Periodontal therapy should NOT be performed in patients who are seen after a stroke

A. For 3 months
B. For 6 months
C. For 9 months
D. For 12 months

166. Peripheral buttressing bone formation is called as

A. Ledging
B. Hemisepta
C. Crater
D. Lipping

167. Periostat is

A. 20 mg capsule of doxycycline hyclate
B. 40 mg capsule of doxycycline hyclate
C. 100 mg capsule of doxycyline hyclate
D. 200 mg capsule of doxycycline hyclate

168. The prime etiological candidate for dental plaque is

A. Streptococcus sanguis
B. Streptococcus milleri
C. Streptococcus mutans
D. Streptococcus mitis

CONS AND ENDO

169. The apico-occlusal taper of the preparation for a cast restoration should be

A. 15°–30°
B. 40°–45°
C. 2°–5°
D. 70°–100°

170. An example of exploring instrument

A. Reamer
B. Smooth broach
C. File
D. Barbed broach

171. **Lining cement used is**
   A. Zinc–oxide Eugenol
   B. Zinc–phosphate cement
   C. Calcium hydroxide
   D. Alginate

172. **The most common cause of flap injury is**
   A. Insufficient extension of releasing incisions
   B. Excessive extension of releasing incision
   C. Using undermining elevation
   D. Improper retractor positioning

173. **The most important aspect of irrigation of canal is**
   A. Aspiration of solution
   B. The irrigating needle use
   C. Chelating action of solution
   D. Volume of solution

174. **The bleaching agent prescribed for night guard bleaching technique is**
   A. Hydrogen peroxide–2%
   B. Sodium hypochlorite–5.25%
   C. Hydrochloric acid
   D. Carbamide peroxide 15%

175. **Fourth canal in a maxillary first molar is most commonly present in**
   A. Palatal root
   B. Mesio buccal root
   C. Mesio lingual root
   D. Disto buccal root

176. **Tip angle of an endodontic instrument should be**
   A. $70 + 10^{\circ}$
   B. $75 + 15^{\circ}$
   C. 70 ± 50
   D. 70 ± 150

177. **K flex files are manufactured from**
   A. Diamond shaped blank
   B. Cylindrical blank
   C. Square blank
   D. Triangular blank

178. **Zone of irritation is characterized by**
   A. Polymorpho nuclear leucocytes
   B. Round cells infiltration
   C. Macrophages and osteoclasts
   D. Fibroblasts and osteoblasts

179. **When a calcified root canal be located or instrumented**
   A. Extraction is the treatment of choice
   B. Retrograde and re–plantation procedure should be considered
   C. The dentist must proceed with the understanding that an unexplored or unfilled canal is worse than perforations
   D. It is not longer accessible to bacterial Infection

180. **When the spread of caries along DEJ exceeds the caries in the contiguous enamel it is termed as**
   A. Forward caries
   B. Residual caries
   C. Rampant caries
   D. Backward caries

181. **Which of the following is NOT present in original GV Black's classification of caries**
   A. Class IV lesion
   B. Class II lesion
   C. Class III lesion
   D. Class VI lesion

182. **The second number in the instrument formula of a gingival marginal trimmer indicates**
   A. Length of the blade
   B. Width of the blade
   C. Primary cutting edge angle
   D. Blade angle

183. **Smear layer debris in root canal is best removed by**
   A. Citric acid
   B. 17% EDTA + 25% NaOCl
   C. 5.20% NaOCl only
   D. 17% EDTA only

184. Most common organism causing caries

A. *Streptococcus faecalis*
B. *Streptococcus viridians*
C. *Streptococcus mutans*
D. *Staphylococcus albus*

185. The most important organism to initiate dental caries is

A. *Streptococcus pyogenes*
B. *Streptococcus viridans*
C. *Streptococcus mutans*
D. *Streptococcus pneumoniae*

186. Samples from root canal can be collected by

A. Swab
B. Syringe and needle
C. Trocar
D. Sterile paper points

ORAL SURGERY

187. Tachyphylaxis during local anesthesia is brought about through the following factors EXCEPT

A. Increased PH of the tissues
B. Hypernatremia
C. Transudation
D. Localised hemorrhage

188. Level V nodes in neck lymph nodes refer to

A. Anterior compartment nodes
B. Posterior triangle nodes
C. Sub mandibular nodes
D. Sub lingual nodes

189. Le Fort I fracture is also known as

A. Pyramidal fracture
B. Suprazygomatic fracture
C. Guerin fracture
D. Guardman's fracture

190. The nerve most likely to get injured during incision placement in wisdom tooth surgery is

A. Lingual nerve
B. Inferior dental nerve
C. Mylohyoid nerve
D. Mental nerve

191. Role of sodium metabisulfite in local anesthetic solution is

A. To maintain isotonicity of solution
B. Antioxidant for vasoconstrictor
C. Preservative
D. Antioxidant for local anesthetic agent

192. The new immature bone that forms during distraction osteogenesis is known as

A. Regenerate
B. Osteoid
C. Callus
D. Osteointegrate

193. In bilateral parasymphyseal fractures of the mandible the fractured segment is displaced posteriorly under the influence of

A. Mylohyoid and geniohyoid
B. Masseter and medial pterygoid
C. Buccinator and posterior belly of digastric
D. Genioglossus, geniohyoid and posterior belly of digastric

194. Abducent nerve paralysis is the earliest finding in the case of

A. LeFort III fracture
B. Naso orbito ethmoid fracture
C. Zygomatic fracture
D. Cavernous sinus thrombosis

195. Dental extraction when indicated in controlled hemophiliacs can be done with

A. Nerve block like inferior alveolar
B. Endotracheal general anesthesia
C. Field block
D. Periodontal ligament injection of LA

196. The technique of doing the incision and drainage of an abscess is known as

A. Andrew's method
B. Hilton's method
C. Nilaton's method
D. Killey's method

197. In children fracture mandible which has not been perfectly reduced but has become firm with slight imperfection the choice of the management would be

A. Arch bar and elastic traction
B. Accept the slight imperfection and allow for later remodeling
C. Re-fracture and plating
D. Re-fracture and interosseous wiring

198. The minimum required distance recommended between implant and superior aspect of inferior alveolar canal is

A. 1 mm
B. 2 mm
C. 4 mm
D. 6 mm

199. 'Wand' is the name of equipment used for

A. Jet injection
B. Electron dental anesthesia
C. Computer controlled local anesthesia
D. General anesthesia

200. Sodium bisulphate used in dental local anesthetic acts as

A. Antibacterial for lignocaine
B. Antibacterial for adrenaline
C. Antioxidant for methylparaben
D. Antioxidant for adrenaline

ANSWERS

HUMAN ANATOMY

1. **Ans: D**

   Ref: BD Chaurasia, 1/E, p. 269

   Explanation
   - At the anterior border of the hyoglossus, the duct is crossed by the lingual nerve

2. **Ans: C**

   Ref: BD Chaurasia, 1/E, p. 335

   Explanation
   - Inferior meatus–largest–opening of the nasolacrimal duct guarded by hasner's valve
   - Middle meatus–maxillary sinus, frontal sinus, middle ethmoidal sinus

3. **Ans: C**

   Ref: BD Chaurasia, 1/E, p. 204

4. **Ans: D**

   Ref: BD Chaurasia, 1/E, p. 139

   Explanation
   - M – Mandibular nerve
   - A – Accessory nerve
   - L – Lesser petrosal nerve
   - E – Emissary vein connecting the cavernous sinus with pterygoid plexus of veins

5. **Ans: A**

   Ref: Di Fiore's Atlas of Histology, 11/E, p. 80

   Explanation
   - Concentric lamellae surround the canals with blood vessels, nerves and connective tissue called the Osteons

6. **Ans: C**

   Ref: BD Chaurasia, 1/E, p. 320

   Explanation
   - Levator veli Palatini is a muscle of soft palate supplied by pharyngeal plexus of accessory nerve

7. **Ans: B**

   Ref: BD Chaurasia, 1/E, p. 358

   Explanation

   Mastoid air sinus is surrounded by:
   - *Superiorly* – tegmen tympani and temporal lobe of cerebrum
   - *Inferiorly* – mastoid process containing mastoid air cells
   - *Anteriorly* – epitympanic recess through auditory meatus
   - *Posteriorly* – sigmoid sinus
   - *Medially* – petrous temporal bone
   - *Laterally* – squamous part of temporal bone

8. **Ans: C**

   Ref: BD Chaurasia, 8/E, p. 154

PHYSIOLOGY

9. **Ans: A**

   Ref: Ganong's, 23/E, p. 02

10. **Ans: C**

    Ref: Ganong's, 23/E, p. 168

    Explanation

Fast pain	*Slow pain*
Sharp	Dull
Localized	Diffuse
Neurotransmitter Glutamate	Substance P
Transmitting by Aδ fibres	C fibres

11. **Ans: B**

    Ref: Sembulingam, 4/E, p. 659

Explanation

- Cyanosis usually occurs only when the quantity of reduced hemoglobin is about 5–7 g%. But in anemia, the Hb content itself is less so, cyanosis cannot occur

12. **Ans: A**

    Ref: Sembulingam, 4/E, p. 546

    Explanation

    - Normal vessel – streamline/laminar flow
    - High velocity of blood – turbulent flow

13. **Ans: A**

    Ref: Guyton, 11/E, p. 249

14. **Ans: C**

    Ref: Sembulingam, 4/E, p. 372

    Explanation

    - Para follicular cells secrete the protein hormone calcitonin
    - It reduces the blood calcium level by decreasing bone resorption

15. **Ans: C**

    Ref: Sembulingam 4/E, p. 107

BIOCHEMISTRY

16. **Ans: D**

    Ref: U. Sathyanarayana and U Chakrapani, 3/E, p. 21

    Explanation

    - Glycogen is the carbohydrate reserve in animals
    - Present in high concentration in liver followed by muscle, brain, etc.
    - It is also found in plants that do not possess chlorophyll (E.g.: yeast, fungi)

17. **Ans: A**

    Ref: U. Sathyanarayana and U Chakrapani, 3/E, p. 395

    Explanation

    - HGPRT (Hypoxanthene Guanine Phosphoribosyl Transferase) is an enzyme of purine salvage pathway and its defect causes Lesch Nyhan syndrome

18. **Ans: A**

    Ref: U. Sathyanarayana and U Chakrapani, 3/E, p. 349

19. **Ans: B**

    Ref: U. Sathyanarayana and U Chakrapani, 3/E, p. 21

GENERAL PATHOLOGY

20. **Ans: A**

    Ref: Robbin's Pathologic Basis of Disease, 7/ E, p. 91

    Explanation

    - *Labile cells* – Continuously dividing tissues; For example: Surface epithelia lining mucosa of excretory ducts
    - *Quiescent or stable cells* – have a low level of replication; e.g.: fibroblasts, endothelial cells, smooth muscles, chrondrocytes, osteocytes
    - *Non dividing or permanent cells* – Neurons, Cardiac muscle cells

MICROBIOLOGY

21. **Ans: B**

    Ref: Oral Microbiology and Infectious Diseases, Schustee & Burnett, 2/E, p. 174

22. **Ans: C**

    Ref: Ananthanarayan and Panicker's Text Book of Microbiology, 8/E, p. 251

23. **Ans: A**

    Ref: Ananthanarayan and Panicker's Text Book of Microbiology, 8/E, p. 20

24. **Ans: D**

    Ref: Ananthanarayan and Panicker's Text Book of Microbiology, 8/E, p. 34

25. **Ans: D**

Ref: Ananthanarayan and Panicker's Text Book of Microbiology, 8/E, p. 8

26. **Ans: C**

Ref: Ananthanarayan and Panicker's Text Book of Microbiology, 8/E, p. 60

Explanation

- Plasmids are circular DNA molecules present in the cytoplasm of bacteria, capable of autonomous replication
- By their ability to transfer genes from one cell to anther by conjugation, they have become important vectors in genetic engineering

27. **Ans: A**

Ref: Ananthanarayan and Panicker's Text Book of Microbiology, 8/E, p. 98

Explanation

- IgG is the only maternal immunoglobulin that is normally transported across placenta and provides natural passive immunity in New born

28. **Ans: B**

Ref: Ananthanarayan and Panicker's Text Book of Microbiology, 8/E, p. 234

Explanation

- Diphtheria toxin acts by inhibiting protein synthesis, specifically; fragment A inhibits polypeptide chain elongation in the presence of NAD by inactivating the elongation factor, EF – 2

PHARMACOLOGY

29. **Ans: C**

Ref: K.D Tripathi, 6/E, p. 742

Explanation

- Ethambutol causes loss of visual acuity/colour vision, field defects due to optic neuritis. Because young children may be unable to report early visual impairment, it should not be used below 6 years of age
- Rifampicin – Hepatitis
- Isoniazid – peripheral neuritis
- Pyrazinamide – hepatotoxicity

30. **Ans: C**

Ref: K.D Tripathi, 6/E, p. 24

Explanation

Prodrug	*Active form*
Levodopa	Dopamine
Enalapril	Enalaprilate
Dipivefrine	Epinephrine
Sulindac	Sulfide metabolite
Proguanil	Cycloguanil
Prednisone	Prednisolone
Bacampicillin	Ampicillin
Sulfasalizine	5–Aminosalicylic acid
Cyclophosphamide	Aldophosphamide
Phamide	Phosphoramide mustard Acrolein
Fluorouracil	Fluorouridine monophosphate
Mercaptopurine	Methylmercaptopurine ribonucleotide
Acyclovir	Acyclovir triphosphate

31. **Ans: B**

Ref: K.D Tripathi, 6/E, p. 136

Explanation

- Cardioselective (beta1) blockers–metoprolol, atenolol, acebutolol, bisoprolol, esmolol, betaxolol, celiprolol, nebivolol

32. **Ans: C**

Ref: K.D Tripathi, 6/E, p. 719

Explanation

Aminoglycosides

- *Systemic* – streptomycin, gentamicin, kanamycin, tobramycin, Amikacin, sisomicin, Netilmicen
- *Topical* – Neomycin, Framycetin
- Erythromycin is a macrolide antibiotic

33. Ans: C

Ref: K.D Tripathi, 6/E, p. 369

34. Ans: D

Ref: K.D Tripathi, 6/E, p. 758

Explanation

- Amphoterecin B inhibits dermatophytes in vitro, but concentrations of AMB attained in infected skin are low and ineffective

35. Ans: D

Ref: K.D Tripathi, 6/E, p. 406, 349

36. Ans: A

Ref: K.D Tripathi, 6/E, p. 837

GENERAL MEDICINE

37. Ans: D

Ref: Davidson, 20/E, p. 665

38. Ans: A

Ref: Davidson, 20/E, p. 801

39. Ans: D

Ref: Harrison, 17/E, Vol. 2, p. 2002

40. Ans: C

Ref: Davidson, 20/E, p. 1182

Explanation

Causes of Asterixis:

- Renal failure
- Liver failure
- Hypercapnia
- Drug toxicity (e.g. phenytoin)
- Acute focal parietal or thalamic lesions

41. Ans: A

Ref: Davidson, 20/E, p. 621

Explanation

- Mitral valve prolapse is also known as 'floppy' mitral and is one of the more common causes of mild mitral regurgitation
- It is caused by congenital anomalies or degenerative myxomatous changes and is sometimes a feature of connective tissue disorders such as marfan's syndrome

42. Ans: C

Ref: Davidson, 20/E, p. 608

Explanation

- In more than 95% of cases, a specific underlying cause of hypertension cannot be found such patients are said to have essential hypertension

43. Ans: A

Ref: Davidson, 20/E, p. 947

44. Ans: D

Ref: Davidson, 20/E, p. 321

Explanation

- Hosts – rodents especially common rat (Rattus norvegicus)
- Particular leptospiral serogroups are associated with characteristic animal hosts
  - Rats – L. icterohaemorrhagiae
  - Dogs – L. canicola
  - Cattles – L. hebdomadis
  - Pigs L. Pomona
- Leptospires can enter their human hosts through intact skin or mucous membranes but entry is facilitated by cuts and abrasions

45. Ans: B

Ref: Davidson, 20/E, p. 358

46. Ans: D

Ref: Davidson, 20/E, p. 633

47. Ans: D

Ref: Davidson, 20/E, p. 1061

Explanation

Causes of bleeding in liver disease

1. Local anatomical abnormalities

2. Reduced hepatic synthesis E.g.: Factors II, VII, IX, X
3. Fibrinogen
4. Reduced clearance of plasminogen activator
5. Thrombocytopenia secondary to hypersplenism
6. Reduced vitamin K absorption (cholestatic jaundice)

48. Ans: C

Ref: Davidson, 20/E, p. 616

Explanation

- Rheumatic fever is a condition triggered by an immune mediated delayed response to infection with specific strains of group A streptococci that possess antigens which may cross react with cardiac myosin and sacrolemmal membrane protein
- Antibodies produced against the streptococcal antigens mediate inflammation in the endocardium myocardium and pericardium as well as the joints and skin

49. Ans: B

Ref: Davidson, 20/E, p. 1052

GENERAL SURGERY

50. Ans: A

Ref: S Das, 5/E, p. 665

51. Ans: D

Ref: S. Das, 5/E, p. 132

52. Ans: B

Ref: S. Das, 5/E, p. 594

53. Ans: C

Ref: S. Das, 5/E, p. 664

54. Ans: B

Ref: S. Das, 5/E, p. 626

55. Ans: D

Ref: S. Das, 5/E, p. 623

DADH

56. Ans: C

Ref: Orban's, 12/E, p.315

57. Ans: A

Ref: Orban's, 12/E, p. 287

58. Ans: C

Ref: Wheeler's, 8/E, p. 430

59. Ans: A

Ref: Wheeler's, 8/E, p. 227

Explanation

- Mesial developmental groove – Maxillary 1st premolar
- Mesiolingual developmental groove – mandibular 1st premolar
- Lingual developmental groove – Mandibular 2nd premolar

DENTAL MATERIALS

60. Ans: C

Ref: Phillip's, 11/E, p. 129

Explanation

- *Softening heat treatment* – Casting is placed in an electric furnace for 10 min at a temperature of 700°C and then it is quenched in water
- *Hardening heat treatment* – Soaking or aging the casting at a specific temperature for 15–30 min before it was water quenched

61. Ans: C

Ref: Phillip's, 11/E, p. 215

Explanation

Type I – 83%

Type II – 77%

Type III – 75%

Type IV – 56%

62. **Ans: B**

Ref: Phillip's 11/E, p. 61

Explanation

- It occurs when combination of dissimilar metals are in direct physical contact

63. **Ans: B**

Ref: Phillip's, 11/E, p. 648

Explanation

NiTi wires

- There is complete transformation from the martensitic NiTi structure to the austentitic NiTi structure at temperature higher than that of oral environment
- Superior spring back

64. **Ans: D**

Ref: Phillip's, 11/E, p. 517

Explanation

- Corrosion process is more limited because the η phase is less susceptible to corrosion than the γ_2 phase of traditional amalgams

65. **Ans: B**

Ref: Phillip's, 11/E, p. 244

66. **Ans: B**

Ref: Phillip's, 11/E, p. 570

Explanation

Alloy type	Total noble metal content
High Noble	≥40 wt% Au
	≥60 wt% Noble metal elements
Noble	≥25 wt% Noble metal elements
Predominantly base metal	< 25wt% Noble metal elements

67. **Ans: D**

Ref: Phillip's, 11/E, p. 198

68. **Ans: B**

Ref: Phillip's, 11/E, p. 551

Explanation

- Maximum particle size – 74 mm
- Average particle size – 15 mm

69. **Ans: C**

Ref: Phillips 11/E p. 261

Explanation

- As the reaction proceeds some of the excess water is taken up in forming dehydrates so that the mix loses its gloss.
- This loss of gloss occurs at approx 9 min

70. **Ans: D**

Ref: Phillip's, 11/E, p. 640

Explanation

- Sensitization – Austentitic stainless steel may lose its resistance to corrosion if it is heated between 400°C–900°C depending on its carbon content caused by precipitation of CrC_3 (chromium carbide) Stabilization–Introduction of one or two elements that form carbide precipitates in preference to chromium thus preventing sensitization E.g.: Niobium or titanium + tantalum

71. **Ans: A**

Ref: Phillip's, 11/E, p. 242

Explanation

- The best method to control gelation time is by the use of retarders. But it is best regulated by the manufacturer
- Gelation time can be altered by altering the W/P ratio but it imparts the physical characteristics of the gel
- The best method to control setting time is by altering the temperature of water Higher the temperature shorter is the setting time, i.e. 1 min reduction in setting time occurs for each 10°C of temperature

72. **Ans: C**

Ref: Phillip's, 11/E, p. 80

Explanation

- MOE – Rigidity or stiffness of a material
- Young's modulus = Stress/Strain
- Unit – Mpa/Psi/force per unit area

ORAL PATHOLOGY AND ORAL MEDICINE

73. **Ans: B**

Ref: Shafer's, 6/E, p. 247

74. **Ans: B**

Ref: Shafer's, 6/E, p. 85

Explanation

- In junctional nevus, the overlying epithelium is usually thin, irregular and shows cells apparently crossing the junction and growing down into the connective tissue – the so called abtropfung or dropping off effect

75. **Ans: A**

Ref: Shafer's, 6/E, p. 569

76. **Ans: D**

Ref: Nevile 3/E, p. 42

77. **Ans: A**

Ref: Shafer's, 6/E, p. 543

78. **Ans: D**

Ref: Shafer's, 6/E, p. 48, 49

79. **Ans: B**

Ref: Regezi, 4/E, p.124

80. **Ans: D**

Ref: Shafer's, 6/E, p. 324

81. **Ans: C**

Ref: Shafer's, 6/E, p. 110

Explanation

- Ca of tongue comprises between 25 – 50% of all intraoral cause

82. **Ans: D**

Ref: Anil Ghom Text book of pathology,1/E, p. 103

83. **Ans: B**

Ref: Shafer's, 6/E, p. 48

84. **Ans: A**

Ref: Shafer's, 6/E, p. 716

85. **Ans: A**

Ref: Shafer's, 6/E, p. 110

86. **Ans: A**

Ref: Wood & Goaz, 5/E, p. 400

87. **Ans: B**

Ref: Shafer's, 6/E, p. 40

88. **Ans: A**

Ref: Shafer's, 6/E, p. 92

89. **Ans: A**

Ref: Neville, 2/E, p. 404

90. **Ans: B**

Ref: Shafer's, 6/E, p. 341

91. **Ans: C**

Ref: Shafer's, 6/E, p. 492

Explanation

- The medullary spaces are filled with inflammatory exudates chiefly PMNs

92. **Ans: C**

Ref: Shafer's, 6/E, p. 508

93. **Ans: B**

Ref: Shafer's, 6/E, p. 340

Explanation

- Acute lymphonodular pharyngitis – Coxsackie virus A10
- Hand, foot and mouth disease - Coxsackie virus A6

94. **Ans: C**

Ref: Shafer's, 6/E, p. 319

95. **Ans: D**

Ref: Shafer's, 6/E, p. 544

Explanation

- The common involvement of the submandibular gland and duct is thought to be due to the tenacity of the submandibular saliva, which, because of its high mucin content, adheres to any foreign particle. The submandibular duct is also long and irregular in its course

96. **Ans: C**

Ref: Shafer's, 6/E, p. 354

97. **Ans: D**

Ref: Shafer's, 6/E, p. 222

98. **Ans: C**

Ref: Shafer's, 6/E, p. 248

Explanation

- A major complicating factor in patients with Sjogren's syndrome is the development of pseudolymphoma and malignant lymphoma

99. **Ans: D**

Ref: Shafer's, 6/E, p. 641, 777

100. **Ans: C**

Ref: Shafer's, 6/E, p. 276

ORAL RADIOLOGY

101. **Ans: D**

Ref: White and Pharoah, 6/E, p. 28

102. **Ans: A**

Ref: White and Pharoah, 6/E, p. 6

Explanation

- X – ray tube is evacuated
- To facilitate movement of electrons by preventing collision of electrons with gas molecules this would significantly reduce their speed
- This also prevents oxidation and "burnout" of the filament

103. **Ans: D**

Ref: White and Pharoah, 6/E, p. 9

104. **Ans: D**

Ref: White and Pharoah, 6/E, p. 56

ORTHODONTICS

105. **Ans: A**

Ref: Bhalaji, 3/E, p. 225

106. **Ans: D**

Ref: Bhalaji, 3/E, p. 396

Explanation

Mild: 0 – 2.5 mm
Moderate: 2.5 – 5 mm
Severe: > 5 mm

107. **Ans: A**

Ref: Bhalaji, 3/E, p. 283

108. **Ans: B**

Ref: Proffit, 4/E, p. 362

109. **Ans: C**

Ref: Orofacial Myology: International Perspectives, 2/E, p.19

110. **Ans: C**

Ref: Graber, 2/E, p. 224

111. **Ans: C**

Ref: Bhalaji, 3/E, p. 13

Explanation

- The use of implants to study bone growth was first introduced by Bjork in 1969

112. **Ans: D**

Ref: Bhalaji, 3/E, p. 43

Explanation

- For transition of end on molar relation to a class I molar relation, the lower molar has to move forward by about 3–5 mm relative to the upper molar by utilization of physiological spaces and leeway space in the lower arch and by differential forward growth of the mandible

113. Ans: A

Ref: Bhalaji, 3/E, p. 357

114. Ans: A

Ref: Bhalaji, 3/E, p. 10

115. Ans: C

Ref: Bhalaji, 3/E, p. 357

116. Ans: A

Ref: Bhalaji, 3/E, p. 428

117. Ans: A

Ref: Orthodontics, Prep Manual for Undergraduates, Sridhar Premkumar, p. 79

118. Ans: B

Ref: Bhalaji, 3/E, p. 48

PEDODONTICS

119. Ans: B

Ref: Shobha Tandon, 1/E, p. 318

120. Ans: B

Ref: Mc Donald, 8/E, p. 45

121. Ans: B

Ref: Mc Donald, 8/E, p. 206

122. Ans: A

Ref: Shobha Tandon, 1/E, p. 542

123. Ans: A

Ref: Shobha Tandon, 1/E, p. 233

124. Ans: C

Ref: Shobha Tandon, 1/E, p. 4

125. Ans: B

Ref: Mc Donald, 8/E, p. 401

Explanation

- Garcia – Godoy
- Buckley – Formacresol soln
- Starkey – Complete pulpectomy technique
- Sweet – Formacresol pulpotomy technique
- Hobson – Beachwood cresol pulpotomy

126. Ans: C

Ref: Shobha Tandon, 1/E, p. 377

P AND SD

127. Ans: A

Ref: Soben Peter, 3/E, p. 109

Explanation

- The government of India introduced on 1st April 1976 "The Cigarettes Act of 1975" requires all manufactures to display "cigarette smoking is injurious to health" on all cartons/packets

128. Ans: C

Ref: Park, 20/E, p. 817

Explanation

30th January – Anti leprosy day
11th July – World population day
2nd October – Anti drug addiction day
11th December – UNICEF day

129. Ans: A

Ref: Soben Peter, 3/E, p. 333

130. Ans: B

Ref: Park, 20/E, p. 67

131. Ans: D

Ref: Park, 20/E, p. 320

132. Ans: A

Ref: Park, 20/E, p. 8

Explanation

- Distinct phases of public health

- Disease control phase (1880–1920)
- Health promotional phase (1920–1960)
- Social engineering phase (1960–1980)
- Health for all phase (1981–2000)

133. Ans: C

Ref: Soben Peter, 3/E, p. 794

Explanation

- Denturists are dental laboratory technicians who are permitted in United States Canada and some other countries to fabricate dentures directly for patients without a dentist's prescription

134. Ans: B

Ref: Soben Peter, 3/E, p. 665

Explanation

- *To do good* – Beneficence
- *To do no harm* – Non-maleficence

135. Ans: C

Ref: Park, 20/E, p. 16

Explanation

Physical quality of life index

- It consolidates these indicators, infant mortality life expectancy at age one and literacy
- Scale of 0 – 100 where O represents – worst performance 100 – represents – best performance
- The ultimate objective is to attain a PQLI of 100

136. Ans: C

Ref: Park, 20/E, p. 606

Explanation

- COPRA – Consumer Protection Act It is a piece of comprehensive legislation and recognizes six rights of the consumer namely
  1. Right to safety
  2. Right to be informed
  3. Right to be choose
  4. Right to heard
  5. Right to seek redressal
  6. Right to consumer education

137. Ans: B

Ref: Soben Peter, 3/E, p. 362

Explanation

- Developed by Grainger in 1965
- Interpretation – change in pH of buccal swab after incubation is read by color comparator
  - PH 4.1 and < 4.1 – Marked caries activity
  - PH 4.2 to 4.4 – Active
  - PH 4.5 to 4.6 – Slightly active
  - PH 4.6 and over – High caries activity

138. Ans: A

Ref: Park, 20/E, p. 59

139. Ans: B

Ref: Soben Peter, 3/E, p. 294

Explanation

- Duraphat–contains 22,600 ppm fluoride
- Fluor protector–Contains 7,000 ppm fluoride
- Carex–contains 1.8%/18,000 ppm fluoride

140. Ans: B

Ref: Soben Peter, 3/E, p. 341

Explanation

Fluoride compounds in water fluoridation

- Fluorspar–85–98% CaF_2
- Sodium fluoride
- Silicofluorides
- Sodium silicofluoride
- Hydroflurosilicic acid
- Ammonium silicofluoride

141. Ans: C

Ref: Park, 20/E, p. 748

PROSTHODONTICS

142. Ans: D

Ref: Nallaswamy, 1/E, p. 625

143. Ans: D

Ref: Heartwell, 4/E, p. 313

144. Ans: A

Ref: Zarb and Bolender, 12/E, p. 10

Explanation

- Maximum biting force of natural teeth: 44 lb (20 kg)
- Maximum biting force of artificial teeth: 13–16 lb (6–8 kg)
- Maximum biting force appear to be 5–6 times less for complete Denture wearers:

145. Ans: B

Ref: Nallaswamy, 1/E, p. 87

146. Ans: B

Ref: Nallaswamy, 1/E, p. 87

147. Ans: A

Ref: Nallaswamy, 1/E, p. 406

148. Ans: A

Ref: Rosensteil, 4/E, p. 325

149. Ans: A

Ref: Rosensteil, 4/E, p. 329

150. Ans: A

Ref: Nallaswamy, 1/E, p. 347

151. Ans: B

Ref: Nallaswamy, 1/E, p. 512

152. Ans: A

Ref: Nallaswamy, 1/E, p. 360

PERIODONTICS

153. Ans: B

Ref: Carranza, 10/E, p. 770

Explanation

Function	*Angulation*
Subgingival insertion	0°
Scaling and root planing	45–90°
Gingival curettage	>90°
Sharpening	70–80°

For scaling and root planning

- Angulation of <45° cutting edge will slide over the calculus, smoothening or burnishing it
- Angulation of >90° lateral surface of blade rather than cutting edge will be against the tooth; calculus may not be removed and become burnished

154. Ans: A & C

Ref: Carranza, 10/E, p. 780

155. Ans: A

Ref: Carranza, 10/E, p. 1019

Explanation

- By Langer and Langer in 1985

156. Ans: B

Ref: Carranza, 10/E, p. 933

Explanation

1. *Horizontal mattress suture* – used for interproximal areas of diastema or wide interdental spaces to adapt the interproximal papilla properly against the bone
2. *Continuous independent slight suture* – used when there is both facial and lingual flap involving many teeth
3. *Anchor suture* – closing of a flap mesial or distal to a tooth
4. *Closed anchor suture* – closing a flap located in an edentulous area mesial or distal to a tooth
5. *Periosteal suture* – to hold in place apically displaced partial thickness flaps

157. Ans: D

Ref: Carranza, 10/E, p. 886

158. Ans: A

Ref: Carranza, 10/E, p. 153

Explanation

Given by Walter Loesche in 1976

1. *Non specific plaque hypothesis* – periodontal disease results from "elaboration of noxious products by the entire plaque flora"
2. *Specific plaque hypothesis* – only certain plaque is pathogenic and its pathogenicity depends on the presence or increase in specific microorganisms

159. Ans: A

Ref: Carranza, 10/E, p. 345

Explanation

1. Periotron – to measure amount of GCF
2. Periotest – to measure endosseus implant rigidity
3. Perioscan – to detect microorganisms using BANA test
4. Perioscope – Microscopes used to look directly at the inner surfaces of the periodontal pockets

160. Ans: A

Ref: Carranza, 10/E, p. 750

Explanation

- Transgingival rounding may further define the anatomy of the furcation defect

161. Ans: D

Ref: Carranza, 10/E, p. 1023

Explanation

- Frenectomy – complete removal of frenum including its attachment to underlying bone
- Frenotomy – incision of the frenum

162. Ans: C

Ref: Carranza, 10/E, p. 1194

163. Ans: A

Ref: Carranza, 10/E, p. 974

Explanation

Actions of citric acid

- Accelerated healing and new cementum formation
- Demineralization and exposure of collagen fibres after root planning
- Removes smear layer exposing dentinal tubules
- Eliminates endotoxins and bacteria from diseased tooth surface

164. Ans: A

Ref: Carranza, 10/E, p. 733

165. Ans: B

Ref: Carranza, 10/E, p. 657

166. Ans: D

Ref: Carranza, 10/E, p. 459

Explanation

- *Ledging* – plateau like bone margins caused by resorption of thickened bony plates
- *Hemisepta* – one wall vertical defect
- *Crater* – concavities in the crest of interdental bone confined within the facial and lingual wall

167. Ans: A

Ref: Carranza, 10/E, p. 806

168. Ans: A

Ref: Carranza, 10/E, p. 141

CONS AND ENDO

169. Ans: C

Ref: Sturdevant, 5/E, p. 850

170. Ans: B

Ref: Grossman, 11/E, p. 191

171. Ans: C

Ref: Sturdavent, 5/E, p. 175

172. Ans: D

Ref: Grossman, 12/E, p. 403

173. Ans: D

Ref: Grossman, 12/E, p. 270

174. Ans: D

Ref: Grossman, 12/E, p. 347

175. Ans: B

Ref: Grossman, 12/E, p. 508

176. Ans: B

Ref: Grossman, 12/E, p. 226

177. Ans: A

Ref: Grossman, 12/E, p. 230

178. Ans: A

Ref: Grossman, 12/E, p. 137

Explanation

- Fish established 4 well defined zones of reaction
  1. *Zone of infection* – PMNs
  2. *Zone of contamination* – Round cells infiltration
  3. *Zone of irritation* – macrophages and osteoclasts
  4. *Zone stimulation* – fibroblasts and osteoclasts

179. Ans: C

Ref: Grossman, 12/E, p. 149

180. Ans: D

Ref: Sturdavent, 5/E, p. 289

Explanation

- *Backward caries* – when the spread of caries along the DEJ exceeds the caries in the contiguous enamel
- *Forward caries* – Caries cone in enamel is larger or same size as that in dentin

181. Ans: D

Ref: Sturdavent, 5/E, p. 295

182. Ans: C

Ref: Sturdavent, 5/E, p. 329

183. Ans: B

Ref: Grossman, 12/E, p. 269

Explanation

- The recommended regimen for irrigation is to employ 17% EDTA for 1 minute followed by a final rinse with NaOCl

184. Ans: C

Ref: Sturdavent, 5/E, p. 69

185. Ans: C

Ref: Sturdavent, 5/E, p. 93

186. Ans: D

Ref: Grossman, 12/E, p. 238

Explanation

- Streptococcus mutans are probably the most important organisms in the initiation of enamel caries and actinomyces viscosus is the most likely to initiate root caries. Lactobacilli are involved in the progression of dentinal caries

ORAL SURGERY

187. Ans: A

Ref: Malamed Local Anesthesia, 5/E, p. 25

188. Ans: B

Ref: Neelima malik, 2/E, p. 736

189. Ans: C

Ref: Neelima Malik, 2/E, p. 354

Explanation

- Le Fort I fracture is also called *Horizontal fracture or Guerin's fracture or Floating fracture*

190. Ans:A

Ref: Neelima Malik, 2/E, p. 130

191. Ans: B

Ref: Malamed Local Anesthesia, 5/E, p. 111

192. Ans: B

Ref: Neelima Malik, 2/E, p. 736

193. Ans: D

Ref: Killey's, 4/E, p. 14

194. Ans: D

Ref: Neelima Malik, 2/E, p. 360

195. Ans: D

Ref: Monheims, 7/E, p. 75

196. Ans: C

Ref: Neelima Malik, 2/E, p. 592

Explanation

- Hilton's method of drainage ensures that no blood vessel or nerve in the vicinity is damaged

197. Ans: B

Ref: Killey's, 4/E, p. 109

198. Ans: B

Ref: Bhalaji, 1/E, p. 309

199. Ans: C

Ref: Malamed Local Anesthesia, 5/E, p. 92

200. Ans: D

Ref: MalamedLocal Anesthesia, 5/E, p. 19

Explanation

- LA with epinephrine may get oxidized if not used immediately turning to a reddish brown color. To avoid this rapid oxidation antioxidants like sodium bisulfite is added in a concentration of 0.05 – 0.1%

5

KCET 2007

HUMAN ANATOMY

1. The preganglionic parasympathetic fibers for otic ganglion commence at

A. Superior salivatory nucleus
B. Inferior salivatory nucleus
C. Nucleus of tractus solitarius
D. Lacrimatory nucleus

2. Medial pterygoid muscle is supplied by

A. Branch from trunk of mandibular nerve
B. Branch from anterior division of Mandibular nerve
C. Branch from posterior division of mandibular nerve
D. Branch from maxillary nerve

3. Facial vein communicates with the cavernous sinus through

A. Retromolar vein and internal jugular vein
B. External jugular vein and internal jugular vein
C. Internal jugular vein and retromandibular vein
D. Superior ophthalmic vein and pterygoid venous plexus

4. The maxillary air sinus opens into middle meatus at

A. Infundibulum
B. Summit of infundibulum
C. Bulla ethmoidalis
D. Hiatus semilunaris

5. 'Wry neck' deformity is due to the damage of

A. Platysma
B. Sternohyoid
C. Sternocleidomastoid
D. Omohyoid

6. Schwann cells are derived from

A. Neural crest cells
B. Mesoderm
C. Endoderm
D. Ectoderm

PHYSIOLOGY

7. Cephalic phase of gastric secretion can be demonstrated by the following experiment

A. Heidenhan's pouch
B. Condition reflex
C. Pavlov
D. None of the above

8. 'P' wave in ECG recording is caused due to

A. Atrial depolarization
B. Atrial repolarization
C. Ventricular depolarization
D. Ventricular repolarization

9. Factor V is

A. Stable factor
B. Christmas factor
C. Hageman's factor
D. Labile factor

10. Trypsin is an activator of all of the following enzymes EXCEPT

A. Chymotrypsinogen
B. Pepsinogen
C. Proelastase
D. Procolipase

11. **Delta waves of electroencephalogram have frequency of**
    A. More than 14 cycles per second
    B. Between 8 and 13 cycles per second
    C. Less than 3.5 cycles per second
    D. Between 4 and 7 cycles per second

12. **Parathyroid hormone increases the blood level of**
    A. Copper
    B. Calcium
    C. Iron
    D. Sodium

13. **Glycosylated haemoglobin assay is helpful in the monitoring of patient with**
    A. Addison's disease
    B. Diabetes Mellitus
    C. Cushing's disease
    D. Grave's disease

14. **The tissue macrophages are derived from the**
    A. Neutrophil
    B. Eosinophil
    C. Monocyte
    D. All of above

BIOCHEMISTRY

15. **Enzymes increase reaction rates by**
    A. Altering the free energy of the action
    B. Decreasing the energy of activation
    C. Enhancing the forward reaction
    D. Inhibiting the backward reaction

16. **Von Gierke's disease is associated with a deficiency of**
    A. Glucose–6–phosphate dehydrogenase
    B. Glucose–6–phosphatase in liver
    C. Phosphorylase in muscle
    D. Glutamine

17. **Ammonia produced by brain is trapped as**
    A. Urea
    B. Uric acid
    C. Creatinine
    D. Glutamine

18. **Dietary fiber is rich in**
    A. Starch
    B. Cellulose
    C. Collagen
    D. Inulin

GENERAL PATHOLOGY

19. **Bleeding time and prothrombin time is prolonged in**
    A. DIC
    B. Thrombocytopenia
    C. Hemophilia
    D. Von Willebrand's disease

20. **The peripheral smear picture in Iron deficiency anaemia will be**
    A. Macrocytic, hypochromic
    B. Leukoerythroblastic
    C. Normocytic, normochromic
    D. Microcytic, hypochromic

21. **An increase in the number of cells in an organ or tissue is**
    A. Hypertrophy
    B. Hyperplasia
    C. Aplasia
    D. Metaplasia

22. **Severe generalized edema is called as**
    A. Myxoedema
    B. Pitting edema
    C. Anasarca
    D. Dependent edema

23. **Transfusion transmitted diseases are all EXCEPT**
    A. HIV
    B. Hepatitis C
    C. CMV
    D. Tuberculosis

MICROBIOLOGY

24. **Phycomycete causing infection in man**
    A. Rhizopus
    B. Mucor

C. Absidia
D. All

25. Sterilization by moist heat is used in
A. Autoclave
B. Hot air oven
C. Filteration
D. Incineration

26. The small non–particulate protein leading to enhanced replication of HBV as well as HIV is
A. HBc Ag
B. HBs Ag
C. HBe Ag
D. HBx Ag

27. The gram negative bacteria most numerous in the oral cavity are
A. Streptococci
B. Veillonellae
C. Salmonella
D. Eikenella

28. Antiseptic technique in surgery was first introduced by
A. Joseph Lister
B. Louis Pasteur
C. Robert Koch
D. Antony Van Leeuwenhock

29. Which component of the cell wall is responsible for endotoxic activity
A. Region I
B. Region II
C. Region III
D. Bovine antigen

30. Immunoglobulin molecule which mediates in anaphylaxis is
A. Ig M
B. Ig G
C. Ig E
D. Ig A

31. Infectious mononucleosis is caused by the virus
A. CMV
B. EBV
C. HIV
D. Herpes simplex

PHARMACOLOGY

32. A hemophiliac patient has rheumatoid arthritis. Which drug might be prescribed to relieve the pain?
A. Acetaminophen
B. Acetylsalicylic acid
C. Phenylbutazone
D. Naproxen

33. The sialogogues used in Xerostomia is
A. Hyoscine
B. Pilocarpine
C. Hyaluronidase
D. Vitamin C

34. For Arsenic poisoning antidote is
A. Penicilamine
B. Des ferroxamine
C. EDTA
D. BAL

35. Following administration, nitrous oxide will become saturated in blood within
A. 3–5 mins
B. 10 mins
C. 10–15 mins
D. 6–8 min

36. Which of these is NOT glycoside?
A. Digoxin
B. Digitoxin
C. Ergotoxin
D. Gitoxin

37. Immune mediated qualitative drug intolerance is called
A. Super sensitivity
B. Idiosyncrasy
C. Hyper sensitivity
D. Hyper acidity

38. The statement NOT true of selective Cox – 2 inhibitor is
A. The analgesic and anti–inflammatory effects identical to that of non–selective NSAIDs

B. They do not offer the cardio protective effect
C. Safe in patients with renal insufficiency
D. Fewer incidence of gastrointestinal side effects

GENERAL MEDICINE

39. The manifestations of congenital syphilis include
A. Lympadenophathy
B. Condyloma Lata
C. Hepatosplenomegaly
D. All of the above

40. Outright or full–blown AIDS is characterized by
A. CD4 T–cells 800 cells/mm^3
B. CD4 T–cells 400 cells/mm^3
C. CD4 T–cells 600 cells/mm^3
D. CD4 T–cells <200 cells/mm^3

41. In hemophilia, abnormality is found in
A. Total leukocyte count
B. Platelet count
C. Red blood cell count
D. Activated partial thromboplastin time

42. The treatment of choice for trigeminal neuralgia is
A. Carbamazepine
B. Morphine
C. Aspirin
D. Ibuprofen

43. Most specific histological lesion in diabetic nephropathy is
A. Widening of glomerular basement membrane
B. Generalized mesangial thickening
C. Occlusion of glomeruli with fibrin caps
D. Hyalinization of afferent arterioles and Kimmelstein–Wilson bodies

44. Infectious disease causing cirrhosis of the liver are
A. Viral hepatitis
B. Toxoplasmosis
C. EB virus
D. All of the above

45. Portal hypertension is characterized by all of the following EXCEPT
A. Splenomegaly
B. Variceal bleeding
C. Dilated veins over the abdomen
D. Gynecomastia

46. Causes of a transudate ascites include all the following EXCEPT
A. Tuberculosis
B. Nephritic syndrome
C. Hypoproteinaemia
D. Congestive cardiac failure

47. Gas gangrene infection is caused by
A. Staphylococcus aureus
B. Pseudomonas
C. Clostridium perfringens
D. E. coli

GENERAL SURGERY

48. Branchial cyst develops from vestigial remnants of
A. Fourth branchial cleft
B. 2nd branchial cleft
C. 3rd branchial cleft
D. 1st branchial cleft

49. Following one is NOT true of carcinoma of lip
A. Most common on vermilion of lower lip
B. A 90% cure rate is possible with surgery or radiotherapy
C. Initially tumor spreads laterally rather than infiltrating deeply
D. Up to one third of the lip cannot be Removed

50. The common site of glomangioma is
A. Head and neck
B. Nail bed
C. Chest wall
D. Retroperitoneal

51. **Commonest cause of cellulitis is**
   A. Staphylococcus
   B. Pseudomonas
   C. Streptococcus
   D. Pneumococcus

52. **Marjolin's ulcer is**
   A. Squamous cell carcinoma from scar
   B. Trophic ulcer
   C. Tuberculous ulcer
   D. Rodent ulcer

53. **In 3rd degrees burns, all are seen EXCEPT**
   A. Vesicles are absent
   B. Painful
   C. Leathery skin
   D. Charred and black

54. **Which of the following statements is true for MEN type I**
   A. There is hyperplasia of parathyroid gland
   B. Chromophobe adenoma of pituitary gland may result in acromegaly
   C. Pancreatic tumours may produce gastrin, insulin, glucagon, somatostatin
   D. All of the above

55. **Rule of 9 to estimate surface area of burns patient was introduced by**
   A. Mortiz Kaposi
   B. Alexander and Wallace
   C. Lister
   D. Barclay

56. **Squamous cell carcinoma has tendency to metastasize through**
   A. Blood stream
   B. Lymphatic system
   C. Direct contact
   D. None of the above

DENTAL MATERIALS

57. **Currently available composites undergo polymerization at a wavelength of**
   A. 474 nm
   B. 470 nm
   C. 460 nm
   D. 464 nm

58. **Thickness of the die spacer should be**
   A. 10–20 μm
   B. 20–40 μm
   C. 30–60 μm
   D. 25–50 μm

59. **Steel is an alloy of iron in which the carbon content is**
   A. Less than 18%
   B. Less than 2%
   C. More than 8%
   D. None of the above

60. **The % of free monomer in a heat–cured acrylic resin is**
   A. 3% to 5%
   B. 8% to 10%
   C. 0.2% to 0.5%
   D. 0.6% to 0.8%

61. **Liquid used in polycarboxylate cement is**
   A. Poly acrylic acid
   B. Phosphoric acid
   C. Eugenol
   D. Methacrylic acid

62. **The total copper content in admixed alloy ranges from approximately**
   A. 1 to 6 weight percent
   B. 9 to 20 weight percent
   C. 30 to 40 weight percent
   D. 45 to 55 weight percent

63. **For dental amalgam, the elastic modulus and tensile strength is**
   A. 40 Gpa and 60–100 MPa
   B. 21 Gpa and 27–55 MPa
   C. 350 Gpa and 110–120 MPa
   D. 360 GPa and 125–130 MPa

64. **The Knoop hardness number of microfilled composite restorative material ranges from**
   A. 50–60 KHN
   B. 25–35 KHN
   C. 15–20 KHN
   D. 40–48 KHN

65. In air abrasive technology, the abrasive particles used are

A. Iron oxide
B. Tin oxide
C. Aluminium oxide
D. Silicon oxide

66. Finer the particle size of silica

A. Slower the hygroscopic expansion
B. Greater the hygroscopic expansion
C. Normal setting expansion
D. No setting expansion

67. The minimum film thickness for luting a single crown

A. 20 μm
B. 25 μm
C. 35 μm
D. 45 μm

68. Putty wash technique (two stage)

A. Light body and putty used at the same time
B. Putty used first and light body used next
C. Light body first and putty later
D. None of the above

DADH

69. Roots of the permanent mandibular 1st molar are

A. Mesio buccal, distobuccal and lingual
B. Mesiolingual, distolingulal and buccal
C. Mesial and distal
D. Buccal and lingual

70. Mixed dentition period lasts from

A. 6–9 years
B. 8–9 years
C. 6–12 years
D. 2–12 years

71. Longest root in the permanent maxillary molar is

A. Buccal
B. Lingual
C. Mesio buccal
D. Distobuccal

72. Eruption of maxillary permanent canine takes place at the age of

A. 9 to 10 years
B. 11 to 12 years
C. 13 to 14 years
D. 8 to 9 years

ORAL PATHOLOGY AND ORAL MEDICINE

73. Carnoy's solution is used in the treatment of

A. Odontogenic Keratocyst
B. Ameloblastoma
C. Dentigerous cyst
D. Mucocele

74. Post extraction bleeding in a leukemic patient is due to

A. Increase in leukocytes
B. Low calcium level
C. Platelet disorder
D. Deficiency of clotting factors

75. The benign neoplasm of 'brown fat' noted in oral/pharyngeal region is

A. Lipoma
B. Hibernoma
C. Teratoma
D. Brown tumor

76. Commonest site for ectopic salivary gland tumor is

A. Tongue
B. Cheek
C. Palate
D. Neck

77. Specimens for a biopsy should be taken from

A. Necrotic area
B. Subdermal layer
C. Border of an ulcerated area
D. Center of an ulcerated area

78. The drug of choice in trigeminal neuralgia is

A. Phenytoin sodium
B. Carbamazepine

C. Gabapentin
D. Sodium Valproate

79. Which of the following viruses appears to be involved in the pathogenesis of Kaposi's sarcoma?

A. Human herpes virus 3
B. Human herpes virus 1
C. Human herpes virus 8
D. Human herpes virus 4

80. Candidal hyphae can be stained using

A. Van Gieson's stain
B. Periodic acid Schiff stain
C. Masson trichrome stain
D. Toluidine blue stain

81. Monro's abscess is seen in the histological picture of

A. Darriers disease
B. Psoriasis
C. Systemic lupus erythematosus
D. Behcets disease

82. 'Canker sore' is otherwise commonly known as

A. Recurrent aphthous ulcer
B. Recurrent herpetic gingivitis
C. Acute necrotizing ulcerative gingivitis
D. Recurrent herpes labialis

83. Generalized microdontia is often associated with

A. Pituitary dwarfism
B. Pituitary gigantism
C. Hereditary ectodermal dysplasia
D. All of the above

84. Which of the following is NOT a feature of Hutchinson's triad?

A. Gumma
B. Hypoplasia of incisors and molars
C. Eighth nerve deafness
D. Interstitial keratitis

85. Venous malformations involving the leptomeninges of the cerebral cortex is a salient feature of

A. Rendu–Osler–Weber disease
B. Maffuci's syndrome
C. Angio–osteohypertrophy syndrome
D. Sturge Weber syndrome

86. Peripheral giant cell granuloma occurs most commonly on the

A. Gingiva
B. Alveolar ridge
C. Palate
D. Floor of the mouth

87. The term 'pulse granuloma' suggests reaction towards the fragments of foreign material like

A. Cotton fibers
B. Black silk
C. Silver amalgam
D. Legumes

88. A patient of 18 years age with sebaceous cysts on the scalp and back of the neck, an osteoma on the right mandible; radiographs reveal multiple impacted supernumerary teeth in both jaws. These findings suggest

A. Cleidocranial dysostois
B. Ectodermal dysplasia
C. Gardener's syndrome
D. Osteogenesis imperfecta

89. Of the following syndromes, taurodontism is associated with

A. Rubinstein–Taybi syndrome
B. Klinefelter syndrome
C. Ascher's syndrome
D. Gardener's syndrome

90. Absence of cementum is a feature of

A. Vitamin D resistant rickets
B. Hypocalcaemia
C. Hypophosphatasia
D. Osteoporosis

91. 'Chemical mumps' is synonymous with

A. Epidemic parotitis
B. Nutritional mumps
C. Iodine mumps
D. Nonspecific mumps

92. Epstein Barr virus is believed to cause
A. Burkitt's Lymphoma
B. Nasopharyngeal carcinoma
C. Oral hairy leukoplakia
D. All of the above

93. The most common neoplasm among HIV positive homosexual males
A. Non–Hodgkin's lymphoma
B. Glomus tumor
C. Kaposi's sarcoma
D. None of the above

94. Topical antifungal agent in candidiasis is
A. Clotrimazole
B. Clotrimoxazole
C. Ornidazole
D. Propanolol

95. One of the following lesions has extremely high rate of malignant transformation
A. Verrucous leukoplakia
B. White sponge nevus
C. Nodular leukoplakia
D. Target or iris lesion

96. The oral lesion called mucous patches is usually multiple, grayish white plaque associated with
A. Pain
B. No pain
C. Itching
D. Burning sensation

97. Antinuclear antibodies are seen in
A. SLE
B. RAS
C. Leukoplakia
D. Noma

ORAL RADIOLOGY

98. Hair–on–end appearance of skull is seen in
A. Sickle cell anemia
B. Fibrous dysplasia
C. Iron deficiency anemia
D. Megaloblastic anemia

99. Ground glass appearance is seen in
A. Fibrous epulis
B. Fibrous dysplasia
C. Ossifying fibroma
D. Crouzon syndrome

100. The optical density of gross film fog typically is
A. 0.6 to 3.0
B. 0.2 to 0.3
C. 0.2 to 0.4
D. 0.6 to 4.0

101. Fixed post mitotic cells are
A. Spermatocytes
B. Fibroblasts
C. Endothelial cells
D. Muscle

102. Clearing agent in fixer solution is
A. Ammonium chloride
B. Ammonium thio sulfate
C. Ammonium sulfate
D. Ammonium oxalate

103. Units of radiation exposure is
A. Rad
B. Roentgen
C. Rem
D. Seivert

ORTHODONTICS

104. Adenoid facies is seen in
A. Mouth breathing habit
B. Bruxism
C. Sub mandibular lymphadenitis
D. Thumb sucking habit

105. Distal shoe guiding appliance is
A. Habit breaking appliance
B. Space regainer
C. Helps in eruption of first permanent molar
D. It is a type of pulpectomy procedure

106. Anterior open bite and maxillary constriction is caused by
A. Thumb sucking
B. Nail biting

C. Bruxism
D. None

107. Site at which ossification stops in the mandible

A. Mandibular lingula
B. Coronoid process
C. Symphysis
D. Angle of the mandible

108. Adams clasps for premolar is made using the following diameter wire

A. 0.8 mm
B. 0.7 mm
C. 0.6 mm
D. 0.5 mm

109. Transposition of teeth is most commonly seen in the region of

A. Maxillary central and lateral incisors
B. Mandibular canine and first premolar
C. Maxillary lateral incisor, canine and premolar
D. Mandibular first and second premolars

110. An expansion appliance made with an expansion screw is an example of

A. Simple anchorage
B. Reciprocal anchorage
C. Multiple anchorage
D. Reinforced anchorage

111. The Optimal orthodontic force per square centimeter of the root surface area is held to be

A. 18–22 gms
B. 18–16 gms
C. 20–26 gms
D. 26–30 gms

112. All of the following are considered micro–skeletal units of the mandible as per the matrix theory EXCEPT

A. Chin
B. Glenoid fossa
C. Coronoid process
D. Angle of the mandible

113. An example of a tissue–borne appliance among the following is

A. Activator
B. Bionator
C. Frankel's functional regulator
D. Twin block

114. The three main vertical pillars of trajectories of force arising from the alveolar process and ending in the base of the skull are all EXCEPT

A. Canine pillar
B. Zygomatic pillar
C. Pterygoid pillar
D. Condylar pillar

115. The activator appliance was introduced by

A. Robin
B. Andresen
C. Clark
D. Andrews

116. "Baker's anchorage" refers to the use of

A. Intramaxillary elastics
B. Intermaxillary elastics
C. Anterior vertical elastics
D. Cross elastics

117. The kind of force that is best suited for orthodontic tooth movement

A. Light continuous forces
B. Intermittent forces
C. Interrupted continuous forces
D. Heavy continuous forces

118. Functional matrix theory suggests that the determinant growth of skeletal tissues resides in

A. Skeletal tissues
B. Sutures
C. Cartilages
D. Non–skeletal tissues

119. Gingivectomy of which of the fibers can reduce the relapse of orthodontically moved teeth

A. Gingival fibers
B. Alveolar crest fibers
C. Transseptal
D. None

PEDODONTICS

120. Which of the following is NOT a type of cerebral palsy?

A. Spasticity
B. Autism
C. Ataxia
D. Athetosis

121. Tell–show–do technique was introduced by

A. Addleston
B. Craig
C. Christopher
D. Keith more

122. According to Stanford–Binet, non–trainable type of mental retardation has IQ of

A. Below 20
B. Between 36–51
C. Above 51
D. 130

123. Which of the following molar relationship is the most common in primary dentition

A. Mesial step
B. Distal step
C. Flush terminal plane
D. Can't say

124. The type of space maintainer advised when there is bilateral loss of teeth in same arch

A. Distal shoe
B. Band and loop
C. Band and Bar
D. Lingual arch holding appliance

P AND SD

125. The SCAN index is generally used as a

A. Malocclusion index
B. Treatment need index
C. Treatment change index
D. Treatment of priority index

126. Fluoride in any form is contraindicated in

A. Chronic renal failure
B. Osteoporosis
C. Hypertension
D. Thyrotoxicosis

127. 'Crippling Fluorosis' is characterized by

A. Blockage of blood vessels
B. Chipping of teeth
C. Rigid spine
D. Calcification of blood vessels

128. Interruption of transmission of disease

A. Disease control
B. Disease elimination
C. Disease eradication
D. Disability limitation

129. Which is the first study on water fluoridation?

A. Grand rapids (Michigan) and Muskegon
B. Newberg and Kingston
C. Brantford and Sarnia
D. Evanston and Park

130. The lethal dose of fluoride for 70 kg adult is

A. 32–64 mg of fluoride/kg body weight
B. 50–60 mg of fluoride/kg body weight
C. 30–70 mg of fluoride/kg body weight
D. 60–80 mg of fluoride/kg body weight

131. Who introduced APF?

A. Muhler
B. Bibby
C. Brudevold
D. More

132. In which year 1st Fluoride dentrifice was accepted by ADA?

A. 1920
B. 1984
C. 1994
D. 1964

133. What is the percentage of fluoride present in APF gel

A. 1.23%
B. 2%
C. 1.85%
D. 0.2%

134. Where was atraumatic restorative treatment first introduced?

A. Tanzania
B. China
C. U.S.A
D. New Zealand

135. What is the function of humectants in dentifrices?

A. Liquefies the dentifrice
B. Prevents water loss and hardening on exposure to air
C. Flavors the tooth paste
D. Cleans tooth surface effectively

136. The model of web of causation of disease was first suggested by

A. Pettenkofer
B. Mac Mohan and Pugh
C. John M. Last
D. CEA Winslow

137. DMFT Index in 1938 was not developed by

A. Dean H. T
B. Henry T. Klein
C. Knutson. J. W
D. Carole E. Palmer

138. "Disability limitation" is a mode of intervention in

A. Primary level of prevention
B. Secondary level of prevention
C. Tertiary level of prevention
D. Primordial prevention

139. The personnel involved in Integrated Child Development Services (ICDS) scheme initiated by Government of India is

A. Dhai
B. Anganwadi worker
C. Village health volunteers
D. School health teacher

140. The caking (drying) of dentifrice is prevented by adding

A. Cellulose
B. $CaCO_3$
C. Water
D. Silica

141. Opaque white areas covering more than 25% but less than 50% of the tooth surface is given the dean's score of

A. 1
B. 2
C. 3
D. 4

PROSTHODONTICS

142. A ferrule is

A. A rule governing gold inlay cavity preparation
B. A mechanical rapid tooth separator
C. An encircling band to metal that increases fracture resistance of the tooth
D. An electronic measuring device for determination of the length of tooth during root canal treatment

143. The biting force at molar region during mastication is

A. 20 to 55 N
B. 30 to 75 N
C. 50 to 75 N
D. 90 to 200 N

144. The theory of matching teeth to face forms was advanced by

A. Hanau
B. Frush and Fisher
C. J. Leon Williams
D. Schiffman

145. Common indication for a hygienic pontic is in

A. Maxillary anteriors
B. Mandibular anteriors
C. Mandibular posteriors
D. Maxillary premolars

146. The–I Bar RPD was introduced by

A. Berg and caputo
B. Kratochvil
C. McDowell
D. Krol

147. Anatomic teeth should have a cusp angle of

A. 30°
B. 31°
C. 32°
D. 33°

148. Ovate pontics are used in

A. Well rounded ridges
B. Knife edge ridges
C. Recently extracted tooth sockets
D. Flat ridges

149. A high tracing device is used for

A. Extra oral graphic tracings
B. Intra oral graphic tracings
C. Cephalometric tracings
D. Determining local forms

150. Functional cusp bevel is given for

A. Marginal integrity
B. Structural durability
C. Retention and resistance form
D. To improve the geometry of tooth Surfaces

151. Osseointegration was first defined by

A. Bothe and Coworkers
B. Greenfield
C. Strock
D. Branemark

152. The average inter condylar distance which is adequate for complete dentures is

A. 110 mm
B. 120 mm
C. 115 mm
D. 140 mm

153. Name the muscle group which opposes the buccinator's mechanism

A. Medial pterygoid
B. Lateral pterygoid
C. Masseter
D. Tongue muscles

154. The superior border of lingual bar major connector should be located below the gingival margin by a minimum of

A. 2 mm
B. 4 mm
C. 5 mm
D. 1 mm

155. Two or more parallel vertical surfaces of abutment teeth shaped to direct the prosthesis during placement and removal, are known as

A. Orientation plane
B. Parallel block out
C. Survey lines
D. Guiding planes

156. The relationship of mandible to the maxilla when the teeth are in maximum occlusal contact irrespective of the position or alignment of the condyle distal assemblies is known as

A. Centric occlusion
B. Centric relation
C. Plane of occlusion
D. Curve of Spee

157. Vibrating line is present on

A. Hard palate
B. Junction of hard and soft palate
C. Soft palate
D. Junction of muscularis mucosa and palatine muscle

PERIODONTICS

158. Rotten apple smell of breath is associated with

A. Liver insufficiency
B. Kidney insufficiency
C. Unbalanced insulin dependent diabetes
D. Respiratory problems

159. Bacterial plaque can effectively induce bone loss (radius of action) of about

A. 1 mm
B. 1.5–2.5 mm
C. 3–5 mm
D. 6–8 mm

160. ANUG is frequently associated with deficiency of

A. Thiamine

B. Riboflavin
C. Niacin
D. Pyridoxine

161. Which of the following is a root–conditioning agent?
A. Hydrogen peroxide
B. Citric acid
C. Benzoic acid
D. Sodium hypochlorite

162. After curettage how long does it take for reepithelialization to occur?
A. 2–7 days
B. 4–5 weeks
C. 1–3 days
D. 1–2 weeks

163. When occlusal forces exceed the adaptive capacity of the tissue injury results. The resultant injury is called
A. Traumatic occlusion
B. Bruxism
C. Trauma from occlusion
D. Tissue injury

164. Splitting of two rooted tooth into two separate portions is called
A. Root resection
B. Hemisection
C. Furcation
D. Recession

165. Current concepts of evaluating health care require a scientific basis for treatment referred as
A. Evidence based therapy
B. Periodontal maintenance
C. Tooth mortality
D. Prevention of loss of attachment

166. Periodontitis is caused by
A. Malnutrition
B. Supra gingival plaque
C. Bio–film
D. Faulty tooth brushing

167. Dental floss is used to prevent
A. Discoloration of teeth
B. Caries in teeth
C. Sensitivity in teeth
D. Inter proximal plaque formation

168. Regeneration in periodontal therapy aims at
A. Bone refill
B. Repair of the bony defect
C. Reconstitution of the lost periodontium
D. Removal of the diseased bone

169. Pellicle formation on enamel starts with
A. Absorption of glycoprotein from saliva
B. Focal areas of mineralization
C. Bacterial colonization
D. Absorption of endotoxins

170. An enzyme present in saliva which causes cell wall lysis
A. Lysozyme
B. Peroxidase
C. Lactoferrin
D. Hyaluronidase

171. In the concept of biological width, the value of biological width is
A. 1 mm
B. 2 mm
C. 3 mm
D. 4 mm

CONS AND ENDO

172. Which of the following is used for 'Figure of eight' wiring for stabilization of subluxated teeth in alveolar injuries?
A. 0.23 mm stainless steel wire
B. 0.35 mm stainless steel wire
C. 0.45 mm stainless steel wire
D. 0.55 mm stainless steel wire

173. The matrix retainer where in anatomy Adaptation is possible without wedges is
A. Tofflemire
B. Steele's siqveland
C. Ivory no. 1
D. Ivory no. 8

174. R C Prep is

A. EDTA
B. EDTA and urea peroxide
C. EDTA and carbamide peroxide
D. EDTA and Cetavlon

175. Self etching primers

A. Simultaneously etches and prime dentin and enamel
B. Etches enamel only
C. Only bonds to enamel
D. Only removes smear layer

176. The most practical method to disinfect gutta percha prior to obturation is

A. Submerge in 5% solution of NaOCl
B. Submerge in Ethyl Alcohol
C. Submerge in 5% NaOCl and rinse with ethyl alcohol
D. Rinse with 3% hydrogen peroxide

177. The compressive strength of dentine is approximately

A. 468 MPa
B. 162 MPa
C. 350 MPa
D. 266 MPa

178. The bleaching material used in night guard vital tooth bleaching is

A. Superoxol
B. Anesthetic ether and hydrochloric acid
C. Sodium bicarbonate
D. Carbamide peroxide

179. Powdered gold is

A. Made by a combination of chemical precipitation and atomization
B. Made by electrolytic precipitation
C. Made by beating pure gold at high temperatures
D. Made by milling pure gold ingots

180. Stielglitz pliers is

A. Used to contour matrix bands
B. Used to hold the silver point
C. Used to remove roots during hemisection
D. Used to place rubber dam clamp on the tooth

181. Which among the following root canal irrigant removes the smear layer?

A. Sodium hypochlorite
B. EDTA
C. Hydrogen peroxide
D. Chlorhexidine

182. The ideal marginal metal for cast inlay restoration should be

A. 20–30 degree
B. 30–40 degree
C. 40–50 degree
D. More than 50 degree

183. All the following criteria contribute to a successful direct pulp capping procedure EXCEPT

A. Hemorrhage from the exposure site is easily controlled
B. The exposure site is small, less than 0.5 mm in diameter
C. Exposure site is the consequence of infected dentin extending into the pulp
D. Exposure occurred in a clean uncontaminated field

184. The maximum head diameter of ISO Gates Glidden drill # 1 is equivalent to

A. No 50 file at D_0
B. No 40 file at D_0
C. No 60 file at D_0
D. No 80 file at D_0

185. The instrument that has four unit formula

A. Gingival margin trimmer
B. Enamel hatchet
C. Hoe
D. Chisel

186. Rubber dam was introduced by

A. Tom Hanks
B. SC Barnum
C. Hedstorm
D. GV Black

187. The simplest form of pulp therapy is

A. Apicoectomy
B. Pulp capping

C. Pulpectomy
D. Pulpotomy

ORAL SURGERY

188. Phleboliths are seen in

A. Dental pulp
B. Salivary gland duct
C. Cavernous haemangioma
D. Subepithelial bulla

189. Gut suturing material is absorbed by

A. Oxidation
B. Hydrolysis
C. Fibrinolysis
D. Proteolysis

190. In modified radical neck dissection following structure is preserved

A. Submandibular gland
B. Internal jugular vein
C. Fat tissue
D. Greater auricular nerve

191. The maximum dosage of local anesthetic agent like lidocaine must be reduced when used in combination with a CNS and/ respiratory depressant because, it may result in

A. Seizures
B. Coma
C. Death
D. All of the above

192. The most common reason for removal of impacted mandibular third molars

A. Referred pain
B. Orthodontic treatment
C. Recurrent pericoronitis
D. Chronic periodontal disease

193. Enbloc resection of the segment of the bone

A. Compete resection of the jaw bone
B. Resection of half of the affected jaw
C. Resection of the tumor only
D. The entire tumor is removed intact with a rim of uninvolved bone while maintaining continuity of jaw

194. The intercanthal distance suggestive of traumatic telecanthus is

A. 30 mm
B. 32 mm
C. 25 mm
D. 40 mm

195. Frey's syndrome can occur following

A. Sagittal split osteotomy
B. Caldwel–luc operation
C. Parotidectomy
D. Marsupialization

196. Which of the following infection is the cause for multiple sites of osteomyelitis of the jaws

A. Peritonsillar abscess
B. Local trauma
C. Hematogenous infection
D. Buccal space infection

197. The oral cleft problem occurs between the period of

A. 1st and 2nd weeks of embryo–fetal life
B. 6th and 10th week of embryo–fetal life
C. 3rd week of embryo–fetal life
D. None of the above

198. Cavernous sinus thrombosis can occur due to spread of odontogenic infection via

A. Tissue spaces
B. Lymphatic route
C. Hematogenous route
D. All of the above

199. The least difficult impaction to remove surgically is

A. Vertical
B. Mesioangular
C. Distoangular
D. Horizontal

200. The distance from the apical end of the implant and superior aspect of Inferior alveolar canal should be minimum of

A. 2 mm
B. 4 mm
C. 6 mm
D. 5 mm

ANSWERS

ANATOMY

1. **Ans: B**

   Ref: BD Chaurasia, 1/E, p. 245

2. **Ans: A**

   Ref: BD Chaurasia, 1/E, p. 253

   Explanation

Muscles of mastication	*Nerve supply*
Masseter nerve	Masseteric nerve, branch anterior division mandibular nerve
Temporalis	2 deep temporal branches from anterior division of mandibular nerve
Lateral pterygoid	A branch of anterior division of mandibular nerve
Medial pterygoid	Branch of main trunk of mandibular nerve

3. **Ans: D**

   Ref: BD Chaurasia, 1/E, p. 177

   Explanation
   - Facial vein communicates with the cavernous sinus through superior ophthalmic vein and pterygoid plexus. Infections from the face can spread in a retrograde direction and cause thrombosis of the cavernous sinus.
   - This is especially likely to occur in infection in the upper lip, cheeks and in the lower part of the nose. This area is called dangerous area of face.

4. **Ans: D**

   Ref: BD Chaurasia, 1/E, p. 337

5. **Ans: C**

   Ref: BD Chaurasia, 1/E, p. 190

6. **Ans: A**

   Ref: Inderbir Singh, 8/E, p. 272

PHYSIOLOGY

7. **Ans: C**

   Ref: Sembulingam, 4/E, p. 210

   Explanation

   Cephalic phase:
   - Unconditioned reflex - sham feeding
   - Conditioned reflex – Pavlov's pouch bell dog experiment

   Gastric phase:
   - Pavlov's pouch, Heidenhain's pouch, Bickel's pouch
   - Intestinal phase – Farrell and Ivy pouch Bickel's pouch
   - Inter digestive phase – Farrell and Ivy pouch, Bickel's pouch
   - Theta waves are seen generally in children below 5 years

8. **Ans: A**

   Ref: Guyton, 11/E, p.123

9. **Ans: D**

   Ref: Guyton, 11/E, p.459

10. **Ans: B**

    Ref: Sembulingam, 4/E, p. 216, 217

11. **Ans: C**

    Ref: Sembulingam, 4/E, p. 834

12. **Ans: B**

    Ref: Sembulingam, 4/E, p. 374

    Explanation
    - Blood calcium level is inversely proportional to PTH secretion

13. **Ans: B**

Ref: Sembulingam, 4/E, p. 391

14. **Ans: C**

Ref: Ganong's, 23/E, p. 63

BIOCHEMISTRY

15. **Ans: B**

Ref: U.Sathyanarayana and U.Chakrapani, 3/E, p. 98

Explanation
- The energy required by the reactants to undergo the reaction is known as Activation energy
- Enzymes reduce the activation energy thereby making the reaction go faster

16. **Ans: B**

Ref: U.Sathyanarayana and U.Chakrapani, 3/ E, p. 269

17. **Ans: D**

Ref: U.Sathyanarayana and U.Chakrapani, 3/ E, p. 336

Explanation
- Glutamine is a storehouse of NH_3
- Ammonia is removed from brain predominantly as glutamine

18. **Ans: B**

Ref: U.Sathyanarayana and U.Chakrapani, 3/ E, p. 508

Explanation
- The complex carbohydrates that are not digested by the human enzymes are called as Dietary fibres
- These include cellulose, hemicellulose, pectin, lignin, gums and mucin

GENERAL PATHOLOGY

19. **Ans: A**

Ref: Harsh Mohan, 3/E, p. 513

20. **Ans: D**

Ref: Robbins, 7/E, p. 646

21. **Ans: B**

Ref: Harsh Mohan, 3/E, p. 231

Explanation
- Hypertrophy – increase in size of the cells
- Aplasia – absence of development of an organ
- Metaplasia – reversible change of one type of cell to another type in response to abnormal stimuli

22. **Ans: C**

Ref: Harsh Mohan 3/E, p. 188

23. **Ans: D**

Ref: Harsh Mohan, 3/E, p. 515

Explanation
- Diseases transmitted by transfusion are:
  1. Hepatitis (HBV, HCV)
  2. CMV
  3. Syphilis
  4. Malaria
  5. Toxoplasmosis
  6. EBV
  7. Brucellosis
  8. AIDS (HIV)

MICROBIOLOGY

24. **Ans: D**

Ref: Ananthanarayan and Panicker's Text Book of Microbiology, 8/E, p. 613

25. **Ans: A**

Ref: Ananthanarayan and Panicker's Text Book of Microbiology, 8/E, p. 32

Explanation
- Dry heat: Hot air oven
- Moist heat: Autoclave

26. Ans: D

Ref: Ananthanarayan and Panicker's Text Book of Microbiology, 8/E, p. 540

Explanation

- HBx Ag and its antibodies are seen in severe chronic hepatitis and hepatocellular carcinoma

27. Ans: B

Ref: Ananthanarayan and Panicker's Text Book of Microbiology, 8/E, p. 266

28. Ans: A

Ref: Ananthanarayan and Panicker's Text Book of Microbiology, 8/E, p. 4

Explanation

- Joseph lister used carbolic acid for antiseptic technique

29. Ans: C

Ref: Ananthanarayan and Panicker's Text Book of Microbiology, 8/E, p. 18

Explanation

- The lipopolysaccharide present on the cell walls of gram negative bacteria consists of 3 regions
  1. Region I – polysaccharide portion determining antigen specificity
  2. Region II – core polysaccharide
  3. Region III – glycolipid portion responsible for endotoxins activities

30. Ans: C

Ref: Ananthanarayan and Panicker's Text Book of Microbiology, 8/E, p. 100

31. Ans: B

Ref: Ananthanarayan and Panicker's Text Book of Microbiology, 8/E, p. 475

Explanation

EBV causes:

1. Infectious mononucleosis
2. Burkitt's lymphoma
3. Lymphomas in AIDS
4. Transplant patients
5. Nasopharyngeal carcinoma

PHARMACOLOGY

32. Ans: A

Ref: Tripathi, 6/E, p. 199

33. Ans: B

Ref: K. D. Tripathi (Essentials for Dentistry, 1/E, p. 73

34. Ans: D

Ref: Satoskar, 20/E, p. 1046

Explanation

- In severe case of arsenical and gold poisoning, administration of specific antidote, dimercaprol (British anti Leuisite) 3 mg/kg, IM at 4 hrs interval for first 2 days, at 6 hr interval on the 3rd day and twice daily for the next 10 days

35. Ans: A

Ref: Satoskar, 20/E, p. 98

36. Ans: C

Ref: K.D.Tripathi, 6/E, p. 493

Explanation

- Cardiac glycosides–digoxin, digitoxin, gitoxin, gitalin, strophanthin-G (Quabain), proscillaridin-A, thevetin, convallotoxin, bufotoxin
- Ergotoxine is a competitive α– adrenergic blocker

37. Ans: C

Ref: K.D.Tripathi, 6/E, p. 81

Explanation

- Super sensitivity – increased response
- Idiosyncrasy – genetically determined abnormal sensitivity to a chemical

38. Ans: C

Ref: K.D.Tripathi, 6/E, p. 197

GENERAL MEDICINE

39. **Ans: D**

Ref: Davidson, 20/E, p. 412

40. **Ans: D**

Ref: Davidson, 20/E, p. 383

41. **Ans: D**

Ref: Harrison, 17/E, Vol – 1, p. 726

42. **Ans: A**

Ref: Davidson, 20/E, p. 1164

43. **Ans: D**

Ref: Davidson, 20/E, p. 842

44. **Ans: D**

Ref: Davidson, 20/E, p. 954, 962

45. **Ans: D**

Ref: Davidson, 20/E, p. 957

Explanation

Clinical features of portal hypertension:

- Portal venous congestion and collateral vessel formation
- Splenomegaly – cardinal finding
- Thrombocytopenia
- Leucopenia
- Variceal bleeding

46. **Ans: A**

Ref: Davidson, 20/E, p. 937

47. **Ans: C**

Ref: Davidson, 20/E, p. 316.

GENERAL SURGERY

48. **Ans: B**

Ref: S.Das, 5/E, p. 622

49. **Ans: D**

Ref: S.Das, 5/E, p. 594

Explanation

- More than 1/3 of lip can be removed if required, but flap reconstruction may be necessary. E.g.: Abbe flap, Estlander's flap.

50. **Ans: B**

Ref: S. Das, 5/E, p. 96

51. **Ans: C**

Ref: S. Das, 5/E, p. 68

52. **Ans: A**

Ref: S.Das, 5/E, p. 108

53. **Ans: B**

Ref: S. Das, 5/E, p. 51

Explanation

- In third degree burns, there is a complete destruction of the epidermis and dermis with irreversible destruction of dermal appendages and epithelial elements including the sensory nerves
- Pain is absent

54. **Ans: D**

Ref: S. Das, 5/E, p. 678

Explanation

- MEN-I – Werner's syndrome
- MEN-II – Sipple's syndrome

55. **Ans: B**

Ref: Manipal Manual of Surgery, 2/E, p.101

56. **Ans: B**

Ref: Manipal Manual of Surgery, 2/E, p.193

Explanation

- Sarcomas – Haemtogenous spread
- Carcinomas – Lymphatic spread

DENTAL MATERIALS

57. **Ans: A**

Ref: Philips, 11/E, p. 412

58. **Ans : B**

Ref: Phillips, 11/E, p. 317

Explanation

- Die spacers used are Resins model paint, Nail polish, etc.
- Die spacer applied in several coats to within 0.5mm of the preparation finish line to provide relief for the cement luting agent and to ensure complete seating.

59. **Ans: B**

Ref: Phillips, 11/E, p. 636

Explanation

- Carbon steel exists in 3 forms

Type	*Crystal Lattice*	*Carbon content (%wt)*
Ferrite	BCC	0.02
Austenite	FCC	2.1
Martensite	BCT	

- Carbon content of stainless steel–0.15–0.2%

60. **Ans: C**

Ref: Phillips, 11/E, p. 736

Explanation

Chemical activation: 3–5%
Heat activation: 0.2–0.5%

61. **Ans: A**

Ref: Phillips, 11/E, p. 466

Explanation

- Phosphoric acid – zinc phosphate cement
- Eugenol – zinc oxide eugenol cement
- Methyl methacrylate – acrylic dental resins (monomers)

62. **Ans: B**

Ref: Phillips, 11/E, p. 505

Explanation

- Low copper alloy – <6% wt
- Admixed alloy – 9–20% wt
- High copper alloy – >6% wt
- Single composition alloy – 13–30% wt

63. **Ans: B**

Ref: Phillips, 11/E, p. 512

Explanation

For Amalgam,

- Tensile strength: 48–70 MPa
- Compressive strength–310 MPa
- Elastic modulus –21 GPa

64. **Ans: B**

Ref: Phillips, 11/E, p. 419

65. **Ans: C**

Ref: Phillips, 11/E, p. 373

66. **Ans: B**

Ref: Phillips, 11/E, p. 302

Explanation

- Normal setting expansion – 0.4 to 0.6%
- Normal Hygroscopic expansion – 1.2 to 2.2%

67. **Ans: B**

Ref: Phillips, 11/E, p. 451

Explanation

- According to ADA specification No. 8, thickness of luting cement should be 25 μm

68. **Ans: B**

Ref: Phillips, 11/E, p. 221

Explanation

- 2 approaches for putty wash technique
  1. Two stage putty wash technique/ Reline technique–Putty used first and light body second
  2. Single stage–Wash material is syringed first and then the unset putty is placed

DADH

69. **Ans: C**

Ref: Wheelers, 8/E, p. 297

Explanation

Characteristic features of mandibular first molar:

- Largest tooth in mandibular arch

- Occlusal form–Hexagonal
- 5 well developed cusps – 2 buccal, 2 lingual and 1 distal
- Developmental viewpoint:
  - Mandibular molars – 4 major cusps 1 minor cusp
  - Maxillary molars – 3 major cusps
- Roots–Mesial and distal and sometimes a third supernumerary tooth may be present–Radix enteromolaris

70. Ans: C

Ref: Wheelers, 8/E, p. 1

Explanation

- The transition or mixed dentition period begins with the emergence of first permanent molars shedding of the deciduous incisors and emergence of the permanent incisors

71. Ans: B

Ref: Wheelers, 8/E, p. 265

Explanation

Characteristic features of maxillary molars

- Largest tooth in maxillary arch
- 4 well formed cusps and fifth cusp-cusp of Carabelli present on mesio lingual cusp
- 3 roots–1 Lingual 2 buccal
  - Lingual root is longest
- Bifurcation area–4 mm (Buccally), 3 mm (mesially) and 5 mm (distally)
- Occlusal aspect–rhomboidal
- Oblique ridge–between mesiolingual (largest cusp) and distobuccal cusp
- Maxillary molar primary cusp – mesiolingual, mesiobuccal and distobuccal

72. Ans: B

Ref: Wheelers, 8/E, p. 53

ORAL PATHOLOGY AND ORAL MEDICINE

73. Ans: A

Ref: Neville, 3/E, p. 686

74. Ans: C

Ref: Shafer, 6/E, p. 777

75. Ans: B

Ref: Shafer's, 6/E, p.138

76. Ans: C

Ref: Neville, 5/E, p. 497

77. Ans: C

Ref: Shafer's, 6/E, p. 594

78. Ans: B

Ref: Burkitts, 11/E, p. 280

79. Ans: C

Ref: Naville, 3/E, p. 557

80. Ans: B

Ref: Naville, 3/E, p. 219

81. Ans: B

Ref: Shafer's, 6/E, p. 804

82. Ans: A

Ref: Shafer's, 6/E, p. 662

83. Ans: A

Ref: Shafer's, 6/E, p. 649

Explanation

- Pituitary gigantism – Macrodontia
- Hereditary ectodermal dysplasia–anodontia or oligodontia

84. Ans: A

Ref: Shafer's, 6/E, p. 324

85. Ans: D

Ref: Shafer's, 6/E, p. 140

86. Ans: A

Ref: Shafer's, 6/E, p. 131

87. Ans: D

Ref: Shafer's, 6/E, p. 485

Explanation

- The foreign material in periapical granuloma, sometimes resembling vegetable matter such as legumes suggesting the term "pulse granuloma"

88. Ans: C

Ref: Shafer's, 6/E, p. 47

Explanation

Gardener's syndrome is a disease complex consisting of

1. Multiple polyposis of large intestine
2. Osteomas of the bone including long bones, skull and joints
3. Multiple epidermoid or sebaceous cysts of the skin, particularly on the scalp and back
4. Occasional occurrence of desmoid tumours
5. Impacted supernumerary and permanent teeth

89. Ans: B

Ref: Shafer's, 6/E, p. 44

Explanation

- It is also seen in trichodento osseous syndrome

90. Ans: C

Ref: Shafer's, 6/E, p. 699

Explanation

- Histological examination of the teeth reveals a decrease in cementum, which varies with the severity of the disease.
- This is presumably as a result of failure of cementogenesis, so that there is no sound functional attachment of the tooth to bone by periodontal ligament accounting to the loosening and premature loss of deciduous teeth

91. Ans: C

Ref: Shafer's, 6/E, p. 180, 85

92. Ans: D

Ref: Shafer's, 6/E, p. 354

Explanation

- Bilateral swelling of the salivary glands occasionally accompanied by administration of either organic or inorganic iodine is referred to as "iodine mumps"

93. Ans: C

Ref: Shafer's, 6/E, p. 163

Explanation

- Approximately 40% of homosexual AIDS patients will develop Kaposi's sarcoma often as an early sign of the disease

94. Ans: A

Ref: Shafer's, 6/E, p. 353

Explanation

- Candidiasis can be effectively treated by topical application of antifungal agents like Nystatin or Clotrimazole
- The systemic antifungals used are fluconazole or itraconazole

95. Ans: C

Ref: Burkitt, 11/E, p. 86

96. Ans: B

Ref: Shafer's, 6/E, p. 323

Explanation

- The oral lesions in secondary syphilis called mucous patches are usually multiple painless, grayish white plaques overlying an ulcerated surface
- They occur most frequently on the tongue gingiva or buccal mucosa

97. Ans: A

Ref: Shafer's, 6/E, p. 827

98. Ans: B

Ref: Shafer's, 6/E, p. 708

ORAL RADIOLOGY

99. Ans: A

Ref: White and Pharoah, 6/E, p. 469

Explanation

- Hair on end appearance is sometimes also seen in Thalassemia

100. Ans: B

Ref: White and Pharoah, 6/E, p. 58

Explanation

- An unexposed film when processed shows some density. This is caused by inherent density of the base and added tint and the development of unexposed silver halide crystals. This minimal density is called gross fog or base plus fog. The optimal density of gross fog is 0.2–0.3

101. Ans: D

Ref: White and Pharoah, 6/E, p. 22

102. Ans: B

Ref: White and Pharoah, 6/E, p. 68

103. Ans: B

Ref: White and Pharoah, 6/E, p. 16

ORTHODONTICS

104. Ans: A

Ref: Bhalaji, 3/E, p. 104

Explanation

- The type of malocclusion most often associated with mouth breathing is called 'long face syndrome' or 'classic adenoid Facies'

105. Ans: C

Ref: Bhalaji, 3/E, p. 224

Explanation

- Also known as intraalveolar appliance
- Given by Willet

106. Ans: A

Ref: Bhalaji, 3/E, pp. 99 and 100

Explanation

- Labial tipping of maxillary anterior teeth
- Over jet increases due to proclination of maxillary anteriors
- Anterior open bite
- Narrow maxillary arch
- Hypotonic upper lip and hyperactive mentalis

107. Ans: A

Ref: Bhalaji, 3/E, p. 28

108. Ans: B

Ref: Bhalaji, 3/E, p. 280

Explanation

- Adam's/universal/liverpool/modified arrowhead clasp is constructed using 0.7 mm wire/28mil/22 guage stainless steel wires

109. Ans: C

Ref: Proffit, 4/E, p. 457

110. Ans: B

Ref: Bhalaji, 3/E, p. 206

111. Ans: C

Ref: Bhalaji, 3/E, p. 186

Explanation

- The optimum orthodontic force is equivalent to the pulse pressure which is 20–26 gm/sq cm. of root surface area

112. Ans: B

Ref: Bhalaji, 3/E, p. 18

Explanation

Micro skeletal units of

a. Maxilla–orbital, pneumatic, palatal and basal

b. Mandible–alveolar, angular, condylar, gonial, mental, coronoid and basal

113. Ans: C

Ref: Bhalaji, 3/E, p. 330

Explanation
- Teeth borne passive–activator, bionator, Herbst
- Teeth borne active–expansion screws, springs
- Tissue borne passive–functional regulator of frankel

114. Ans: D

Ref: Bhalaji, 3/E, p. 53

115. Ans: B

Ref: Bhalaji, 3/E, p. 338

116. Ans: B

Ref: Bhalaji, 3/E, p. 207

Explanation
- Class II elastic traction–b/w lower molar and upper anteriors
- Class III elastic traction–b/w upper molar and lower anteriors

117. Ans: A

Ref: Bhalaji, 3/E, p. 201

118. Ans: D

Ref: Bhalaji, 3/E, p. 17

Explanation
- Functional matrix theory was put forth by Melvin Moss

119. Ans: A

Ref: Bhalaji, 3/E, p. 454

PEDODONTICS

120. Ans: B

Ref: Shobha Tandon, 1/E, p. 542

Explanation Types of cerebral palsy

a. Spastic–70%-cerebral cortex is affected
b. Athetosis 15%-basal ganglia is affected
c. Ataxia 5%-cerebellum
d. Mixed 10%
e. Tremors-basal ganglia
f. Rigidity-basal ganglia

121. Ans: A

Ref: Shobha Tandon, 1/E, p. 148

122. Ans: A

Ref: Mc Donald, 8/E, p. 37

123. Ans: C

Ref: Shobha Tandon, 1/E, P. 110

124. Ans: D

Ref: Shobha Tandon, 1/E, p. 394

P AND SD

125. Ans: B

Ref: Soben Peter, 3/E, p. 216

Explanation
- Standardized continuum of Aesthetic Need (SCAN) scale was used for the development of the aesthetic component

126. Ans: A

Ref: Soben Peter, 3/E, p. 329

Explanation
- Kidney is the chief organ of excretion of fluoride
- Renal clearance rate of fluoride is 35 ml/min
- 30% fluoride - excreted in 6 hours
- 60% fluoride - excreted in 24 hours

127. Ans: C

Ref: Soben Peter, 3/E, p. 327

Explanation
- Pathologic skeletal fluorosis–20 to 80 mgF/day for 10–20 years

Features:
- Rigid spine
- Stiff joints
- Immobilization of patient

128. **Ans: B**

Ref: Park, 20/E, p. 38

Explanation

- Disease elimination – interruption of transmission of disease
- Disease eradication – termination of all transmission of infection by extermination of the infectious agent

129. **Ans: A**

Ref: Soben Peter, 3/E, p. 335

Explanation

- First community water fluoridation scheme–began in Grand Rapids, USA in 1945

130. **Ans: A**

Ref: Soben Peter, 3/E, p. 326

Explanation

- Chronic lethal dose–32–64 mg F/kg
- Acute lethal dose–5–10 g F/kg

131. **Ans: C**

Ref: Soben Peter, 3/E, p. 301

Explanation

- Bibby – First Clinical trial of fluoride dentrifice in 1942
- Muhler – Fluoride application

132. **Ans: D**

Ref: Soben Peter, 3/E, p. 312

133. **Ans: A**

Ref: Soben Peter, 3/E, p. 302

Explanation

- APF gel- pH 4–5, Fluoride concentration – 1.23%

134. **Ans: A**

Ref: Soben Peter, 3/E, p. 390

135. **Ans: B**

Ref: Soben Peter, 3/E, p. 313

Explanation

- Commonly used humectants are glycerol, sorbitol and propylene glycol

136. **Ans: B**

Ref: Park, 20/E, p. 32

Explanation

- Pettenkofer – Multifactorial causation

137. **Ans: A**

Ref: Soben Peter, 3/E, P. 177

Explanation

- DMFT-Henry. T. Klein, Carrole. E. Palmer and Knutson.W in 1934
- Modified DMFT – Joseph.Z.Anaise in 1983

138. **Ans: C**

Ref: Soben Peter, 3/E, p. 253

Explanation

Levels of Prevention

a. Primary prevention – health promotion specific protection
b. Secondary prevention – early diagnosis and prompt treatment
c. Tertiary prevention – disability limitation rehabilitation

139. **Ans: B**

Ref: Park, 20/E, p. 509

140. **Ans: A**

Ref: Soben Peter, 3/E, p. 313

Explanation

- Binding or thickening agents are hydrophilic substances that stabilize dentifrice formulations and prevent the separation of solid and liquid phases

141. **Ans: B**

Ref: Soben Peter, 3/E, p. 205

PROSTHODONTICS

142. **Ans: C**

Ref: Rosenstiel, 4/E, p. 375

143. **Ans: D**

Ref: Zarb & Bolender, 12/E, p.10

144. **Ans: C**

Ref: Winkler, 2/E, p. 206

145. **Ans: C**

Ref: Rosensteil, 4/E, p. 627, 626

146. **Ans: B**

Ref: Nallaswamy, 1/E, p. 365

147. **Ans: D**

Ref: Winkler, 2/E, p. 223

Explanation

- The first anatomic porcelain teeth were designed by Alfred Gysi of Switzerland

148. **Ans: C**

Ref: Rosensteil, 4/E, p. 629

149. **Ans: A**

Ref: Nallaswamy, 1/E, p. 148

150. **Ans: B**

Ref: Rosensteil, 4/E, p. 260

151. **Ans: D**

Ref: Zarb and Bolender, 12/E, p. 484

Explanation

- Ossointegration was first defined by Per Ingvar Branemark

152. **Ans: A**

Ref: Boucher's, 9/E, p. 313

153. **Ans: D**

Ref: Nallaswamy, 1/E, p. 381

Explanation

- A balance is usmally maintained between the buccinators and the tongue. This balance results in a dead zone of nil force. This zone is called neutral zone or zone of minimal conflict of zone of equilibrium

154. **Ans: B**

Ref: Nallaswamy, 1/E, p. 337

155. **Ans: D**

Ref: Mc Crackens, 11/E, p. 85

156. **Ans: B**

Ref: Zarb and Bolender, 12/E, p. 18

157. **Ans: C**

Ref: Zarb and Bolender, 12/E, p. 217

PERIODONTICS

158. **Ans: C**

Ref: Carranza, 10/E, p.335

Explanation

Odour	*Etiology*
Rotten egg smell	Volatile sulphur compounds
Dead mice small	Liver insufficiency, volatile sulphur compounds and aliphatic compounds
Fishy odour	Kidney insufficiency, trimethylaminuria
Rotten onion	Arsenic
Melon odour	Eucalyptus

159. **Ans: B**

Ref: Carranza, 10/E, p. 456

Explanation

- Range of effectiveness of about 1.5–2.5 mm within which bacterial plaque can induce bone loss. Beyond 2.5 mm there is no effect

160. **Ans: C**

Ref: Carranza, 10/E, p. 397

Explanation

Vitamin deficiency Periodontal manifestation

- Vitamin A: Hyperkeratosis, hyperplasia of gingiva, increased pocket formation

- Vitamin D: Osteoclastic resorption of alveolar bone
- Niacin: Necrosis of gingiva
- Riboflavin: Severe lesions of the gingiva and periodontal tissues
- Folic acid: Necrosis of gingiva, periodontal ligament and alveolar bone without inflammation
- Vitamin C: Haemorrhage, collagen destruction and edema of gingiva (boggy gums) interference with bone formation and retarded healing

161. Ans: B

Ref: Carranza, 10/E, p. 973

Explanation

- Citric acid, fibronectin and tetracyclines are used in biomodification of root surface

162. Ans: A

Ref: Carranza, 10/E, p. 912

Explanation

After curettage

a. Re epithelialization–2–7 days
b. Restoration of junctional epithelium–5 days
c. Immature collagen fibers appear–21 days

163. Ans: C

Ref: Carranza, 10/E, p. 467

Explanation

- Traumatic occlusion–is an occlusion that produces tissue injury

164. Ans: B

Ref: Carranza, 10/E, p. 996

Explanation

a. Hemisection–splitting of a 2 rooted tooth into 2 separate portions
b. Bicuspidization–if the 2 parts are separated and preserved
c. Root resection–one of the roots is removed after hemisection procedure, often involves the distobuccal root of maxillary first molar

165. Ans: A

Ref: Carranza, 10/E, p. 1206

166. Ans: C

Ref: Carranza, 10/E, p. 138

167. Ans: D

Ref: Carranza, 10/E, p. 735

168. Ans: C

Ref: Carranza, 10/E, p. 632

Explanation

- *Regeneration* – is the biologic process by which architecture and function of lost tissues are completely restored by formation of new periodontal ligament and cementum
- *Repair* – is healing of tissues without completely restoring the last tissues
- *New attachment* – is a reunion of connecting tissue with the root surface that has been pathologically exposed

169. Ans: A

Ref: Carranza, 10/E, p. 141

Explanation

- Formation of enamel pellicle occurs by relative adsorption of macromolecules
- The mechanisms involved in enamel pellicle formation include electrostatic, vanderwaal's and hydrophobic forces

170. Ans: A

Ref: Carranza, 10/E, p. 349

Explanation

Function of saliva

1. Lubrication
2. Physical protection
3. Cleansing
4. Buffering
5. Tooth integrity maintenance
6. Antibacterial action.

171. Ans: B

Ref: Carranza, 10/E, p. 1044

Explanation

- Biologic width (2.04 mm) = Junctional epithelium (0.97 mm) + Connective tissue (1.07 mm)

CONS AND ENDO

172. Ans: B

Ref: Ingle, 5/E, p. 823

173. Ans: B

Ref: Review of Operative Dentistry and Endodontics, Nisha Garg and Amith Garg, 1/E, p. 171

174. Ans: B

Ref: Cohen, 9/E, p. 322

175. Ans: A

Ref: Sturdavent, 5/E, p. 257

Explanation

- The bonding mechanism of self etching primer is based on the simultaneous etching and priming of enamel and dentin forming a continuum in the substrate and incorporating smear plugs into the resin tags

176. Ans: C

Ref: Ingle, 6/E, p. 1057

177. Ans: D

Ref: Sturdavent, 5/E, p. 28

Explanation

Dentin:

- Compressive strength – 266 MPa
- Tensile strength – 40 MPa
- Modulus of elasticity – 1.67×10^6 Psi

178. Ans: D

Ref: Sturdavent, 5/E, p. 645

Explanation

- Carbamide peroxide is used in dentist prescribed home applied technique (i.e. night guard breaching)
- It degrades into 3% H_2O_2 (active ingredient) and 7% urea
- Bleaching materials with carbopol are recommended because it thickens the bleaching solution and extends the oxidation process

179. Ans: A

Ref: Sturdavent , 5/E, p. 920

180. Ans: B

Ref: Grossman, 12/E, p. 281

181. Ans: B

Ref: Ingle, 6/E, p. 1000

182. Ans: B

Ref: Sturdavent , 5/E, p. 859

Explanation

- A cavosurface design with 30–40° marginal metal on the inlay helps to seal and protects the margins and results in a strong enamel margin with an angle of 140– 150° degrees

183. Ans: C

Ref: Grossman, 12/E, p. 315

184. Ans: A

Ref: Grossman, 12/E, p. 233

185. Ans: A

Ref: Sturdavent, 5/E, p. 332

186. Ans: B

Ref: Sturdavent, 5/E, p. 463

Explanation

- Rubber dam was first developed by SC Barnum in 1864

Types – based on thickness

- Thin 0.006 inch/0.15 mm
- Medium 0.008 inch/0.2 mm

- Heavy 0.10 inch/0.25 mm
- Extra heavy 0.12 inch/0.30 mm
- Special heavy 0.14 inch/0.35 mm

187. Ans: B

Ref: Grossman, 12/E, p. 312

ORAL SURGERY

188. Ans: C

Ref: Laskin, Vol. 2, p. 524

189. Ans: D

Ref: Neelima. S. Malik,2/E, p. 64

190. Ans: B

Ref: Neelima. S. Malik,2/E, p. 738

191. Ans: D

Ref: Malamed Local Anesthesia, 5/E, p. 313

192. Ans: C

Ref: Neelima Malik, 2/E, p. 123

193. Ans: D

Ref: Neelima Malik, 2/E, p. 474

Explanation

- Enbloc resection allows complete excision of the tumour, but at the same time a continuity of the jaw bone is retained and thus deformity, disfigurement and the need for secondary cosmetic surgery and prosthetic rehabilitation are avoided

194. Ans: D

Ref: Bhalaji, 1/E, p. 632

Explanation

- Detachment of the medial canthal attachment of the eye may occur in severe naso – ethmoidal injuries, giving rise to Traumatic telecanthus widening of inter canthal distance > 35 mm is indicative of Traumatic Telecanthus.

195. Ans: C

Ref: Neelima Malik, 2/E, p. 238

196. Ans: C

Ref: Neelima Malik 2nd edn p. 640

Explanation

- Haematogenous infections may cause multiple sites of OML. The organisms enter the blood stream through a minor wound in the skin or infection of upper respiratory tract or infection of middle ear

197. Ans: B

Ref: Neelima Malik, 2/E, p. 547

198. Ans: C

Ref: Neelima Malik, 2/E, p. 635

199. Ans: B

Ref: Neelima Malik, 2/E, p. 133

Explanation

- Most difficult impaction – Distoangular
- Least difficult impaction – Mesioangular

200. Ans: A

Ref: Peterson, 4/E, p. 320

Explanation

Structure	*Minimum required distance between implant and indicated structure*
Buccal plate	0.5 mm
Lingual plate	1 mm
Maxillary sinus	1 mm
Nasal cavity	1 mm
Incisive canal	Avoid midline maxilla
Inter implant distance	3 mm between outer edge of implants
Inferior alveolar canal	2 mm from superior aspect of bony canal
Mental nerve	5 mm from anterior or bony foramen
Inferior border	1 mm
Adjacent natural tooth	0.5 mm

6

KCET 2008

HUMAN ANATOMY

1. Fascial sheath for thyroid gland is provided by

A. Investing layer of deep cervical fascia
B. Prevertebral fascia
C. Pretracheal fascia
D. Carotid sheath

2. Depression of the mandible during the opening of the mouth is caused by

A. Medial pterygoid
B. Lateral pterygoid
C. Temporalis
D. Masseter

3. All the following structures are contents of the carotid sheath EXCEPT

A. Vagus nerve
B. Internal jugular vein
C. Common carotid artery
D. Sympathetic trunk

4. Posterior belly of digastric muscle is supplied by

A. Mandibular nerve
B. Maxillary nerve
C. Ansa cervicalis
D. Facial nerve

5. Palatine tonsil develops from

A. Dorsal part of II pharyngeal pouches
B. Ventral part of II pharyngeal pouches
C. Dorsal part of III pharyngeal pouches
D. Ventral part of I pharyngeal pouches

PHYSIOLOGY

6. Normal glomerular filtration rate is

A. 125 mL/day
B. 650 mL/min
C. 180 mL/min
D. 125 mL/min

7. Gastrointestinal hormone in the following is

A. Pepsin
B. Ptyalin
C. Cholecystokinin
D. Trypsin

8. Shift of the oxygen dissociation curve to right is caused by the following factors except

A. Increased 2, 3, BP.
B. Increased temperature
C. Increased concentration of carbon-dioxide
D. Increased concentration of oxygen

9. All of the following are endogenous corticosteroids released by the adrenal cortex except

A. Cortisol
B. Cortisone
C. Dexamethasone
D. Aldosterone

BIOCHEMISTRY

10. Energy expenditure during normal breathing

A. 25%–50% of total energy spent

B. 50%–75% of total energy spent
C. 15%–20% of total energy spent
D. 2%–3% of total energy spent

11. One molecule of beta–carotene gives rise to

A. One unit of vitamin A
B. Two units of vitamin A
C. Three units of vitamin A
D. Four unit of vitamin A

12. Which of the following acts as lung surfactant?

A. Lysolecithin
B. Cephalin
C. Dipalmitoyl lecithin
D. Phosphoditylinositol

13. Which vitamin is synthesized by intestinal bacteria?

A. Vitamin A
B. Vitamin K
C. Vitamin D
D. Vitamin E

14. Inactive precursors of enzymes are known as

A. Apoenzymes
B. Coenzymes
C. Proenzymes
D. Holoenzymes

15. One of the symptoms of Vitamin A deficiency is

A. Nyctalopia
B. Xerophthalmia
C. Bitot's spot
D. Keratomalacia

16. Scurvy is caused by deficiency of

A. Vitamin C
B. Vitamin D
C. Vitamin B
D. Vitamin K

GENERAL PATHOLOGY

17. Features of a benign tumour are all EXCEPT

A. Absence of hyperchromasia of nucleus
B. Retained basal polarity
C. Slow growth
D. Presence of local invasion

18. Lipofuscin is an insoluble endogenous pigment, also known as

A. Lipochrome
B. Wear and tear pigment
C. Aging pigment
D. All of the above

MICROBIOLOGY

19. The process of 'phagocytosis' was discovered by

A. Celsus
B. Elie Metchinkoff
C. Virchow
D. None of the above

20. Which of the following immunoglobulin is responsible for allergic reactions

A. IgG
B. IgE
C. IgM
D. IgD

21. Infectious mononucleosis is caused by

A. Bacterial infection
B. Varicella zoster virus infection
C. HIV infection
D. Epstein-Barr (EB) virus infection

22. Cell wall deficient bacteria are

A. *Escherichia coli*
B. *Staphylococci*
C. *Spirochetes*
D. *Mycoplasma*

23. Lowenstein Jensen medium is selectively used to cultivate

A. *Vibrio cholera*
B. *Mycobacterium tuberculosis*
C. *Salmonella typhi*
D. *Treponema pallidum*

24. The commoly used fluorescent dye in the detection of tubercle bacilli

A. Acridine orange
B. Thioflavin
C. Congo red
D. Auramine and rhodamine

25. **Endotoxin is released from**
    A. C. albicans
    B. S. Sanguis
    C. Gram negative bacteria
    D. Actinomyces viscosus

26. **Leucopenia is characteristic of**
    A. Appendicitis
    B. Enteric fever
    C. Meningitis
    D. Myocardial Infarction

27. **Bence Jones protein found in the urine may be suggestive of**
    A. Hyperparathyroidism
    B. Hodgkins disease
    C. Multiple myeloma
    D. Christian's syndrome

28. **The earliest identifiable cells of T-cell lineage during maturation are**
    A. CD7+Pro-T-cells
    B. CD4+Pre-T-cells
    C. CD8+Pro-T-cells
    D. CD8+Pre-T-cells

29. **Group A carbohydrate of Str. Pyogenes cross reacts with human**
    A. Synovial fluid
    B. Myocardium
    C. Cardiac valves
    D. Vascular intima

PHARMACOLOGY

30. **The drug of choice in the management of patient with acute anaphylaxis is**
    A. Dexamethasone
    B. Adrenaline
    C. Aminophylline
    D. Morphine

31. **Penicillin exerts its effect on bacterial by infecting with**
    A. Cellular respiration
    B. Cellular oxidation
    C. Cell wall synthesis
    D. Cellular division

32. **Which of the following synthetic steroid shows predominantly mineralocorticoid action?**
    A. Hydrocortisone
    B. Spironolactone
    C. Dexamethasone
    D. Fludrocortisone

33. **An anxiolytic, not interacting with GABAergic system and used in generalized anxiety is**
    A. Alprazolam
    B. Buspiron
    C. Diazepam
    D. Phenobarbital

34. **The toxic effect of Beta receptor antagonists includes all the following except**
    A. Hypoglycemic episodes in diabetes
    B. Worsening of preexisting asthma
    C. Ischemic cardiac episode on abrupt discontinuation
    D. Precipitate migrainic effect

35. **Sublingual route of administration**
    A. Has a slow onset of action
    B. Does not produce systemic effect
    C. Decreases drug excretion
    D. Bypasses first pass metabolism

36. **Clopidogrel is an**
    A. Anti hypertensive
    B. Antidiabetic
    C. Antiplatelet
    D. Anticoagulant

GENERAL MEDICINE

37. **AIDS is a disease of the immune system primarily affecting**
    A. Granulocytes
    B. Immunoglobulins
    C. Opsonins
    D. T lymphocytes

38. **Renal papillary necrosis is seen in**
    A. Sickle cell anemia
    B. Gouty nephropathy

C. Chronic glomerulo nephritis
D. Hypercalcaemia

39. Microalbuminuria is defined as albumin

A. <30 microgms/24 hours urine collection
B. 30–300 microgms/24 hours urine collection
C. 300–550 microgms/24 hours urine collection
D. >500 microgms/24 hours urine collection

40. The criteria to diagnose the infective endocarditis are

A. Osler nodes
B. Roth spot
C. Positive blood culture
D. All of the above

41. Sinus tachycardia is seen in

A. Beta blocker therapy
B. Athletes
C. Hypothyroidism
D. Severe anaemia

42. Normal body mass index is between

A. 16.5–20.5
B. 18.5–24.9
C. 25.0–29.9
D. 30.0–39.9

43. Which of the following is indicative of left ventricular failure?

A. Neck vein distension
B. Ascites
C. Anorexia
D. Orthopnoea

44. Secondary prevention of myocardial infarction management therapy includes

A. Antiplatelet therapy
B. A.C.E inhibitor
C. Statins
D. All

45. First priority in management of burn injury is

A. Exposure
B. Fluid resuscitation
C. Circulation
D. Airway control

46. Intention tremor is a feature of

A. Loss of function of thalamus
B. Loss of function of hypothalamus
C. Loss of function of cerebellum
D. Loss of function of basal ganglia

47. Which of the following statement about P24 antigen of HIV is not true?

A. It can be detected during the window period
B. Free P24 antigen disappears after the appearance of lgM response to it
C. Virus load parallels P24 titre
D. It remains during asymptomatic phase

GENERAL SURGERY

48. Lock jaw is due to

A. Clostridium Tetani
B. Pasteurella Tularensis
C. Bordetella Pertussis
D. Steptococcus

49. The commonest organism causing bacterial tonsillitis

A. Staphylococcus aureus
B. Grp-A streptococcus
C. Streptococcus fecalis
D. Methicillin resistant staph aureus

50. Pulsating varicose vein is due to

A. Arterio venous fistula
B. Sapheno femoral incompetence
C. Deep vein thrombosis
D. Abdominal tumour

51. Absolute indication for surgery in hyperparathyroidism is

A. Serum calcium <2.82 m mol^{-1}
B. Increased bone density
C. Urinary tract calculi
D. Patient more than 50 years of age

52. **Cold abscess formation is due to**
   A. Presence of acute inflammation
   B. Formation of caseous pus with signs of acute inflammation
   C. Formation of caseous pus without signs of acute inflammation
   D. Infected cyst

53. **Punched out edge is a characteristic of which type of ulcer**
   A. Tuberculosis
   B. Rodent ulcer
   C. Syphilitic ulcer
   D. Non specific

54. **The commonest thyroid malignancy is**
   A. Anaplastic
   B. Follicular
   C. Papillary
   D. Medullary

DENTAL MATERIALS

55. **The filler size (silica) in homogenous microfilled composites is**
   A. 1–2 μ
   B. 4 μ
   C. 0.04 μ
   D. 0.5 to 3 μ

56. **The inability of the air in the mold to escape through the pores in the investment leads to**
   A. Localised shrinkage
   B. Back pressure porosity
   C. Subsurface porosity
   D. Back pressure porosity

57. **The premature termination of the flow of molten metal during solidification termed is**
   A. Gas inclusion porosity
   B. Subsurface porosity
   C. Localized shrinkage porosity
   D. Back pressure porosity

58. **Of the various glass ionomer products, the highest cumulative release of fluoride after 30 days is from**
   A. Type I glass ionomer
   B. Type II glass ionomer
   C. Glass ionomer liner (conventional)
   D. Glass ionomer liner (light–cure)

59. **The chroma in color is**
   A. Dominant color of an object
   B. Degree of saturation
   C. Type of color
   D. Lightness or darkness of color

60. **Co–efficient thermal expansion of amalgam is**
   A. 6.6 alpha (ppm k-1)
   B. 11.4 alpha (ppm k-1)
   C. 14.0 alpha (ppm k-1)
   D. 25.0 alpha (ppm k-1)

61. **Photosensitizer used in light activated composite resins are**
   A. Organosilane
   B. Benzyl peroxide
   C. Collidal silica
   D. Camphoroquinone

62. **Super abrasive is**
   A. Sand
   B. Silicon carbide
   C. Diamond
   D. Aluminum oxide

63. **Class II stone, densite or improved stone is**
   A. Type III
   B. Type IV
   C. Type V
   D. None of the above

64. **Eames technique for proportioning alloy and mercury is**
   A. 1:1 by volume
   B. 8:5 by weight
   C. 5:8 by volume
   D. 1:1 by weight

65. **Who discovered stainless steel?**
A. Adams CP
B. Schwartz AM
C. Brearley
D. Backofen WA and Gales GF

DADH

66. **Oblique ridge of permanent maxillary first molar connects**
A. Mesiobuccal cusp and distobuccal cusp
B. Distobuccal cusp and mesiolingual cusp
C. Mesiobuccal cusp and distolingual cusp
D. Mesiolingual cusp and distolingual Cusp

67. **Occlusal aspect of the maxillary first premolar is roughly**
A. Octagonal
B. Trapezoidal
C. Hexagonal
D. Rhomboidal

68. **The most accepted theory for dentin sensitivity**
A. Transduction theory
B. Direct neural stimulation
C. Hydrodynamic theory
D. Hydrostatic theory

69. **The term 'Dead tract' in dentin was coined by**
A. Robinson
B. Sir Wilfred Fish
C. Silverman
D. Silverstone

70. **Number of line angles in anterior teeth**
A. 4 line angles
B. 8 line angles
C. 6 line angles
D. 10 line angles

ORAL PATHOLOGY AND ORAL MEDICINE

71. **Vitamin deficiencies which cause enamel hypoplasia are due to**
A. Vitamin B and vitamin C
B. Vitamin A and vitamin C and D
C. Vitamin B and vitamin E
D. Vitamin A and vitamin K

72. **Mucus cyst of the mouth is a .... type of cyst**
A. Implantation
B. Retention
C. Hyper plastic
D. Degenerative

73. **Pleomorphic adenoma is a tumour of**
A. Maxillary sinus
B. Odontogenic epithelium
C. Salivary glands
D. Lymph nodes

74. **In Ludwig's angina there is bilateral involvement of the following spaces**
A. Submandibular, massetric, and retropharyngeal spaces
B. Retropharyngeal, parapharyngeal and buccal spaces
C. Submandibular, submental and sublingual spaces
D. Buccal, parotid and retropharyngeal spaces

75. **Which of the following is a secondary site of spread of odontogenic infection involving pterygomandibular space?**
A. Infratemporal space
B. Canine space
C. Buccal space
D. Sublingual space

76. **Hemosiderin particles are seen histologically in case of**
A. Fibroma
B. Pregnancy tumor
C. Peripheral giant cell granuloma
D. Papilloma

77. **In cleidocranial dysostosis, sometimes the roots of the permanent teeth are**
A. Thin and long
B. Thin and short
C. Thick and short
D. Fused

78. White lesion with definite precancerous potential
A. Leukoplakia
B. Discoid lupus erythematosus
C. Lichen planus
D. All of the above

79. Forensic identification utilizes
A. Lip prints
B. Lip Schutz bodies
C. Lip pits
D. Lip reading

80. Mikulicz disease is usually characterized by
A. Unilateral or bilateral salivary and lacrimal gland swelling
B. Unilateral or bilateral salivary gland swelling and rheumatoid arthritis
C. Malignant transformation of epithelial and lymphocytic component of salivary glands
D. None of the above

81. Nikolsky sign is positive in
A. Pemphigus vulgaris
B. Bechet's disease
C. Herpes simplex
D. All the above

82. Auspitz sign is seen in
A. Fibrous dysplasia
B. Lichen planus
C. Psoriasis
D. Pemphigus

83. The characteristic feature of "Driven snow" appearance is seen in
A. Ameloblastoma
B. Odontoma
C. Primary intra osseous carcinoma
D. Calcifying epithelial odontogenic Tumor

84. The causes of facial palsy are
A. Herpes simplex viral infection
B. Acoustic neuroma
C. Leprosy
D. All of the above

85. Salivary duct calculi
A. Produce pain on eating
B. Are commonest in the parotid ducts
C. Are common cause of acute parotitis
D. Are associated with hypercalcaemic states

86. Lesion showing presence of verocay bodies and having predeliction for occurrence in the tongue
A. Neurilemmoma
B. Neurofibroma
C. Pyogenic granuloma
D. Rhabdomyoma

87. The histological appearance of "lava flowing around boulders in dentin dysplasia" suggests
A. Attempt to repair the defective dentin
B. Abrupt arrest to dentin formation in crown
C. Abnormal dentin formation in a disorganized fashion
D. Cascades of dentin to form root

88. Marble bone disease is a synonym for
A. Osteopetrosis
B. Osteoporosis
C. Osteogenesis imperfecta
D. Osteomyelitis

89. Subepithelial vesicles are characteristic of the all the following except
A. Bullous pemphigoid
B. Cicatricial pemphigoid
C. Pemphigus
D. Epidermoslysis bullosa acquisita

90. Mucin in mucous cells usually demonstrated by
A. PAS stain
B. H and E stain
C. Mucicarmine stain
D. Mallory stain

91. Corps ronds and grains are seen in the histopathologic picture of
A. Darrier's disease
B. Warty dyskeratoma
C. Pemphigus
D. Erythema multiforme

92. Talon cusp may be associated with
A. Cleidocranial dysplasia
B. Grinspan syndrome
C. Rubinstein-Taybi syndrome
D. Acromegaly

93. Intraepithelial micro abscesses are referred as
A. Sub acute inflammation
B. Phoenix abscess
C. Acanthosis
D. Monro's abscess

94. Rubeola is due to
A. Paramyxo virus
B. Pox virus
C. Papilloma virus
D. Herpes virus

95. Noma is also known as
A. Cancrum oris
B. Candidiasis
C. Chancre
D. Pyogenic granuloma

96. Lipschutz bodies are seen in
A. Herpes simplex
B. Herpes zoster
C. Apthous ulcer
D. Cancrum oris

97. Squamous cell carcinoma
A. Spreads through lymphatics
B. Radioresistant
C. Metastasise through blood stream
D. Surgical excision contraindicated

98. The principal causative agent in the initiation of dental caries is
A. In sufficient fluoride exposure
B. Lacto bacillus acidophilus
C. Steptococcus mutans
D. Fermentable carbohydrates

99. Delhi boil refers to
A. Solar keratosis
B. Malignant pustule
C. L.Tropica sore
D. Veneral ulcer

ORAL RADIOLOGY

100. Vertical angulation for IOPA radiograph of the maxillary canine using bisecting angle technique is
A. +40
B. –40
C. +45
D. +50

101. The quantity of X-ray is controlled by
A. Kilovoltage
B. Milliamperage
C. Total filteration
D. Exposure time

102. The fastest dental film currently available has the speed rating of
A. "D" speed
B. "C" speed
C. "F" speed
D. "E" speed

103. Thyroid dose from panoramic radiography is about
A. 22 mGY
B. 34 mGY
C. 51 mGY
D. 0.074 mGY

104. Of the following which is the best projection to study the fracture of zygomatic arch
A. Lateral oblique view
B. PA Caldwell view
C. Submentovertex view
D. Lateral cephalometric view

ORTHODONTICS

105. Ideal age for the use of delaire facemask in the treatment of skeletal maxillary deficiency cases is in the

A. 6 to 8 year old age group
B. 8 to 10 year old age group
C. 10 to 12 year old age group
D. 12 to 14 old age group

106. In cephalostats the distance between the X-ray source and the midsaggital plane of the patient is fixed at

A. 50 inches
B. 55 inches
C. 60 inches
D. 65 inches

107. Cephalometrics was introduced in 1934 by

A. Willam R Proffit
B. Broadbent and Hofrath
C. Robert E Moyers
D. Cecil Steiner

108. The condylar cartilage in the mandible is held to be a

A. Primary cartilage
B. Secondary cartilage
C. Tertiary cartilage
D. Non-growing cartilage

109. The functional cranial component theory was proposed by

A. Melvin moss
B. Van der Klaauw
C. Sicher
D. James Scott

110. The Leeway space of Nance in the maxillary and mandibular arches per side, respectively is

A. 1.7 mm, 3.4 mm
B. 1.7 mm, 0.9 mm
C. 0.9 mm, 1.7 mm
D. 3.4 mm, 1.7 mm

111. The tooth movement that requires the least amount of orthodontic force

A. Extrusion
B. Intrusion
C. Tipping
D. Bodily

112. The major tissue system of the body that is the earliest to complete its growth development in life is

A. Muscular
B. Neural
C. Lymphatic
D. Lymphoid

113. A distinctive clinical manifestation of a successful rapid maxillary expansion is

A. Anterior crossbite
B. Posterior crossbite
C. Midline diastema
D. Open bite

114. Which of the following is not a transient/ self correcting malocclusion?

A. Spaced primary dentition
B. Deep overbite in primary dentition
C. Flush terminal planes in primary dentition
D. Anterior crossbite in primary Dentition

115. Hand wrist radiograph provides a view of

A. 25 bones
B. 27 bones
C. 30 bones
D. 32 bones

116. Dolicocephalic head form and leptoproscopic facial form is associated with

A. Square arch form
B. Round Dental arches
C. Long and Narrow
D. U Shaped arch form

PEDODONTICS

117. In apexification techniques the commonly used material is

A. Zinc oxide eugenol

KCET 2008

B. Gutta Percha
C. Calcium hydroxide
D. Composite resins

118. The best time to begin the counseling of parents and establishing a child's preventive programme actually starts
A. Before the birth of the child
B. Infants (0–2 year)
C. Toddlers (1–3 years)
D. Pre School (3–6 years)

119. In case of conscious sedation for children aged 6 months to 3 years, clear liquids should be stopped.
A. 4 hours before the procedure
B. 6 hours before the procedure
C. 8 hours before the procedure
D. 10 hours before the procedure

120. Which of the following is not a type of mouth breathing?
A. Obstructive
B. Anatomical
C. Physiological
D. Habitual

121. Kanner's syndrome is also known as
A. Autism
B. Osteogenesis imperfecta
C. Trigeminal neuralgia
D. Diabetes mellitus type 1

122. Id, Ego, super ego are part of
A. Erikson's model of personality development
B. Freud's psychoanalytic theory
C. Piaget's theory
D. Frankel's theory

123. Best time to see a 3 year old child in the dental office
A. Early in the morning
B. Just before lunch
C. Just after lunch
D. Any time

124. In class III Ellis fracture
A. Only enamel is involved
B. Enamel and dentine are involved
C. Enamel, dentine and pulp are involved
D. Non-vital pulp

125. The facio-lingual dimension of the Band and loop space maintainer should be approximately
A. 8 mm
B. 10 mm
C. 4 mm
D. 5 mm

126. Occlusal sealants are retained on the enamel surface chiefly by
A. Mechanical retention in deep pit and fissure
B. Chemical bonding between sealant and enamel
C. Mechanical retention by sealant penetration into the etched enamel
D. Chemical bonding between the sealant and etched enamel surface

127. The avulsed tooth should be placed in the socket
A. Within 30 min
B. Within 1 hour
C. 24 hours
D. 2 hours

128. Riga-Fede disease is caused by
A. A saprophytic fungus that normally occurs in nail
B. Immunosuppressive state
C. Abrasion of tongue by the teeth during sucking
D. A recurrent viral infection which remains latent in nerve tissue

P AND SD

129. 'Rural health scheme' in India was launched in the year
A. 1978
B. 1975
C. 1977
D. 1976

130. An attribute or exposure that is significantly associated with the development of a disease is

A. Agent factor
B. Risk factor
C. Exposure factor
D. Risk indicator

131. One of them is not a principle of health education

A. Credibility
B. Feedback
C. Setting an example
D. Utilization

132. List of the charges established or agreed to, by a dentist for specific dental services

A. Table of allowances
B. Fee schedule
C. Reasonable fee
D. Capitation

133. The commonly used theory to predict individual's behavior regarding preventive health care

A. Social cognitive theory
B. Health belief model
C. Transtheoritical model
D. Salutogenic model

134. An ongoing learning opportunity that enables all students (K-12) to be productive learners and to make well considered health decisions throughout their lives

A. Comprehensive school health programme
B. Health promotion
C. Comprehensive school health education
D. Health literacy

135. In one of the principles of health education 'soil, seed, sower', soil is

A. Medium by which facts can be transmitted
B. Health facts that are to be given
C. The people to whom health education is given
D. People who give health education

136. 'Shoe leather survey' was conducted by

A. MC Kay
B. Dr GVBlack
C. Churchill HV
D. Dr Trendley H Dean

137. In Debris index component given by Greene and Vermillion in 1964, extrinsic stains without debris on the index teeth is scored as

A. 0
B. 1
C. 2
D. 3

138. Age group in which NaF applied in Knutson technique

A. 2, 5, 10, 12
B. 4, 6, 10, 12
C. 3, 7, 11, 13
D. No specific age interval

139. Which of the following has higher fluoride content?

A. Bone
B. Cementum
C. Dentin
D. Enamel

140. Navy plaque Index was introduced by

A. Muhlemann
B. Ennever
C. Grossman and Fedi
D. None of the above

141. The number of new cases occurring in a defined population during a specified period of time is

A. Prevalence
B. Incidence
C. Point prevalence
D. Period prevalence

142. Salt fluoridation was pioneered by

A. US public health commission
B. Switzerland
C. New Zealand
D. Singapore

143. "Loss of head" in water purification is related to

A. Filtration capacity
B. Disinfection of water
C. Fluoridation of water
D. Chlorination of water

144. Commonest index used for measuring the plaque on the teeth is

A. Ramfjord index
B. Russel's index
C. Loe and silness index
D. Miller's index

PROSTHODONTICS

145. Jiffy denture is a type of

A. Interim immediate denture
B. Conventional complete denture
C. Fixed partial denture
D. Cast partial denture

146. The mean denture bearing area for the edentulous mandible is

A. 12.25 cm2
B. 22.96 cm2
C. 25.12 cm2
D. 20.96 cm2

147. Niswonger's technique is used to determine

A. Horizontal relation
B. vertical relation
C. Orientation relation
D. Centric relation

148. Trubyte tooth indicator is used for determining

A. Length of the tooth
B. Width of the tooth
C. Thickness of the tooth
D. Form of the tooth

149. Non rigid connectors are indicated for an FPD when

A. It is not possible to prepare two abutments with a common path of placement
B. The abutments are prepared with a common path of placement
C. The abutments have a poor crown to root ratio
D. The abutments have a ideal crown to root ratio

150. The abutment for a proximal half crown has

A. An intact buccal surface
B. An intact lingual surface
C. An intact distal surface
D. An intact mesial surface

151. Combination syndrome is manifested by

A. Maxillary distal extension RPD opposing a mandibular CD
B. Maxillary class IV RPD opposing mandibular distal extension RPD
C. Maxillary CD opposing mandibular class IV RPD
D. Maxillary CD opposing mandibular distal extension RPD

152. The direct retainer of choice when the principle abutment tooth has lost its periodontal support is

A. Embrasure clasp
B. Ring clasp
C. Multiple circlet clasp
D. Onlay clasp

153. The hinge joint articulator was designed by

A. Bonwill
B. Gariot
C. Gysi
D. Hanau

154. A patient with a rational, sensible, calm and composed disposition is

A. An exacting patient
B. A hysterical patient
C. An indifferent patient
D. A philosophical patient

155. For balanced occlusion, the factor that cannot be controlled by the dentist is

A. Incisal guidance
B. Condylar guidance
C. Cuspal heights
D. Plane of occlusion

156. The seat for any occlusal rest on abutment should be

A. Less than 90° to the long axis of the abutment
B. Parallel to the pontic
C. Parallel to the long axis of the abutment
D. On proximal surface of the abutment

157. The cross section of a lingual bar should be

A. Pear shaped
B. Round shaped
C. Half round shaped
D. Half pear shaped

158. The recommended finish line for porcelain jacket crown is

A. Chamfer
B. Knife Edge
C. Shoulder
D. Shoulder with bevel

159. The main drawback of a saddle pontic is

A. It is unhygienic
B. It is unaesthetic
C. It is bulky
D. It does not restore the tooth contours

160. The number of times an individual swallows per day, while awake

A. 600
B. 800
C. 700
D. 900

PERIODONTICS

161. The term curettage is derived from the word "curette" which means

A. To 'penetrate'
B. To 'cleanse'
C. To 'deviate'
D. To 'enucleate'

162. Periodontal screening and recorder system (PSR) is recorded by using periodontal probe which has...............

A. Graduation 1, 2, 3, 4, 5, 6, 7
B. 0.5 mm ball tip with color coded 3.5 ti 5.5 mm
C. Color coded for every 3 mm
D. Graduated 1, 5, 10 and 15 mm

163. A membrane immunoassay has been recently marked as 'Evalusite' it is designated to detect .... microorganism.

A. *Actinomycetemcomitans, P. gingivalis* and *P. intermedia*
B. *Actinomycetemcomitans, T. denticola and B. forsythus*
C. *Strep. sanguinis, Strep. mitis and T. denticola*
D. *P. gingivalis* and *E. corrodens*

164. 'Burtonian' line-seen in the gingiva because of ....intoxication

A. Phosphorus
B. Lead
C. Mercury
D. Chromium

165. Percentage of chlorhexidine used as a mouth wash is

A. 0.1%
B. 0.2%
C. 0.3%
D. 0.4%

166. The use of DNA probe is to

A. Assess the pocket depth
B. Check the bleeding
C. Detect specific microorganisms
D. Detect Furcation involvement

167. Helium-Neon (HeNe) lasers are example for

A. Excimer lasers
B. Gas lasers
C. Diode lasers
D. Solid state lasers

168. .... are fundamentally dual monocular telescopes with side by side lenses convergent to focus on the operative field
A. Loupes
B. Cameras
C. Spectacles
D. Lenses

169. Junctional epithelium
A. Keratinized
B. Non Keratinized
C. Hyper keratinized
D. Para keratinized

170. Plasma cells are mostly seen in one of the stages of gingivitis
A. Initial lesion
B. Early lesion
C. Established lesion
D. Advanced lesion

171. Biological width means
A. Sum of connective tissue and junctional epithelium
B. Distance from the tip of the papilla to the base of the sulcus
C. Distance from marginal gingiva to muco-gingival junction
D. Distance from incisal edge of the tooth to muco-gingival junction

172. Cementum and enamel meet edge to edge in ....% of cases
A. 5–10%
B. 30%
C. 60–65%
D. 100%

173. Crater-like gingival deformities are seen in
A. ANUG
B. Aggressive periodontitis
C. Chronic periodontitis
D. Chronic gingivitis

174. Which of the following antibiotics is not indicated for periodontal therapy?
A. Erythromycin
B. Metronidazole
C. Tetracycline
D. Augmentin

175. 'Chediak-Higashi syndrome' is primarily
A. Leukocyte disorder
B. Platelet disorder
C. RBC disorder
D. Chronic granulomatous disorder

176. The proteins found in attachment plaque
A. Albumin and globulin
B. Amelogenin and enamelin
C. Sialoproteins
D. Desmoplakin and plakoglobin

177. Microorganism which uses steroids as growth factor is
A. *P. ginigivalis*
B. *P. intermedius*
C. *S. sanguinis*
D. *D. mutans*

CONS AND ENDO

178. The temperature of glass bead sterilizer is
A. 425–475°F
B. 218–246°F
C. 325–345°F
D. 250–275°F

179. Affected dentin differs from infected dentin in that, it has
A. Been invaded by organisms
B. They both are precisely same
C. Not been invaded by microorganisms
D. Not been demineralized

180. Hand cutting instruments are composed of
A. Handle and blade
B. Handle, shank and blade
C. Shank and blade
D. Handle, shank and head

181. Crown infarction is
A. Necrosis of pulp following a fracture
B. An incomplete fracture of enamel without loss of tooth structure
C. Fracture of crown en mass
D. Vertical fracture of crown

182. Currently one of the popular root end filling material in great vogue is
A. Calcium hydroxide
B. Glassionmer cement
C. Microfilled composite resin
D. Mineral trioxide-aggregate (MTA)

183. Endodontic instruments most prone to fracture if used improperly in curved canals is
A. K-files
B. K-reamers
C. H-files
D. Nickel titanium files

184. The confirmatory test for pulp vitality is
A. Thermal test
B. Test cavity
C. Analytical technology electrical pulp tester
D. Digital pulp videography

185. Retention in a composite restoration is mainly attained by
A. Chemical adhesion
B. Acid etching and bonding
C. Inverted truncated shape
D. Undercuts

186. Bases provide
A. No thermal insulation
B. Mechanical support for the restoration
C. Expansion space for cast restoration
D. Exothermic heat for increased pulpal blood circulation

187. Degassing means
A. Removal of residual surface contamination
B. Removal of gases
C. Addition of gases
D. Disinfecting

188. According to ISO standardization, root canal files and reamers should have a taper of
A. 0.02 mm per cm
B. 0.02 mm per mm
C. 0.03 mm per cm
D. 0.03 mm per mm

189. One of the purposes of etching beveled enamel surface is to
A. Increase surface energy
B. Produce macro under cut
C. To increase convenience
D. To prevent caries

190. Which of the following principles of the cavity preparation is not considered much in modern methods of restorative dentistry?
A. Extension for prevention
B. Convenient form
C. Removal of the undermined enamel
D. Removal of the carious dentine

191. Digital imaging fiber-optic transillumination (DIFOTI)
A. Is used to detect to dental caries
B. Is used to detect enamel fracture
C. Is used to detect plaque
D. All of the above

ORAL SURGERY

192. In cases of medical emergencies an invasive technique to deal with airway obstruction is
A. Chest thrust
B. Abdominal thrust
C. Mouth to mouth resuscitation
D. Laryngoscopy

193. If a patient is absolutely allergic to LA, the specific drug used in its place
A. Bupivacaine hydrochloride
B. Benzalkonium chloride
C. Diphenhydramine hydrochloride
D. Ketamine hydrochloride

194. The thickness of split thickness skin graft used in maxillofacial surgery ranges from
A. 2 to 3 mm
B. 1 to 2 mm
C. 0.3 to 0.5 mm
D. 1.3 to 1.5 mm

195. The most likely agent in the local anesthetic solution to which patients could be allergic is

A. Lignocaine
B. Epinephrine
C. Thymol
D. Methyl paraben

196. During surgery of submandibular gland following cranial nerve may get injured

A. Glossopharyngeal nerve
B. Accessory nerve
C. Hypoglossal nerve
D. Trigeminal nerve

197. Phleboliths are seen in

A. Dental pulp
B. Salivary gland duct
C. Cavernous hemangiomas
D. Subepithelial bulla

198. The following is not a type of fracture

A. Traumatic
B. Pathological
C. Anatomical
D. Stress

199. The weakest part of the mandible where fracture occurs is

A. Neck of condyle
B. Angle of mandible
C. Canine fossa
D. All of the above

200. Apexogenesis is

A. Physiologic process of root development
B. Inducing the root development
C. Arresting the root development
D. It is a type of pulpectomy procedure

ANSWERS

HUMAN ANATOMY

1. **Ans: C**

   Ref: BD Chaurasia, 1/E, p. 276

2. **Ans: B**

   Ref: BD Chaurasia, 1/E, p. 253

3. **Ans: D**

   Ref: BD Chaurasia, 1/E, p. 277

   Explanation

   Contents of carotid sheath

   - Common carotid artery
   - Internal jugular vein
   - Vagus nerve

     The sympathetic trunk/Ansa cervicalis is a thin nerve loop embedded in the anterior wall of the carotid sheath

4. **Ans: D**

   Ref: BD Chaurasia, 1/E, p. 267

   Explanation

   - *Anterior belly of digastric*–derived form first arch supplied by nerve to mylohoid
   - *Posterior belly of digastric*–derived from second arch supplied by facial nerve

5. **Ans: B**

   Ref: Inderbir Singh Text Book of Embryology, 1/E, p. 110

PHYSIOLOGY

6. **Ans: D**

   Ref: Sembulingam, 4/E, p. 290

7. **Ans: C**

   Ref: Sembulingam, 4/E, p. 256

8. **Ans: D**

   Ref: Sembulingam, 4/E, p. 641

9. **Ans: C**

   Ref: Sembulingam, 4/E, p. 396

BIOCHEMISTRY

10. **Ans: D**

    Ref: U. Sathyanarayana & U. Chakerapani, 3/E, p. 503

11. **Ans: B**

    Ref: U.Sathyanarayana and U.Chakrapani, 3/E, p. 119

12. **Ans: C**

    Ref: U. Sathyanarayana and U. Chakrapani, 3/E, p. 716

    Explanation

    - It is responsible for maintaining the surface tension in the alveoli
    - Surfactant deficiency causes respiratory distress syndrome

13. **Ans: B**

    Ref: U. Sathyanarayana and U.Chakrapani, 3/E, p. 130

14. **Ans: C**

    Ref: U. Sathyanarayana and U. Chakrapani, 3/E, p. 102

    Explanation

    Proenzymes are also called zymogens

15. **Ans: A**

    Ref: U. Sathyanarayana and U.Chakrapani, 3/E, p. 123

    Explanation

    Nyctalopia or night blindness is one of the earliest symptoms of vitamin A deficiency

16. **Ans: A**

    Ref: U. Sathyanarayana and U. Chakrapani, 3/E, p. 134

GENERAL PATHOLOGY

17. Ans: D

Ref: Harsh Mohan, 3/E, p. 238

18. Ans: D

Ref: Harsh Mohan, 3/E, p. 50

Explanation

- Lipofuschin or lipochrome is a yellowish brown intracellular lipid pigment found in atrophied cells of testes and in neurons in senile
- It is seen in the myocardial fibres hepatocytes, leydig cells of testes and in neurons in senile dementia

MICROBIOLOGY

19. Ans: B

Ref: Ananthanarayan and Panicker's Text Book of Microbiology, 8/E, p.6

20. Ans: B

Ref: Ananthanarayan and Panicker's Text Book of Microbiology, 8/E, p. 100

21. Ans: D

Ref: Ananthanarayan and Panicker's Text Book of Microbiology, 8/E, p.475

22. Ans: D

Ref: Ananthanarayan and Panicker's Text Book of Microbiology, 8/E, p. 16

Explanation

- When lysosome acts on gram positive organism in hypertonic solution a protoplast is formed
- Gram negative bacteria–spheroplast differs from protoplast that some cell wall material is retained

23. Ans: B

Ref: Ananthanarayan and Panicker's Text Book of Microbiology, 8/E, p. 672

24. Ans: D

Ref: Ananthanarayan and Panicker's Text Book of Microbiology, 8/E, p. 353

25. Ans: C

Ref: Ananthanarayan and Panicker's Text Book of Microbiology, 8/E, p. 82

26. Ans: B

Ref: Ananthanarayan and Panicker's Text Book of Microbiology, 8/E, p. 297

Explanation

Leucopenia and relative lymphocytosis is characteristic of enteric fever

27. Ans: C

Ref: Ananthanarayan and Panicker's Text Book of Microbiology, 8/E, p. 100

Explanation

- Bence Jones protein is an abnormal immunoglobulin found in multiple myeloma
- It can be identified in urine by its characteristic property of coagulation when healed to 50°C but re dissolving at 70°C

28. Ans: A

Ref: Ananthanarayan and Panicker's Text Book of Microbiology, 8/E, p. 128

29. Ans: C

Ref: Ananthanarayan and Panicker's Text Book of Microbiology, 8/E, p. 208

Explanation

- Antigenic relationships of streptococcus pyogenes have been demonstrated between
  - Capsular hyaluronic acid and human synovial fluid
  - Cell wall protein and myocardium
  - Group A carbohydrate and cardiac valves
  - Cytoplasmic membrane antigens and vascular intima
  - Peptidoglycans and skin antigens

PHARMACOLOGY

30. **Ans: B**

Ref: KD Tripathi, 6/E, p. 130

31. **Ans: C**

Ref: KD Tripathi, 6/E, p. 694

32. **Ans: D**

Ref: KD Tripathi, 6/E, p. 282

33. **Ans: B**

Ref: KD Tripathi, 6/E, p. 451

Explanation

Buspirone is the first azapirone, a new class of anti anxiety drugs to retrieve mild to moderate anxiety

- Does not produce significant sedation or cognitive/full impairment
- Does not interact with BZD receptor or modify GABA ergic transmission
- Does not produce tolerance or physical dependence
- Dose not suppress BZD or barbiturate withdrawl syndrome
- Has no muscle relaxant or anticonvulsant activity

34. **Ans: D**

Ref: KD Tripathi, 6/E, p. 139

35. **Ans: D**

Ref: KD Tripathi, 6/E, p. 7

36. **Ans: C**

Ref: KD Tripathi, 6/E, p. 610

GENERAL MEDICINE

37. **Ans: D**

Ref: Davidson, 20/E, p. 383

38. **Ans: A**

Ref: Davidson, 20/E, p. 1037

Explanation

- Ocular–retinopathy, vitreous bleed
- Pulmonary infection–sickle chest syndrome
- CNS–cerebrovascular accident, subarachnoid bleed, epilepsy
- Cardiac–sickle myocardium, cardiomegaly, transfusional iron load
- Renal–eneuresis, haematuria, papillary necrosis, chronic renal failure
- Osteomyelitis
- Choleolithiasis
- Splenic infarction
- Verterbral, collapse, osteoporosis
- Dactylitis
- Arthropathy
- Priapism
- Leg laceration

39. **Ans: B**

Ref: Davidson, 20/E, p. 842

40. **Ans: D**

Ref: Davidson, 20/E, p. 631

41. **Ans: D**

Ref: Davidson, 20/E, p. 561

Explanation

Some pathological causes of sinus bradycardia and tachycardia

Sinus bradycardia

- Myocardial infarction
- Sinus node disease (Sick sinus syndrome)
- Hypothermia
- Hypothyroidism
- Cholestatic jaundice
- Raised intracranial pressure
- Drugs, e.g. – β blocker, digoxin verapamil

Sinus tachycardia

- Anxiety
- Fever
- Anaemia
- Heart failure

- Thyrotoxicosis
- Phaeochromocytoma
- Drugs, e.g. adrenoceptor agonists (bronchodilators)

42. Ans: B

Ref: Davidson, 20/E, p. 113

43. Ans: D

Ref: Davidson, 20/E, p. 545

44. Ans: D

Ref: Davidson, 20/E, p. 596, 597

45. Ans: D

Ref: Bailey & Love, 25/E, p. 380

46. Ans: C

Ref: Davidson, 20/E, p. 1182

Explanation

- Intentional tremor is the characteristic oscillation at the end of a movement which occurs in cerebellar disease due to the breakdown of feed back control of targeted movements

47. Ans: D

Ref: Harrison, Vol.1, 20/E, p. 1166

GENERAL SURGERY

48. Ans: A

Ref: Manipal Manual of Surgery, 2/E, p. 30

Explanation

- Trismus or lock jaw occurs due to severe contraction of masseter muscle

49. Ans: B

Ref: Manipal Manual of Surgery, 2/E, p. 366

50. Ans: A

Ref: S. Das, 5/E, p. 205

51. Ans: C

Ref: S. Das, 5/E, p. 674, Davidson, 20/E, p. 776

Explanation

- When hyperparathyroidism is corrected, further stone formation is prevented but pre existing stones need to be removed surgically
- Surgery in hyperparathyroidism is indicated for young patients (<50 years) and those with clear–cut symptoms or documented complications such as peptic ulceration, renal stones, renal impairment or osteopenia

52. Ans: C

Ref: S. Das, 5/E, p. 66

53. Ans: C

Ref: S. Das, 5/E, p. 130

Explanation

- Gummatous ulcer has punched out indolent edge and painless on healing it leaves a "tissue paper scar"

54. Ans: C

Ref: S. Das, 5/E, p. 664

DENTAL MATERIALS

55. Ans: C

Ref: Phillip's, 11/E, p. 418

56. Ans: B

Ref: Phillip's, 11/E, p. 346

57. Ans: C

Ref: Phillip's, 11/E, p. 342

58. Ans: D

Ref: Phillip's, 11/E, p. 481

59. Ans: B

Ref: Phillip's, 11/E, p. 41

60. Ans: D

Ref: Phillip's, 11/E, p. 55

61. **Ans: D**

Ref: Phillip's, 11/E, p. 408

Explanation

- Camphoroquinone (0.2 wt%) is a commonly used photosensitizer that absorbs blue light with wavelengths between 400 and 500 nm

62. **Ans: C**

Ref: Phillip's, 11/E, p. 368

Explanation

- Diamond is called a super abrasive because of its ability to abrade any other known substance

63. **Ans: B**

Ref: Phillip's, 11/E, p. 275

64. **Ans: D**

Ref: Phillip's, 11/E, p. 521

65. **Ans: C**

Ref: Text book of Dental Materials, SharmilaHussain, 1/E, p. 100

DADH

66. **Ans: B**

Ref: Wheeler's, 8/E, p. 277

67. **Ans: C**

Ref: Wheeler's, 8/E, p. 277

68. **Ans: B**

Ref: Orban's, 12/E, p. 96

69. **Ans: B**

Ref: Dental Caries: Etiology, Pathology and Pathogenesis, Leon. M. Silverstone, p. 217

70. **Ans: C**

Ref: Wheeler's, 8/E, p. 14

ORAL PATHOLOGY AND ORAL MEDICINE

71. **Ans: B**

Ref: Shafer's, 6/E, p. 50

72. **Ans: B**

Ref: Shafer's, 6/E, p. 540

73. **Ans: C**

Ref: Shafer's, 6/E, p. 219

Explanation

- Pleomorphic adenoma is a benign tumour of the salivary glands

74. **Ans: C**

Ref: Shafer's, 6/E, p. 508

75. **Ans: A**

Ref: Neelima malik, 2/E, p. 620

76. **Ans: C**

Ref: Shafer's, 6/E, p. 131

Explanation

- Foci of haemorrhage, with liberation of hemosiderin pigment and its subsequent ingestion by mononuclear phagocytes, as well as inflammatory cell infiltration are characteristic features of peripheral giant cell granuloma

77. **Ans: B**

Ref: Shafer's, 6/E, p. 722

78. **Ans: D**

Ref: Burkitt, 11/E, P.. 77

79. **Ans: A**

Ref: Shafer's, 6/E, p. 896

Explanation

- Lip prints – Imprint produced by the grooves in the lip
- Sulci laborum rubrorum – wrinkles and grooves visibile on the lips
- Chieloscopy – examination of lip prints

80. **Ans: A**

Ref: Shafer's, 6/E, p. 245

81. **Ans: A**

Ref: Shafer's, 6/E, p. 817

82. **Ans: C**

Ref: Shafer's, 6/E, p. 803

Explanation

- Psoriasis of the skin is characterized by the occurrence of small sharply delineated, dry papules, each covered by a delicate silvery scale which has been described as resembling a thin layer of mica
- If the deep scales are removed, one or more tiny bleeding points are disclosed, a characteristic feature named "Auspitz sign"
- After removal of the scale, the surface of the skin is red and dusky in appearance

83. **Ans: D**

Ref: Shafer's, 6/E, p. 279

84. **Ans: D**

Ref: Neville, 3/E, p. 860

85. **Ans: A**

Ref: Shafer's, 6/E, p. 544

86. **Ans: A**

Ref: Shafer's, 6/E, p. 200

Explanation

- Verocay bodies are small hyaline structures characteristically present in neurilemmoma

87. **Ans: D**

Ref: Shafer's, 6/E, p. 57

Explanation

- In Type I Radicular Dentin Dysplasia normal dentinal tubule formation appears to have been blocked so that new dentin forms around obstacles and takes on the characteristic appearance described as "lava flowing around boulders"
- Electron microscopy shows that this pattern of "cascades of dentin" results from repetitive attempts to form root structure

88. **Ans: A**

Ref: Shafer's, 6/E, p. 699

Explanation

- Osteopetrosis is also called marble bone disease/Albert–Schonberg disease or osteosclerosis fragilis generalisata

89. **Ans: C**

Ref: Shafer's, 6/E, p. 818

90. **Ans: A**

Ref: Maji jose ,16/E, p. 67

91. **Ans: A**

Ref: Shafer's, 6/E, p. 811

Explanation

- Keratosis follicularis or darrier's disease is characterized by typical cells called crops/ronds/grains
- The corps and ronds are larger than normal squamous cells representing partially keratinized cells

92. **Ans: C**

Ref: Shafer's, 6/E, p. 41

Explanation

- Talon's cusp is also seen in Morris Sturge Weber syndrome

93. **Ans: D**

Ref: Shafer's, 6/E, p. 804

94. **Ans: A**

Ref: Shafer's, 6/E, p. 341

Explanation

- Measles/Rubeola/Morbilli is caused by paramyxovirus which is a RNA virus

95. Ans: A

Ref: Shafer's, 6/E, p. 326

Explanation

- Noma is also known as cancrum oris or gangrenous stomatitis

96. Ans: A

Ref: Shafer's, 6/E, p. 337

Explanation

- Lipschutz bodies are intranuclear inclusions seen in herpex simplex infection
- These are eosinophillic, ovoid, homogenous structures within the nucleus,which tends to displace the nucleolus and nuclear chromatin peripherally

97. Ans: A

Ref: Neville, 3/E, p. 417

98. Ans: C

Ref: Shafer's, 6/E, p. 415

99. Ans: C

Ref: Davidson,20/E, p.298

Explanation

- Delhi boil is an indolent, slow healing Leishmania Tropicalis ulcer

ORAL RADIOLOGY

100. Ans: C

Ref: Pramod John, 1/E, p. 205, White & Pharoah, 6/E, p. 135

Explanation

Different vertical angulations;

Teeth	*Maxillary*	*Mandibular*
Incisors	+40°	–15°
Canines	+45°	–20°
Premolar	+30°	–10°
Molars	+25°	–5°

101. Ans: B

Ref: White and Pharoah, 6/E, p. 7

Explanation

- Quality of X-rays is controlled by KVp

102. Ans: C

Ref: White and Pharoah, 6/E, p. 61

103. Ans: D

Ref: White and Pharoah, 5/E, p.53

104. Ans: C

Ref: White and Pharoah, 6/E, p. 205

ORTHODONTICS

105. Ans: A

Ref: Gurkeerat Singh, 2/E, p. 501

106. Ans: C

Ref: Bhalaji, 3/E, p. 145

Explanation

- The distance between the X–ray rource and mid sagittal plane is fixed–5 feet/ 152.4 cm

107. Ans: B

Ref: Bhalaji, 3/E, p. 143

108. Ans: B

Ref: Bhalaji, 3/E, p. 36

Explanation

- Bone growth follows secondarily at the condyle to maintain constant contact with the cranial base

109. Ans: B

Ref: Bhalaji, 3/E, p. 17

110. Ans: C

Ref: Bhalaji, 3/E, pp. 44, 48

111. Ans: B

Ref: Profit, 4/E, p. 340

112. Ans: B

Ref: Bhalaji, 3/E, p. 10

113. Ans: C

Ref: Bhalaji, 3/E, p. 254

114. Ans: C

Ref: Bhalaji, 3/E, p. 48

115. Ans: C

Ref: Proffit, 4/E, p.103

116. Ans: C

Ref: Bhalaji, 3/E, p. 121

PEDODONTICS

117. Ans: C

Ref: Shobha Tandon, 1/E, p. 360

118. Ans: A

Ref: Shobha Tandon, 1/E, p. 219

119. Ans: A

Ref: Mc Donald's, 8/E, p. 290

Explanation

Dietary instructions before conscious sedation

1. No milk or solids for 6 hours for children aged 6–36 months old for 6–7 hours for children 36 months and older
2. Clear liquids up to 3 hours before the procedure for children aged 6 months and older

120. Ans: C

Ref: Shobha Tandon, 1/E, p. 446

Explanation

Finn has classified mouth breathing into

- Anatomic
- Obstructive
- Habitual

121. Ans: A

Ref: Shobha Tandon, 1/E, p. 554

122. Ans: B

Ref: Shobha Tandon, 1/E, p. 122

123. Ans: A

Ref: Shobha Tandon, 1/E, p. 141

124. Ans: C

Ref: Shobha Tandon, 1/E, p. 500

125. Ans: A

Ref: Shobha Tandon, 1/E, p. 456, Wheeler's, 8/E, p. 75

126. Ans: C

Ref: Shobha Tandon, 1/E, p. 235

127. Ans: C

Ref: McDonald, 8/E, p. 486

128. Ans: C

Ref: McDonald, 8/E, p. 183

P AND SD

129. Ans: C

Ref: Park, 20/E, p. 778

Explanation

- Recommended by Shrivastav committee (1975)
- Accepted by Govt of India in 1977

130. Ans: B

Ref: Park, 20/E, p. 36

131. Ans: D

Ref: Park, 20/E, p. 764

Explanation

Principles of Health Education

1. Credibility
2. Interest
3. Participation
4. Motivation
5. Comprehension
6. Reinforcement
7. Learning by doing
8. Known to unknown
9. Setting an example

10. Good human relations
11. Feedback
12. Leaders

132. Ans: B

Ref: Soben Peter, 3/E, p. 650

Explanation

- Table of allowances–is defined as a list of covered services that assigns to each service a sum that represents the total obligation of the plan but does not necessarily represent a dentist's full fee for service
- Reasonable fee– if the fee is justifiable considering the special circumstances or the particular patient in question
- Capitation–the contrasting provider whether a HMO group practice, IPA or individual dentist receives an established negotiated sum on a monthly or yearly basis for eligible patient

133. Ans: B

Ref: Soben Peter, 3/E, p. 565

134. Ans: C

Ref: Soben Peter, 3/E, p. 557

135. Ans: C

Ref: Soben Peter, 3/E, p. 526

Explanation

- Soil–People to whom health education is given
- Seed–Health facts to be given
- Sower–Media used to transmit the facts

136. Ans: D

Ref: Soben Peter, 3/E, p. 272

137. Ans: B

Ref: Soben Peter, 3/E, p. 133

Explanation

Debris index (DI)

Score Criteria

0 No debris or stain present
1 Soft debris covering not more than one third of the tooth surface and/or presence of extrinsic stains without other debris regardless of surface area covered
2 Often debris covering more than one third, but not more than two thirds, of the exposed tooth surface
3 Soft debris covering more than two thirds of the exposed tooth surface

Calculus Index (CI)

Score Criteria

0 No calculus present
1 Supragingival calculus covering not more than third of the exposed tooth surface
2 Supragingival calculus covering more than one third but no more than two thirds of the exposed tooth surface and/or the presence of individual flecks of subgingival calculus around the cervical portion of the tooth or both
3 Supragingival calculus covering more than two third of the exposed tooth surface and/or a continuous heavy band of subgingival calculus around the cervical portion of the tooth or both

138. Ans: C

Ref: Sober Peter, 3/E, p. 299

Explanation

- The four visit procedure for application of NaF is recommended for ages 3, 7, 11, 13 coinciding with the eruption of different groups of primary and permanent teeth. Thus most of the teeth would be treated soon after their eruption, maximizing the protection afforded by topical application

139. Ans: B

Ref: Soben Peter, 3/E, p. 283

140. Ans: C

Ref: Soben Peter, 3/E, p. 144

Explanation

- Was developed by Grossman F. D and Fedi P. F in 1970
- To assess the plaque control status among naval personnels
- Ennever j. sturzenberger C. P and Radike A. W L in 1961
- Ennever J,etalin 1961 Calculus surface severity index
- Muhlemann H. R and Villa. P 1967 – Marginal line calculus index

141. Ans: B

Ref: Park, 20/E, p. 57

142. Ans: B

Ref: Soben Peter, 3/E, p. 352

143. Ans: A

Ref: Park, 20/E, p. 623

144. Ans: C

Ref: SobenPeter, 3/E, p. 138

Explanation

- Silness and Loe index–plaque index
- Loe and Silness index–gingival index

PROSTHODONTICS

145. Ans: A

Ref: Zarb and Bolender, 12/E, p. 123

Explanation

- It is a type of interim immediate denture
- It differ from IID in that the denture teeth are usually made with tooth colored autopolymerizing acrylic resin

146. Ans: A

Ref: Zarb and Bolender, 12/E, p. 10

Explanation

- Denture bearing area
- Maxilla–22.96 cm^2
- Mandible–12.25 cm^2

147. Ans: B

Ref: Nallaswamy, 1/E, p. 135

148. Ans: D

Ref: Heartwell, 4/E, pp. 313, 317

149. Ans: A

Ref: Rosensteil, 4/E, p. 845

150. Ans: C

Ref: Nallaswamy, 1/E, p. 590

151. Ans: D

Ref: Nallaswamy, 1/E, p. 252

Explanation

- It was identified by Kelly in 1972

152. Ans: C

Ref: Nallaswamy, 1/E, p. 360

153. Ans: B

Ref: Winkler, 2/E, p. 143

Explanation

- Hinge joint articulator is a class I articulator designed by JB Gariot in 1805

154. Ans: D

Ref: Nallaswamy, 1/E, p. 15

155. Ans: B

Ref: Nallaswamy, 1/E, p. 193

156. Ans: A

Ref: Nallaswamy, 1/E, p. 347

Explanation

- If it is more than 90°, the forces acting on the prosthesis will not be transmitted along a long axis of the abutment tooth

157. Ans: D

Ref: Mc Crackens, 11/E, p. 39

158. Ans: C

Ref: Rosensteil, 4/E, p. 220

Explanation

Shoulder finish line

Advantage: Bulk of restorative material

Disadvantage: Less conservative of tooth structure

Indication:

- Facial margin of metal
- Ceramic Crowns
- Complete ceramic crown

159. Ans: A

Ref: Nallaswamy, 1/E, p. 510

160. Ans: B

Ref: Zarb and Bolender, 12/E, p. 9

PERIODONTICS

161. Ans: B

Ref: Carranza, 10/E, p. 909

162. Ans: B

Ref: Carranza, 10/E, p. 558

Explanation

PSR system

- Patients mouth is divided into 6 sextants
- Each tooth is probed, by walking the probes at least 6 points around each tooth

163. Ans: A

Ref: Carranza, 10/E, p. 591

Explanation

- Evalusite–ELISA for Aa, P. and Pi

Note: Abiodent–Periotemp probe

164. Ans: B

Ref: Carranza, 10/E, p. 306

Explanation

- Gingival pigmentation is linear, steel gray and associated with local inflammation

165. Ans: B

Ref: Carranza, 10/E, p. 338

Explanation

- Plaque control – 0.2%
- Post surgical rinsing – 0.12% (peridex, perigard)
- Ultrasonic scaling (prerinsing) – 0.12%
- Subgingival chip – 2.5 mg (periochip)
- Halitosis
  - Chlorhexidine – 0.05%
  - CPC – 0.05%
  - Zinc lactate – 0.14%

166. Ans: C

Ref: Carranza, 10/E, p. 592

167. Ans: B

Ref: Carranza, 10/E, p. 1036

168. Ans: A

Ref: Carranza, 10/E, p. 1030

169. Ans: B

Ref: Carranza, 10/E, p. 53

170. Ans: C

Ref: Carranza, 10/E, p. 359

171. Ans: A

Ref: Carranza, 10/E, p. 1051

Explanation

- Connective tissue attachment + junctional epithelial attachment = Biologic width 1.07 + 0.97 = 2.04

172. Ans: B

Ref: Carranza, 10/E, p. 76

Explanation

- Cementum overlaps enamel 60–65%
- Edge to edge 30%
- Fail to meet 5–10%

173. Ans: A

Ref: Carranza, 10/E, p. 391

174. Ans: A

Ref: Carranza, 10/E, p. 800

KCET 2008

Explanation

- Common antibiotic regimens used to treat periodontal diseases

Regimen	*Dosage/single agent duration*
Amoxicillin	500 mg Three times daily for 8 days
Azithromycin	500 mg Once daily for 4–7 days
Ciprofloxacin	500 mg Twice daily for 8 days
Clindamycin	300 mg Three times daily 10 days
Doxycycline or Minocycline	100–200 mg Once daily for 21 days
Metronidazole	500 mg Three times daily for 8 day

Combination therapy

- Metronidazole + 250 mg of Three times daily for 8 amoxicillin each days
- Metronidazole + 500 mg of Twice daily for 8 days ciprofloxacin each

175. Ans: A

Ref: Carranza, 10/E, p. 298

176. Ans: D

Ref: Carranza, 10/E, p. 140

177. Ans: B

Ref: Carranza, 10/E, p. 241

Explanation

- Increase in hormone levels correlates with increase in the subgingival proportions of prevotella intermedia, a micro-organism that can substitute progesterone or estradiol for vit K as an essential bacterial growth factor

CONS AND ENDO

178. Ans: A

Ref: Grossman, 12/E, p. 174

179. Ans: C

Ref: Sturdavent, 5/E, p. 291

Explanation

Affected dentin	*Infected dentin*
Hard in consistnecy	Soft and leathery
Bacteria absent	Bacteria is present
Dark in colour	Light in colour
Remineralizable	Not remineralizable
Should be preserved	Should be removed

180. Ans: B

Ref: Sturdavent 5/E p. 328

181. Ans: B

Ref: Ingle, 6/E, p. 1330

182. Ans: D

Ref: Cohen, 9/E, p. 278

183. Ans: C

Ref: Grossman, 12/E, p. 230

184. Ans: B

Ref: Grossman, 12/E, p. 70

185. Ans: B

Ref: Sturdavent 5/E p. 245

186. Ans: B

Ref: Sturdavent 5/E p. 174

Explanation

- Bases (1–2 μm) are used to provide thermal protection for the pulp and to supplement mechanical support for the restoration by distributing local stresses from the restoration across the underlying dentin surface

187. Ans: A

Ref: Sturdavent 5/E p. 920

188. Ans: B

Ref: Grossman, 12/E, p. 226

189. Ans: A

Ref: Sturdavent 5/E, p. 240

190. Ans: A

Ref: Sturdavent 5/E, p. 290

191. Ans: A

Ref: Sturdavent 5/E, p. 419

ORAL SURGERY

192. Ans: D

Ref: Neelima Malik, 2/E, p. 156

193. Ans: C

Ref: Malamed LA, 5/E, p. 322

194. Ans: C

Ref: Laskin, Vol. 2, p. 340

195. Ans: A

Ref: Neelima Malik 2/E, p. 620

196. Ans: C

Ref: S. Das, 5/E, p. 609

197. Ans: C

Ref: Laskin, Vol. 2, p. 524

Explanation

- Some hemangiomas contain calcified bodies that may be palpated. These are known as Phleboliths
- When they develop in the cheek, the radiographic findings can be misleading and a diagnosis of parotid sialolith may be made

198. Ans: C

Ref: Killey's, 4/E, p. 524

199. Ans: A

Ref: Neelima Malik, 2/E, p. 379

200. Ans: A

Ref: Shobha Tandon, 1/E, p. 520

Explanation

- Indications of Apexogenesis
  - Relatively large exposure
  - Patients seen within 72 hours
  - Moderate haemorrhage

7

KCET 2009

HUMAN ANATOMY

1. **The following arteries provide a rich blood supply to the face, EXCEPT**
   A. Buccal artery
   B. Mental artery
   C. Posterior auricular artery
   D. Infra orbital artery

2. **Bell's palsy results in the inflammation of one of the following nerves**
   A. Hypoglossal nerve
   B. Accessory nerve
   C. Facial nerve
   D. Glossopharyngeal nerve

3. **Secretomotor fibres for the parotid gland are relayed in one of the following ganglia**
   A. Otic ganglion
   B. Submandibular ganglion
   C. Ciliary ganglion
   D. Pterygopalatine ganglion

4. **Median cleft of the upper lip occurs as result of defective formation of the**
   A. Frontonasal prominence
   B. Lateral nasal prominence
   C. Lens placode
   D. Mandibular prominence

5. **Injury to one of the following arteries results in extradural hematoma**
   A. Middle meningeal artery
   B. Facial artery
   C. Temporal artery
   D. Anterior cerebral artery

6. **Which of the following is a derivative of the second branchial cleft?**
   A. Tympanic cavity
   B. Meckel's cartilage
   C. Palatine tonsil
   D. Tongue base

7. **The mucosa of the posterior third of the tongue is supplied by**
   A. Facial nerve
   B. Trigeminal nerve
   C. Mandibular nerve
   D. Glossopharyngeal nerve

8. **Taste functions are primarily mediated by**
   A. Lingual nerve
   B. Chorda tympani
   C. Hypoglossal nerve
   D. Glossopharyngeal nerve

PHYSIOLOGY

9. **All the following causes the secretion of gastric juice during cephalic phase EXCEPT**
   A. Food in the mouth
   B. Sight of food
   C. Food in the stomach
   D. Thought of food

10. **All of the following features are seen in cerebellar dysfunction EXCEPT**
   A. Static tremor
   B. Dysmetria
   C. Scanning speech
   D. Rebound phenomenon

11. **Lymphocytes are located in each of the following tissues or organs EXCEPT one. The one exception is**
   A. Brain
   B. Spleen
   C. Lymph nodes
   D. Thymus glands

12. **In an emergency which of the following blood groups can be transfused without cross matching**
   A. B +ve
   B. AB +ve
   C. O +ve
   D. O –ve

BIOCHEMISTRY

13. **Haemophilia A is due to the deficiency of factor**
   A. II
   B. V
   C. VIII
   D. IX

14. **Insulin increases the following pathways in the liver EXCEPT**
   A. Fatty acid synthesis
   B. Glycogen synthesis
   C. Protein synthesis
   D. Glucose synthesis

15. **Which of the following fatty acids cannot be synthesized in humans?**
   A. Palmitic acid
   B. Stearic acid
   C. Oleic acid
   D. Linoleic acid

16. **Biotin is required for the activity of**
   A. Pyruvate carboxylase
   B. Lactate dehydrogenase
   C. Succinate thiokinase
   D. Phosphohexose isomerase

17. **Vitamin D**
   A. Absorption requires bile pigments
   B. Synthesis is regulated at the reaction catalyzed by 25–hydroxylase
   C. Deficiency in adults leads to rickets
   D. Along with PTH increases calcium resorption from bone

18. **Bilirubin is formed from**
   A. Cholic acid
   B. Cholesterol
   C. Heme
   D. Purines

GENERAL PATHOLOGY

19. **Increased level of serum alkaline phosphate is seen in**
   A. Osteopetrosis
   B. Fibrous dysplasia
   C. Paget's disease
   D. Ossifying fibroma

20. **The dominant histologic feature of infarction is**
   A. Liquefactive necrosis
   B. Coagulative necrosis
   C. Chronic inflammation
   D. Scar tissue

21. **The type of acute myelogenous leukemia associated with a high incidence of disseminated intra vascular coagulation is**
   A. Acute erythroleukemia
   B. Acute promyelocytic leukemia
   C. Acute megakaryocytic leukemia
   D. Acute myelomonocytic leukemia

22. **Abnormal function of epithelial chloride channel protein is the cause of**
   A. Ehlers Danlos syndrome
   B. Marfan syndrome
   C. Cystic fibrosis
   D. Diabetes insipidus

23. **Free radicals can be inactivated by the following enzymes EXCEPT**
   A. Glutathione peroxidase
   B. Catalase
   C. Superoxide dismutase
   D. Myeloperoxidase

24. The most common site of origin for venous thrombi leading to pulmonary embolism is

A. Ascending aorta
B. Portal vein
C. Deep leg veins
D. Right atrium

MICROBIOLOGY

25. The process of attenuation can be achieved by all EXCEPT

A. Growing bacteria in adverse environment
B. Growing bacteria in unconventional host
C. Serial passage in an experimental host
D. Repeated cultures in artificial media

26. S4. Dane Particle refers to

A. Hepatitis A virus
B. Hepatitis B virus
C. Hepatitis C virus
D. Hepatitis E virus

27. The spirochete which is associated with fusospirochetosis is

A. Treponema pallidum
B. Treponema pertenue
C. Borrelia burgdorferi
D. Borrelia Vincenti

28. Post streptococcal acute glomerulonephritis is an example for

A. Type I hypersensitivity
B. Type II hypersensitivity
C. Type III hypersensitivity
D. Type IV hypersensitivity

29. Biological control used in an autoclave is the spores of

A. Bacillus stearothermophilus
B. Clostridium welchii
C. Bacillus cereus
D. Clostridium histolyticum

30. Recurrent epididymitis is a feature of following infection

A. Wuchereria bancrofti
B. Ascaris lumbricoides
C. Mumps
D. Tuberculosis

31. The cell wall deficient bacteria

A. Rickettesiae
B. Mycoplasma
C. Chlamydiae
D. Escherichia

32. Nonseptate hyphae with a tendency to branch at 90 degree angle is characteristic of

A. Mucor
B. Aspergillosis
C. Cryptococcus neoformans
D. Coccidiodies immiitis

33. Mycobacterium tuberculosis is best demonstrated by

A. Gram's stain
B. H and E stain
C. Ziehl–Neelsen stain
D. PAS Stain

PHARMACOLOGY

34. Which of the following statements about azoles is FALSE?

A. They are fungistatic
B. They are hepatotoxic
C. Resistance to the drug is common
D. They affect the metabolism of drugs such as cyclosporine necessitating an increase in the dosage

35. beta blocker with additional α blocking property is

A. Propanolol
B. Timolol
C. Metoprolol
D. Labetalol

36. The most preferred anti emetic for emesis induced by anticancer drugs is

A. Ondansetron
B. Metoclopromide
C. Chlorpromazine
D. Dicyclomine

37. All of the following glucocorticoids can be given by inhalation EXCEPT

A. Dexamethasone
B. Beclomethasone
C. Budesonide
D. Fluticasone

38. Drugs that exhibit first pass metabolism are all EXCEPT one

A. Morphine
B. Nitroglycerine
C. Propranolol
D. Salicylates

39. Which one of the following is not TRUE of angiotensin converting enzyme inhibitor (ACE inhibitor)?

A. May cause hyperkalemia in diabetic patient
B. Contraindicated in pregnancy
C. Contraindicated in diabetic nephropathy
D. NSAID may impair its hypotensive Effect

40. Most important drug used in the treatment of coronary artery disease is

A. Aspirin
B. Digoxin
C. Streptokinase
D. Nifedipine

41. The sensitive period for tetracycline induced discoloration in the permanent maxillary and mandibular incisors and canines is

A. 3 months postpartum to seventh year of life
B. 4 months in utero to 3 months post partum
C. 5 months in utero to 9 months post partum
D. Birth to seventh year

GENERAL MEDICINE

42. The first heart sound is loud in all the following EXCEPT

A. Mitral stenosis
B. Short PR interval
C. Tachycardia
D. Mitral valve calcification

43. False about risk factor for stroke

A. Diabetes
B. Anemia
C. Heart failure
D. Alcohol

44. A 30 year old highly health conscious woman has been ingesting vitamins and health foods. She is complaining of hair loss, double vision and headache. Her liver function tests are abnormal. She may be suffering from

A. Dry beriberi
B. Hypervitaminosis A
C. Vitamin E deficiency
D. Hypervitaminosis D

45. Test of primary hemostasis

A. Coagulation time
B. Bleeding time
C. Prothrombin time
D. Platelet count

46. Predisposing factors for urinary tract infection are

A. Pregnancy
B. Obstruction to urinary tract
C. Vesicoureteral influx disorder
D. All of the above

47. Haemoptysis is caused by the following

A. Leukaemia
B. Haemophilia
C. Anticoagulant therapy
D. All

48. An attack of cluster headache can be aborted by

A. Morphine administration
B. Breathing oxygen
C. Aspirin administration
D. Sublingual nitroglycerine administration

49. A pulmonary disorder causes the alveoli to break and coalesce into large air spaces. The lungs also lose elasticity and compliance is increased. A person who suffers from this disease will have

A. Increased dead air space
B. Increased vital capacity
C. Decreased PCO_2 in the blood
D. Decreased antero–posterior diameter

50. All the following are features of acute severe asthma EXCEPT

A. Respiratory rate >25
B. Heart rate >110
C. PEF <50% of normal or predicted
D. Temperature >102°F

GENERAL SURGERY

51. Thyrotoxicosis is characterized by

A. Exophthalmos
B. Sinus bradycardia
C. Constipation
D. Slow relaxation of deep tendon reflexes

52. Treatment of choice in cold nodule of thyroid

A. Subtotal thyroidectomy
B. I_{131}
C. Hemithyroidectomy
D. Excision of nodule

53. Commonest site of carcinoma of the tongue

A. Posterior one third
B. Ventral surface
C. Tip of the tongue
D. Lateral margin

54. Commonest site of thyroglossal duct cyst

A. Beneath the foramen caecum
B. Suprahyoid
C. Beneath the hyoid bone
D. At the cricoid cartilage

55. Most common cause of postoperative shock is

A. Hypovolaemia
B. Cardiogenic
C. Septic
D. Air embolism

56. Wound healing is

A. Impaired in anemic patient
B. Not impaired by hypoproteinaemia
C. Stimulated by steroids
D. More rapid in young than in old

57. Cystic hygroma is a

A. Haemangioma
B. Lymphangioma
C. Lung abscess
D. Liver cirrhosis manifestation

DENTAL MATERIALS

58. The effects associated with cold working can be eliminated by a heat treatment called

A. Age hardening heat treatment
B. Annealing heat treatment
C. Homogenization heat treatment
D. Solution heat treatment

59. Which of the following increases castability of base metal alloys?

A. Tin
B. Beryllium
C. Molybdenum
D. Carbon

60. Crocus cloth is

A. Emery
B. Garnet
C. Pumice
D. Rouge

61. Purpose of adding indium to metal alloy in porcelain fused to metal is

A. To improve bonding
B. To increase strength
C. To decrease porosity
D. To match the thermal expansion of metal and porcelain

62. **Which one of the following impression materials is elastic, sets by a chemical reaction and is catalyzed by chloroplatinic acid?**
    A. Condensation silicone
    B. Poly ethers
    C. Poly sulfides
    D. Poly vinyl siloxane

63. **With indirect spruing, which one of the following porosities can be minimized?**
    A. Back pressure porosity
    B. Localized shrinkage porosity
    C. Pin hole porosity
    D. Micro porosity

64. **The main difference between powders of dental plaster and dental stone is**
    A. Chemical composition
    B. Solubility in water
    C. Particle shape and size
    D. Shelf life

65. **In brazing, filler metal has a melting point of**
    A. 250 degree centigrade
    B. below 450 degree centigrade
    C. 80 to 100 degree centigrade
    D. Above 450 degree centigrade

66. **Direct coupling or by the exchange of a hydrogen atom from one growing chain to another in a polymerization chain reaction is termed**
    A. Induction
    B. Propagation
    C. Termination
    D. Chain transfer

67. **Most commonly used initiator for the polymerization of methyl methacrylate is**
    A. Hydrogen peroxide
    B. Benzoyl peroxide
    C. Isopropyl alcohol
    D. Hydroquinone

68. **Which of the following cast gold alloys is used for fabricating partial denture frameworks?**
    A. Type I–soft
    B. Type II–hard
    C. Type III–hard
    D. Type IV–extra hard

69. **The following are the microhardness tests done to check the hardness**
    A. Brinell and Rockwell tests
    B. Knoop and Vickers tests
    C. Shore and Barcol tests
    D. Knoop and Brinell tests

70. **The effect of trituration on strength in an amalgam restoration depends on**
    A. Amalgam alloy
    B. Trituration time
    C. Speed of amalgamator
    D. All the above

DADH

71. **Any one of the three rounded protuberances on incisal ridges of newly erupted incisor is called**
    A. Tubercle
    B. Cusp
    C. Mammelon
    D. Fossa

72. **The high level clear cell present in the oral epithelium**
    A. Melanocyte
    B. Lymphocyte
    C. Merkel cell
    D. Langerhans cell

ORAL PATHOLOGY AND ORAL MEDICINE

73. **Palatal papillary hyperplasia is best treated by**
    A. Cryosurgery
    B. Electrosurgery
    C. Electrocautery
    D. Radiotherapy

74. The plunging ranula is so called because of

A. Its size
B. Lifting of tongue
C. Extension through mylohyoid
D. Involvement of lingual nerve

75. Eagleton criteria is to diagnose

A. Bilateral TMJ ankylosis
B. Ludwig's angina
C. Cavernous sinus thrombosis
D. Oro antral fistula

76. The following lesion is a doubtful pre–malignant lesion for oral malignancy

A. Leukoplakia
B. Chronic hyperplastic candidiasis
C. Erythroplakia
D. Oral lichen planus

77. Chronic periostitis in children is known as

A. Cherubism
B. Garre's osteomyelitis
C. Histiocytosis X
D. Tuberculous osteomyelitis

78. Differential diagnosis of hypercementosis includes all of the foolowing EXCEPT

A. Cemental dysplasia
B. Cemental aplasia
C. Condensing osteitis
D. Focal periapical osteopetrosis

79. One of the following drug is advocated in the management of oral submucous fibrosis

A. Beta carotene
B. Ibuprofen
C. Acyclovir
D. Nystatin

80. Which of the following statements about Sjogren's syndrome is incorrect?

A. MRI shows salt and pepper appearance
B. Lacrimal gland enlargement is common
C. Minor salivary gland biopsy is a diagnostic test
D. Pilocarpine is the most useful and convenient drug in its treatment

81. Definitive dental diagnosis of oral cancer is made by

A. Complete radiographic survey
B. Biopsy
C. Exfoliative cytology
D. Pantograph

82. A radicular cyst is most often caused by

A. Deep restorations
B. Trauma
C. Primary occlusal traumatism
D. Dental caries

83. A bony hard asymptomatic swelling found on the midline of the hard palate, that appears radiopaque on a radiograph is most likely a

A. Odontoma
B. Myxoma
C. Bonecyst
D. Torus palatinus

84. The following lesions are premalignant EXCEPT

A. Bowens disease
B. Solar keratosis
C. Radio keratosis
D. Epidermoid carcinoma

85. Oral lesions of secondary syphilis includes all EXCEPT

A. Snail track ulcers
B. Mucous patches
C. Chancre of tongue
D. Hutchinson's wart

86. A histologic evidence of wide spread formation of globular hypocalcified dentin and high pulp horns reaching the dentinoenamel junction, absence of lamina dura around the teeth in radiograph are the characteristic feature of

A. Vitamin D resistant rickets
B. Hypophosphatasia
C. Hypervitaminosis – A
D. Vitamin A deficiency

87. **Which of the following is not a clinical feature of Pierre-Robin syndrome?**
   A. Micrognathia
   B. Retrognathia
   C. Glossoptosis
   D. Coloboma of lower eyelid

88. **"Ghost cells" are characteristically seen in the epithelial linings of**
   A. Dentigerous cyst
   B. Radicular cyst
   C. Keratocyst
   D. Calcifying odontogenic cyst

89. **Developmental cyst associated with impacted tooth**
   A. Radicular cyst
   B. Dentigerous cyst
   C. Odontogenic keratocyst
   D. Lateral periodontal cyst

90. **Which one of the following feature is not associated with primary hyperparathyroidism?**
   A. Giant cell tumor
   B. Sharply defined radiolucencies of maxilla and mandible
   C. Partial loss of lamina dura
   D. Hypercementosis

91. **Squamous papilloma is induced by**
   A. EBV
   B. HSV
   C. HPV
   D. CMV

92. **Apical cysts having a direct connection with apical foramen have been termed as**
   A. Residual
   B. Bay
   C. Paradental
   D. Collateral

93. **A non–neoplastic hereditary bone lesion, histologically similar to central giant cell granuloma, affects the children and shows a bilateral involvement of the jaws with eye of heaven appearance clinically**
   A. Fibrous dysplasia
   B. Cherubism
   C. Craniofacial dysostosis
   D. Chondro ectodermal dysplasia

94. **Fissured tongue is a component of**
   A. Melkerson–Rosenthal syndrome
   B. Apert's syndrome
   C. Swift's disease
   D. Macroglossia

95. **Acantholysis is pathognomonic of**
   A. Lichen planus
   B. Submucous fibrosis
   C. Pemphigus
   D. Pemphigoid

96. **Presence of Epstein Barr virus in hairy leukoplakia can be demonstrated using following methods EXCEPT**
   A. Tzanck smear
   B. Polymerase chain reaction
   C. In situ hybridization
   D. Electron microscopy

97. **Acute osteomyelitis is commonly caused by**
   A. *Staph aureus*
   B. *S. pyogenes*
   C. *H. influenzae*
   D. *Salmonella*

ORAL RADIOLOGY

98. **Cells are most sensitive to radiation in**
   A. G2 phase
   B. G1 phase
   C. G1 phase and early S phase
   D. G2 phase and late S phase

99. **Which of the following is a device of radiation dose measurement?**
   A. Storage phosphor plate
   B. Ionization chamber
   C. Coolidge tube
   D. Charged couple device

100. **The radiographic appearance of osteosarcoma is**
   A. Soap bubble appearance

B. Onion skin appearance
C. Cotton wool appearance
D. Sunray spicules appearance

ORTHODONTICS

101. Distortion of labiodental sounds occurs in
A. Skeletal class II malocclusion
B. Open bite
C. Skeletal class III malocclusion
D. All of the above feature

102. Mouth breathing with enlarged tonsils and adenoids may be best described as
A. Anatomic
B. Obstructive
C. Physiologic
D. Habitual

103. Serial extractions are indicated when there is
A. No skeletal discrepancy with dental crowding >10 mm
B. No skeletal discrepancy with dental crowding between 5–7 mm
C. Skeletal discrepancy >5 mm with dental crowding <5 mm
D. Skeletal discrepancy >10 mm with dental crowding <5 mm

104. The number of bones seen in a hand wrist radiograph is
A. Twenty five
B. Twenty six
C. Twenty seven
D. Thirty

105. When the diameter of the wire is doubled, the flexibility of the spring
A. Decreases by four times
B. Increases by sixteen times
C. Decreases by sixteen times
D. Remains the same

106. Which one of the following has maximum familial tendency?
A. Protruded maxillary incisors
B. Open bite
C. Deep bite
D. Upper and lower cross bite

107. The type of force exerted by headgears or facemasks is
A. Light force
B. Continuous force
C. Intermittent force
D. Interrupted force

108. A maxillary anterior bite plane appliance is used to correct
A. Anterior cross bite
B. Posterior cross bite
C. Retroclined mandibular anterior teeth
D. Increased anterior over bite or deep Bite

109. In the three planes of space, in both maxilla and mandible, growth is first completed in
A. Width
B. Length
C. Height
D. All at the same time

110. Appliance of choice in cases with anteroposterior Maxillary deficiency is
A. Cervical pull headgear
B. Reverse pull headgear
C. Occipital pull headgear
D. Parietal pull headgear

111. Camouflage treatment is best avoided in
A. Mild to moderate skeletal class II malocclusions
B. Severe skeletal class III malocclusions
C. Good vertical proportions of the face
D. Patients in the age of growth Modulation

PEDODONTICS

112. The best alternative storage medium for avulsed teeth in case transport media are not available is
A. Milk
B. Water
C. Saline
D. Blood

113. The reasons for maxillary permanent canine impaction could be all EXCEPT

A. Long development period
B. Dubious course in eruption
C. Occupies several developmental positions in succession
D. Asymmetrical development

114. Mentally retarded child will have an intelligence quotient (IQ) in the range of

A. 110–119
B. 80–89
C. 69 and below
D. 140 and up

115. Eruption of first permanent molar causes

A. Early mesial shift
B. Late mesial shift
C. Closure of leeway space
D. None of the above

116. According to Ellis and Dewey classification a fracture of 51 involving dentin and associated loss of vitality is classified as

A. Class 2
B. Class 4
C. Class 8
D. Class 9

117. Recently added in the centre of pediatric treatment triangle is

A. Type of treatment
B. Society
C. Child response
D. Facilities in clinic

118. The most aesthetic and frequently placed crown for primary incisors is

A. Stainless steel crowns
B. Open face stainless steel crowns
C. Prefabricated veneered steel crowns
D. Strip crowns

119. The most accepted cause for late incisor crowding is

A. Late mandibular growth
B. Pressure from third molar
C. Lack of normal attrition
D. Lingual eruption of mandibular Incisors

120. Which terminal plane is favourable for E/E to have class I molar relationship?

A. Flush terminal plane
B. Mesial step
C. Distal step
D. None of the above

121. Grooves, which are present in gum pads between the canine and the first molars and relate the upper and lower gum pads are called

A. Gingival groove
B. Vestibular groove
C. Dental groove
D. Lateral groove

122. "Safety valve" mechanism is

A. The anteroposterior increment in the maxilla at 14 years
B. Increase in the mandibular inter canine width at 14 years
C. Increase in the mandibular height at 12 years
D. Increase in the maxillary inter canine width at 12 years

123. A papoose board is used for immobilization of

A. Whole body
B. Extremities only
C. Head only
D. Jaws only

124. Behavior modification includes all of the following EXCEPT

A. Tell show do
B. Desensitization
C. Modeling
D. HOME

125. Obturation of deciduous tooth can be done with

A. Gutta purcha
B. Iodoform paste
C. Silver points
D. Thermoplastisized gutta percha

126. The distal shoe appliance is used

A. When first primary molar is lost prematurely
B. When second primary molar is lost and first permanent molar has erupted
C. When second primary molar is lost first permanent molar has not erupted
D. When first primary molar is lost and first permanent molar has erupted

P AND SD

127. Prophylactic odontotomy was proposed by

A. Hyatt
B. Cvek
C. Louis Ripa
D. Marthaler

128. Percentage of APF used is

A. 1.23%
B. 12.3%
C. 8%
D. 2%

129. Thylstrup Fejerskov Index Opaque white lines are more pronounced and frequently merge to form small cloudy areas scattered over the whole surface', the score given is

A. 2
B. 4
C. 6
D. 7

130. .... is defined as an organization of member agents having social relation amongst themselves

A. Family
B. Society
C. Community
D. Culture

131. Pulp capping is procedure which comes under which level of prevention

A. Primary
B. Secondary
C. Tertiary
D. Both A and C

132. The procedure where carious tooth tissue is removed by hand instruments, and the cavity is restored with a restorative material that 'sticks' to the tooth is

A. Preventive resin restoration
B. Atraumatic restorative treatment
C. Type 4 restoration
D. Pit and fissure sealants

133. Concentration of Stannous Fluoride used in dental office for topical application

A. 2%
B. 8%
C. 1.23%
D. 0.05%

134. Collection of health information, its use and its transmission to other levels of the health system by non professional health workers is

A. Sentinel surveillance
B. Lay reporting
C. Census
D. Survey

135. All of the following are village level workers under primary health care EXCEPT

A. Village health guide
B. Anganwadi worker
C. Clerks
D. Trained birth attendants

136. The CPITN probe was designed for the detection of

A. Supragingival calculus
B. Debris
C. Subgingival calculus
D. Subgingival stains

137. Practices that have been repeated by a number of generation practices that tend to be followed simply because they have been followed in the past. This refers to

A. Habits
B. Beliefs
C. Customs
D. Convention

138. Who introduced Patient Hygiene Performance index (PHP Index)?

A. Podshadley and Haley
B. Green and vermilion
C. Gruebell
D. Quingley and Hein

139. Equitable distribution, community participation, intersectional coordination and appropriate technology are the principles of

A. Primary health care
B. Social science
C. Primary prevention
D. Epidemiology

140. One sub centre cover

A. 1000 population
B. 2000 population
C. 4000 population
D. 5000 population

141. Proteolysis chelation theory was given by

A. Gottlieb
B. Schwatz and Martin
C. Burch and Jackson
D. Pincus

142. The most commonly occurring value in a distribution of data is

A. Mean
B. Median
C. Mode
D. Range

143. Listing conditions in some order of severity without attempting to define any mathematical relation between categories is

A. Nominal scale
B. Ordinal scale
C. Internal scale
D. Ratio scale

PROSTHODONTICS

144. Epulis fissuratum is

A. Pyogenic granuloma
B. Periapical granuloma
C. Inflammatory fibrous hyperplasia
D. Inflammatory gingival hyperplasia

145. Compared with porcelain teeth, acrylic teeth have all of the following EXCEPT

A. Chemical bond to denture
B. Hard and brittle
C. Minimal abrasion of opposing dentition
D. Silent on contact

146. Bi–zygomatic width divided by 16 gives approximately mesio distal width of

A. Upper central incisor
B. Lower central incisor
C. Upper anterior teeth
D. Lower anterior teeth

147. Tissue conditioners are temporary in nature as

A. They cause trauma to the ridge
B. They become hard after sometime
C. They have to be replaced periodically
D. Both B and C

148. Labially inclined anterior teeth preventing conventional clasp designs may be better implemented with the

A. Snow shoe effect
B. Swing lock concept
C. Boucher's concept
D. Kennedy's concept

149. All of the following are advantage of shoulder finish line EXCEPT

A. Good crown contour
B. Less distortion
C. Provide adequate bulk
D. Superior marginal adaptation

150. Which of the following is an anterior deprogramming device?

A. Herbst appliance
B. Hawleys appliance
C. Lucus Jig
D. Lucia Jig

151. Retromylohyoid curtain is formed by all EXCEPT

A. Superior constrictor
B. Palatoglossus muscle

C. Mylohyoid
D. Masseter

152. The posterior plane of occlusion for most complete denture patient is parallel to
A. Interpupillary line
B. Ala tragus line
C. Cantho tragus line
D. Mandibular plane

153. Uniform reduction of the tooth surface may be ensured by the placement of
A. Pins
B. Depth grooves
C. Ledges
D. Bevels

154. Wax addition instrument is
A. PKT no. 2
B. PKT no. 5
C. PKT no. 4
D. PKT no. 3

155. Mechanical methods to determine vertical dimension are
A. Pre extraction records
B. Ridge relation
C. A and B
D. Phonetics

156. The lever action that occurs in distal extension partial dentures is
A. 1st–order lever
B. 2nd–order lever
C. 3rd–order lever
D. 4th–order lever

157. Major connector should be
A. Able to act as indirect retainer
B. Able to function as direct retainer
C. Rigid to connect bilateral components
D. Able to function as stress breakers

158. Group function occlusion is characterized by
A. Disocclusion of posterior teeth when mandible is protruded
B. Working side contacts from canine to all posterior teeth without balancing side contacts
C. Cuspid rise in protrusion
D. Presence of balancing side contacts

PERIODONTICS

159. Good diabetic control is said to be present when glycosylated hemoglobin is
A. 7.9%
B. >13%
C. 10–12%
D. 3–4%

160. Green stain is caused due to
A. Chromogenic bacteria on enamel cuticle
B. Consumption of beetle leaf for more than 1 year
C. Methyl red
D. Stannous fluoride

161. Grafts taken from and individual of same species as the recepient is known as
A. Autograft
B. Isograft
C. Allograft
D. Xenograft

162. Elastic fiber system present in the lamina propria consists all of these EXCEPT
A. Oxytalan
B. Elastin
C. Elaunin
D. Collagen

163. The following parts of gingiva are keratinized EXCEPT
A. Marginal Gingiva
B. Attached Gingiva
C. Interdental papilla in the anterior teeth
D. Interdental col

164. Reticular fibers found in periodontal ligament consists of
A. Type I
B. Type III
C. Type IV
D. Type XII

165. The predominant immune cell in the initial lesion of gingivitis is

A. B cell
B. T cell
C. PMN
D. Plasma cell

166. Life preserver shaped enlargement of the gingival margin is known as

A. Stillman's clefts
B. Birbeck granules
C. Mc Call festoons
D. None of the above

167. These substances plays a major role in regulating cell–cell and cell–matrix interaction in cementum

A. Sharpey's fibers
B. Intrinsic fibers
C. Proteoglycans
D. Phosphoproteins

168. Which stage of gingivitis is also called subclinical gingivitis?

A. Initial stage
B. Advanced stage
C. Early stage
D. Established stage

169. All these factors affects the height and thickness of facial and lingual bony plates EXCEPT

A. Alignment of teeth
B. Angulation of root to the bone
C. Occlusal forces
D. Mesiodistal angulation of crest of interdental septum

170. Which calcium channel blocker can cause excessive growth of gingival tissues?

A. Cyclosporin
B. Nifedipine
C. Phenytoin
D. Corticosteroid

171. Frequent periodontal abscess appear to be an important periodontal feature in

A. Nutritional deficiency
B. Diabetes Mellitus
C. Hormonal imbalance
D. Cardiovascular diseases

172. Professional misconduct or breach of duty that results in injury or damage to an individual is called

A. Negligence
B. Litigation malpractice
C. Malpractice
D. Punitive damages

173. Tooth mobility is not reversible when there is

A. Inflammation in periodontium
B. Trauma from occlusion
C. Loss of alveolar bone
D. Faulty tooth brushing technique

174. Which of the following cell types contain a vasoactive amine that is released in inflammatory process?

A. Plasma cells
B. Mast cells
C. T–lymphocytes
D. B–lymphocytes

175. Coronoplasty should be carried out in patient with

A. Occlusal prematurities
B. Parafunctional habits
C. Signs of trauma from occlusion
D. All of the above feature

176. "Punched out" craterlike necrosis involving the interdental papillae is a diagnostic feature of

A. Plasma cell gingivitis
B. Granulomatous gingivitis
C. Necrotizing ulcerative gingivitis
D. Periodontitis

177. The ability of different species of plaque microorganisms to adhere to one another is

A. Coaggregation
B. Coexistence
C. Symbiosis
D. Selective absorption

178. Which one of the following associated with periodontal disease may not be imaged on a radiograph?

A. Open contacts
B. Calculus
C. Bacterial plaque
D. Over hanging restorative margins

CONS AND ENDO

179. Fluid flow, in or out of the dentinal tubules is proportional to the tubule diameter by

A. Third power of the diameter
B. Sixth power of the diameter
C. Square of the diameter
D. Fourth power of the diameter

180. In preparing an endodontically treated tooth for receiving a cast post, the minimal amount of gutta–percha to be maintained for proper apical seal is

A. 1 mm
B. 8 mm
C. 4 mm
D. 0 mm

181. In cavity preparation line angle is

A. Union of three surfaces
B. Union of four surfaces
C. The junction of two plane surfaces of different orientation along a line
D. Internal boundary of a cavity

182. Turbid dentin in carious tooth is all EXCEPT

A. Zone of bacterial invasion
B. Zone which cannot be remineralized
C. Zone in which collagen is irreversibly denatured
D. Zone that need not be removed before Restoration

183. In molecular biological methods in Endodontics the process of annealing the complementary bases of two single stranded DNA is known as

A. DNA–DNA micro processing
B. DNA–DNA processing
C. DNA–DNA hybridization
D. DNA–DNA coupling

184. Hedstroem file is an instrument used for

A. Canal enlargement
B. Length determination
C. Obturating with Gutta Percha in Mc Spadden technique
D. Endodontic implants

185. The commonly used acid for etching enamel and dentine is

A. Dilute sulphuric acid
B. Phosphoric acid
C. Concentrated acetic acid
D. 37% hydrochloric acid

186. Minor modifications done in the existing tooth contours to improve a smile is termed

A. Cosmetic contouring
B. Smile contouring
C. Micro dentistry
D. Enamel reshaping

187. Myospasm that is involuntary continuous contraction of a muscle due to overstretching which is already strained because of sustained mouth opening during RCT is

A. Charley horse
B. Erces expand
C. Muscle tear
D. Hardy stretch

188. When removing rubber dam, the first step is to

A. Remove to clamp
B. Release the holder
C. Apply lubricant
D. Cut the interseptal rubber with scissors

189. The most frequently used pin for pin retained amalgam restoration is

A. Cemented pin
B. Self threaded pin
C. Friction lock pin
D. Both cemented and friction lock pins

190. The total number of point angles present for class II amalgam restoration is

A. 4
B. 6
C. 8
D. 11

191. Cavitated caries lesions include all EXCEPT

A. Chalkiness of enamel on walls and base of pit and fissure
B. Brown gray discoloration under enamel adjacent to pit or fissure
C. No radiolucency below occlusal enamel
D. Softening at the base of pit or fissure

ORAL SURGERY

192. Protein concentration of cystic fluid is

A. 1–2 gm/dl
B. 5–11 gm/dl
C. 10–20 gm/dl
D. 0–4 gm/dl

193. In a patient suffering from liver disease the main complication encountered during extraction

A. Syncope
B. Post operative infection
C. Prolonged bleeding
D. Convulsions

194. Which of the following is the weakest part of the orbit?

A. Medial wall
B. Lateral wall
C. Floor of the orbit
D. Roof of the orbit

195. Paresthesia over nasal and upper lip following fractured zygoma is because of involvement of

A. Facial nerve
B. Posterior superior alveolar nerve
C. Infraorbital nerve
D. Mental nerve

196. Use of acrylated arch bars for closed reduction of mandible fractures was described by

A. Schuchardt (1956)
B. Risdon (1929)
C. Stanstout (1943)
D. Leonard (1977)

197. Ecchymosis and hematoma are treated with

A. Intermittent ice pack
B. Continuous ice pack
C. Intermittent hot pack
D. Pressure and pack

198. In the functional neck dissection the following structures are preserved

A. Sternomastoid muscle, spinal accessory nerve and internal jugular vein
B. Sternomastoid muscle, external jugular vein and internal jugular vein
C. Submandibular gland, thoracic duct and facial artery
D. Strap muscles, facial artery and facial vein

199. "Moon face" appearance is seen in

A. Isolated Lefort I fracture
B. Lefort II and Lefort III fractures
C. Mandibular fractures
D. Unilateral zygomatic complex fractures

200. TENS therapy is useful in

A. Myofacial pain dysfunction syndrome
B. Trigeminal neuralgia
C. Facial palsy
D. Neurosis

ANSWERS

HUMAN ANATOMY

1. **Ans: C**

Ref: BD Chaurasia, 1/E, p. 176

2. **Ans: C**

Ref: BD Chaurasia, 1/E, p. 173

3. **Ans: A**

Ref: BD Chaurasia, 1/E, p. 245

4. **Ans: A**

Ref: Inderbir Singh, 8/E, p. 132

5. **Ans: A**

Ref: BD Chaurasia, 1/E, p. 212

Explanation

- The frontal or anterior branch is commonly involved
- The haematoma presses on the motor area giving rise to hemiplegia of the opposite side

6. **Ans: C**

Ref: Inderbir Singh, 8/E, p. 10

Explanation

Pouches	*Derivatives*
First pouch	Pharyngo tympanic tube Middle ear cavity Tympanic antrum
Second pouch	Tonsil Tubotympanic recess
Third pouch	Inferior parathyroid gland Thymus
Fourth pouch	Superior parathyroid glands
Fifth pouch	Para follicular cells of thyroid

7. **Ans: D**

Ref: BD Chaurasia, 1/E, p. 273

Explanation

Nerve supply of tongue

- Motor supply–hypoglossal nerve EXCEPT palatoglossus which is supplied by the cranial root of the accessory nerve through pharyngeal plexus
- Sensory supply–anterior 2/3rd–lingual nerve and taste sensation by chorda tympani

Posterior 1/3rd–glossopharyngeal nerve

Posterior most part vagus nerve.

8. **Ans: B**

Ref: BD Chaurasia, 1/E, p. 273

PHYSIOLOGY

9. **Ans: C**

Ref: Sembulingam, 4/E, p. 210

Explanation

- Secretion of gastric juice by the stimuli arising from head region is called cephalic phase
- During this phase, the gastric secretion occurs even without the presence of food in the stomach

10. **Ans: A**

Ref: Sembulingam, 4/E, p. 790

11. **Ans: A**

Ref: Sembulingam, 4/E, p. 95

12. **Ans: D**

Ref: Sembulingam, 4/E, p. 119 and 121

Group	*Antigen in RBC*	*Antibody in serum*
A	A	Anti B
B	B	Anti A
AB	A and B	No antibody
O	No antigen	Anti A and Anti B
O	–ve is universal donor	
AB	+ve is universal recipient	

BIOCHEMISTRY

13. **Ans: C**

Ref: U. Sathyanarayana, U. Chakrapani, 3/ E, p. 193

14. **Ans: D**

Ref: U. Sathyanarayana, U. Chakrapani, 3/ E, p. 671

15. **Ans: D**

Ref: U. Sathyanarayana, U. Chakrapani, 3/ E, p. 31

Explanation

- The fatty acids that cannot be synthesized by the body and should be supplied in the diet are known as essential fatty acids, chemically, they are PUFA namely linoleic acid and linolenic acid

16. **Ans: A**

Ref: U. Sathyanarayana, U. Chakrapani, 3/ E, p. 147

Explanation

- The conversion of pyruvate to oxaloacetate by biotin dependent pyruvate carboxylase is essential for the synthesis of glucose from many non–carbohydrate sources

17. **Ans: D**

Ref: U. Sathyanarayana, U. Chakrapani, 3/ E, p. 125

Explanation

- Calcitriol along with PTH increases the mobilization of calcium and phosphate from the bone. This causes calcium resorption from bone causing elevation in plasma calcium and phosphate levels

18. **Ans: C**

Ref: U. Sathyanarayana, U. Chakrapani, 3/ E, p. 215

Explanation

- Cholic acid–synthesis of bile acids
- Cholesterol–bile acids, steroid hormones, vitamin D

GENERAL PATHOLOGY

19. **Ans: C**

Ref: Harsh Mohan, 3/E, p. 422

Explanation

- Serum alkaline phosphatase–high
- Serum Ca–normal to high

20. **Ans: B**

Ref: Harsh Mohan, 3/E, p. 223

Explanation

- All infarcts are coagulative necrosis EXCEPT cerebral infarct. The pathognomonic cytologic change of which shows characteristic liquefactive necrosis

21. **Ans: B**

Ref: Harsh Mohan, 3/E, p. 493

22. **Ans: C**

Ref: Robbin's Pathologic Basis of Disease, 7/ E, p. 490 – 491

23. **Ans: D**

Ref: Harsh Mohan, 3/E, p. 32, 31

Explanation

Antioxidants are endogenous or exogenous substance which inactivate the free radicals. They are:

- Vitamins-E, A and C
- Sulfhydryl containing compounds e.g.: cysteine and glutathione
- Serum proteins, e.g.: ceruloplasmin and transferrin
- Enzyme–superoxide dismutase, catalase, glutathione peroxidase

24. **Ans: C**

Ref: Harsh Mohan, 3/E, p. 215

MICROBIOLOGY

25. Ans: C

Ref: Ananthanarayan and Panicker's Text Book of Microbiology, 8/E, p. 78

Explanation

Reduction of virulence is known as attenuation. This can be achieved by:

- Passage through unfavourable hosts
- Repeated cultures in artificial media
- Growth in high temperature
- In the presence of weak antiseptic
- Prolonged storage in culture

26. Ans: B

Ref: Ananthanarayan and Panicker's Text Book of Microbiology, 8/E, p. 539

27. Ans: D

Ref: Ananthanarayan and Panicker's Text Book of Microbiology, 8/E, p. 380

Explanation

- Borrelia vincenti is almost always associated with fusiform bacilli (fuso-bacterium fusiforme)
- This symbiotic, infection is known as fusospirochetosis, e.g.: Vincent's angina

28. Ans: C

Ref: Ananthanarayan and Panicker's Text Book of Microbiology, 8/E, p. 210

Explanation

- In acute glomerulonephritis, the pathogenesis may be due to antigenic cross relations/antibodies formed against streptococci cross react with glomerular basement membrane and result in damage. It is more often an immune complex disease. This is clearly type III hyper sensitivity reaction.

29. Ans: A

Ref: Ananthanarayan and Panicker's Text Book of Microbiology, 8/E, p. 34

30. Ans: A

Ref: Satish Gupte, 8/E, p. 405

31. Ans: B

Ref: Ananthanarayan and Panicker's Text Book of Microbiology, 8/E, p. 16

32. Ans: A

Ref: Ananthanarayan and Panicker's Text Book of Microbiology, 8/E, p. 614

33. Ans: C

Ref: Ananthanarayan and Panicker's Text Book of Microbiology, 8/E, p. 348

Explanation

- They appear as red acid fast bacilli in blue background of pus cells and epithelial cells

PHARMACOLOGY

34. Ans: D

Ref: KD Tripathi, 6/E, p. 799

35. Ans: D

Ref: KD Tripathi, 6/E, p. 137

36. Ans: A

Ref: K D Tripathi, 6/E, p. 646

Explanation

- Ondansetron is a 5 – HT3 antagonist

37. Ans: A

Ref: KD Tripathi, 6/E, p. 224

Explanation

- Dexamethasone–used for inflammatory and allergic conditions – 0.5 – 5 mg/ day orally
- Shock, cerebral edema etc 4–20 mg/day IV/IM
- Also used topically

38. Ans: D

Ref: KD Tripathi, 6/E, p. 28

39. Ans: C

Ref: K D Tripathi, 6/E, p. 487

Explanation

- Prolonged ACE inhibitor therapy, prevents or delays end stage renal disease in type I as well as type II diabetes

40. Ans: A

Ref: K D Tripathi, 6/E, p. 190, 191

Explanation

- By inhibiting platelet aggregation aspirin lowers the incidence of reinfarction. TXA2 synthesis in platelets is inhibited at low doses

41. Ans: A

Ref: KD Tripathi, 6/E, p. 714

GENERAL MEDICINE

42. Ans: D

Ref: Davidson, 20/E, p. 558

43. Ans: B

Ref: Davidson, 20/E, p. 1202

Explanation

Stroke risk factors:

Modifiable

- High blood pressure
- Heart disease (atrial fibrillation, heart failure, endocarditis)
- Diabetes mellitus
- Hyperlipidaemia
- Smoking
- Excess alcohol consumption
- Polycythaemia
- Oral contraceptives
- Social deprivation

44. Ans: B

Ref: Davidson, 20/E, p. 121

45. Ans: D

Ref: Davidson, 20/E, p. 1007

46. Ans: D

Ref: Davidson, 20/E, p. 467

Explanation

Risk factors for urinary tract infection

Incomplete bladder emptying

- Bladder outflow obstruction
- Neurological problems (e.g. multiple sclerosis, diabetic neuropathy)
- Gynaecological abnormalities (e.g. uterine prolapse)
- Vesico – ureteric reflux

Foreign bodies:

- Urethral catheter or ureteric stent.

Loss of host defences:

- Atrophic urethritis and vaginitis in post – menopausal women
- Diabetes mellitus

47. Ans: D

Ref: Davidson, 20/E, p. 663

Explanation

Causes of haemoptysis

Bronchial disease

- Carcinoma*
- Bronchial adenoma
- Bronchiectasis*
- Acute bronchitis*
- Foreign body

Parenchymal disease

- Tuberculosis *
- Trauma
- Suppurative pneumonia
- Actinomycosis
- Lung abscess
- Mycetoma
- Parasites (e. g. hydatid disease, flukes)

Lung vascular disease

- Pulmonary infarction *
- Indiopathic pulmonary
- Polyarteritis nodosa
- Haemosiderosis
- Goodpasture's syndrome

Cardiovascular disease:

- Acute left ventricular failure *
- Mitral stenosis
- Aortic aneurysm

Blood disorders:

- Leukaemia
- Anticoagulants
- Haemophilia

* More common causes

48. Ans: B

Ref: Davidson, 20/E, p. 1163

49. Ans: A

Ref: Davidson, 20/E, p. 679

50. Ans: D

Ref: Davidson, 20/E, p. 677

Explanation

Immediate assessment of acute severe

Acute severe asthma

- PEF 33–50% predicted (< 200 I / min)
- Respiratory rate – 25/min
- Heart rate – 110/min
- Inability to complete sentences in 1 breath

GENERAL SURGERY

51. Ans: A

Ref: S. Das, 5/E, p. 655

52. Ans: C

Ref: S. Das, 5/E, p. 653

53. Ans: D

Ref: S. Das, 5/E, p. 588

Explanation

- Carcinoma tongue is most common in the anterior
- 2/3 of the tongue near the edges

54. Ans: C

Ref: S. Das, 5/E, p. 626

55. Ans: D

Ref: S. Das, 5/E, p. 9

Explanation

- It is a haemorrhagic shock caused due to sudden loss of blood volume or loss of fluid from the vascular space

56. Ans: D

Ref: S. Das, 5/E, p. 6

Explanation

- Protein depletion causes impairment of granulation tissue and collagen formation Thereby impaired wound healing
- Excess corticosteroid administration inhibits granulation tissue formation

57. Ans: B

Ref: S. Das, 5/E, p. 224

DENTAL MATERIALS

58. Ans: B

Ref: Phillips, 11/E, p. 633

Explanation

- The effects associated with cold working, e.g. strain hardening, decreased ductility and distorted grains – can be reversed simply by heating the metal to an appropriate elevated temperature. This process is called annealing
- The more severe the degree of cold working, the more rapidly the effects can be reversed by annealing
- 3 stages of annealing:
  1. Recovery
  2. Crystallization
  3. Grain growth

59. Ans: B

Ref: Phillips, 11/E, p. 599

60. Ans: D

Ref: Phillips, 11/E, p. 370

61. **Ans: A**

Ref: Phillips, 11/E, p. 581

Explanation

- Adding less than 1% of oxide forming elements such as iron, indium and tin to high gold contact alloy , the porcelain metal bond strength improves

62. **Ans: D**

Ref: Phillips, 11/E, p. 215

63. **Ans: B**

Ref: Phillips, 11/E, p. 342

64. **Ans: C**

Ref: Phillips, 11/E, p. 257

Explanation

- The differences between α and β hemi-hydrates are a result of differences in crystal size, surface area and degree of lattice perfection
- α–form/dental plaster – large form consisting of large irregularly shaped orthorhombic crystal particles with capillary pores
- β–form/dental stone–smaller regularly shaped crystalline particles in the form of rods or prisms

65. **Ans: D**

Ref: Phillips, 11/E, p. 608

Explanation

- Brazing requires a heating temperature above 450°C/840°F

66. **Ans: C**

Ref: Phillips, 11/E, p. 158

Explanation

Stages in polymerization

- Induction – activation of free radicals which in turn initiate growing polymer chains
- Propagation – stage of polymerization during which polymer chains continue to grow to high molecular weights
- Chain transfer – a stage of polymerization in which the growing end of a chain is transferred to another molecule, initiating further chain growth
- Termination – stage of polymerization were polymer chains cease to grow

67. **Ans: B**

Ref: Phillips, 11/E, p. 407

68. **Ans: D**

Ref: Phillips, 11/E, p. 571

69. **Ans: B**

Ref: Phillips, 11/E, p. 98

70. **Ans: D**

Ref: Phillips, 11/E, p. 524

DADH

71. **Ans: C**

Ref: Wheeler's, 8/E, p. 13

72. **Ans: A**

Ref: Orban's, 12/E, p. 221

ORAL PATHOLOGY AND ORAL MEDICINE

73. **Ans: C**

Ref: Burkit, 11/E, p.133

74. **Ans: C**

Ref: Shafer's, 6/E, p.543

75. **Ans: C**

Ref: A Practical Guide to Hospital Dentistry, K. George Varghese, 1/E, 150

Explanation

Eagleton's Criteria

- Known site of injection
- Evidence of blood stream injection
- Early signs of venous obstruction in the retina, conjunctiva or eyelid

- Paresis of 3rd, 4th and 6th cranial nerves
- Abscess formation in the neighbouring tissue
- Evidence of meningeal irritation

76. Ans: D

Ref: Shafer's, 6/E, p. 803

Explanation

- Although there seems to be a slightly higher incidence of oral squamous cell carcinoma in patient with oral lichen planus than in general population. The actual overall frequency of malignant transformation is very low (0.3 – 3%)

77. Ans: B

Ref: Shafer's, 6/E, p. 497

78. Ans: B

Ref: Shafer's, 6/E, p. 585

79. Ans: A

Ref: Shafer's, 6/E, p. 100

80. Ans: A

Ref: Shafer's, 6/E, p. 247

81. Ans: B

Ref: Shafer's, 6/E, p. 593

82. Ans: D

Ref: Shafer's, 6/E, p. 268

Explanation

- Islands of squamous epithelium which have developed from Odontogenic rests of Malassez can be found in a periapical granuloma without cystic transformation endodontists refer to these granulomas as "bay cyst"

83. Ans: D

Ref: Shafer's, 6/E, p. 154

84. Ans: D

Ref: Shafer's, 6/E, p. 88

85. Ans: C

Ref: Shafer's, 6/E, p. 323

Explanation

- Chancre of tongue is seen in primary Syphilis
- Tertiary syphilis–Gumma

86. Ans: A

Ref: Shafer's, 6/E, p. 714

87. Ans: D

Ref: Shafer's, 6/E, p. 717

88. Ans: D

Ref: Shafer's 6/E p. 292

89. Ans: B

Ref: Shafer's, 6/E, p. 255

90. Ans: D

Ref: Shafer's, 6/E, p. 651

91. Ans: C

Ref: Shafer's, 6/E, p. 80

92. Ans: B

Ref: Shafer's, 6/E, p. 268

93. Ans: B

Ref: Shafer's, 6/E, p. 713

94. Ans: A

Ref: Shafer's, 6/E, p. 21

Explanation

- Melkerson Rosenthal syndrome – chelitis with facial palsy and plicated tongue

95. Ans: C

Ref: Shafer's, 6/E, p. 818

96. Ans: A

Ref: Shafer's, 6/E, p. 818

97. Ans: A

Ref: Shafer's, 6/E, p. 492

ORAL RADIOLOGY

98. **Ans: C**

Ref: White & Pharoah, 6/E, p. 19

99. **Ans: B**

Ref: Karjodkar, 2/E, p. 73

100. **Ans:**

Ref: White & Pharoah, 6/E, p. 414

ORTHODONTICS

101. **Ans: A**

Ref: Bhalaji, 3/E, p. 397

102. **Ans: B**

Ref: Bhalaji, 3/E, p. 104

Explanation

Mouth breathing may be classified as

1. Anatomic
2. Obstructive
   - i. Short upper lip
   - ii. Deviated nasal septum
   - iii. Nasal polyps
   - iv. Chronic inflammation of nasal mucosa
   - v. Localized benign tumours
   - vi. Allergic reaction of nasal turbinates
   - vii. Allergic reaction of nasal mucosa
   - viii. Obstructive adenoids

103. **Ans: A**

Ref: Gurkeerat Singh, 2/E, p. 568

104. **Ans: D**

Ref: Profit, 4/E, p. 103

105. **Ans: C**

Ref: Bhalaji, 3/E, p. 289

Explanation

- Flexibility of spring to a large extent, depends on the diameter of the wire used $F \alpha D^4/L^3$

106. **Ans: C**

Ref: Bhalaji, 3/E, p. 433

107. **Ans: D**

Ref: Bhalaji, 3/E, p. 202

Explanation

- Interrupted forces of approx 200–300 gms, for 10–14 hours a day

108. **Ans: D**

Ref: Bhalaji, 3/E, p. 437

109. **Ans: A**

Ref: Profit, 4/E, p. 45, 46

110. **Ans: B**

Ref: Bhalaji, 3/E, p. 371

111. **Ans: B**

Ref: Bhalaji, 3/E, p. 402

PEDODONTICS

112. **Ans: A**

Ref: Shobha Tandon, 2/E, p. 598

113. **Ans: D**

Ref: Mc Donald, 8/E, p. 663

114. **Ans: B**

Ref: Shobha Tandon, 1/E, p. 538

115. **Ans: B**

Ref: Shobha Tandon 1/E, p. 114

Explanation

- Early mesial shift – due to eruptive force of permanent molars
- Late mesial shift – due to exfoliation of primary molars and mesial migration of permanent molars

116. **Ans: D**

Ref: Shobha Tandon, 1/E, p. 500

Explanation

- Ellis class 9 is fracture of deciduous teeth

117. Ans: B

Ref: Shobha Tandon, 2/E, p. 5

118. Ans: D

Ref: Pinkham, 4/E, p. 366

119. Ans: A

Ref: Shobha Tandon, 1/E, p. 116

120. Ans: B

Ref: Shobha Tandon, 1/E, p. 11, 113

Explanation

Primary	*Permanent*
Flush terminal plane	End to end
Mesial step	Class I, Class III
Distal step	Class II

121. Ans: D

Ref: Shobha Tandon, 1/E, p. 53

Explanation

- Gingival groove – separates the gum pad from the palate
- Transverse groove – divides each gum pad into 10 segments
- Lateral sulcus – is a deepened groove separating the canine and deciduous first molar segments

122. Ans: D

Ref: Orthodontics Preparation Manual for Undergraduates, 1/E, Kumar, p. 10

123. Ans: A

Ref: Shobha Tandon, 1/E, p. 152

Explanation

Passive restraint, i.e. with the aid of restraining device can be classified as

For body	*Pedi wrap*
	Papoose board sheets
	Beanbag with straps
	Towel and tapes
For extremities	Velcro straps
	Posey straps
	Towel and drapes
For the head	Head positioner
	Forearm body support
Mouth	Mouth blocks
	Banded tongue blades
	Mouth props

124. Ans: D

Ref: Shobha Tandon, 1/E, p. 151

Explanation

- This is an aversive conditioning technique for a child who displays a negative behavior and does not respond to moderate behavior modification

125. Ans: B

Ref: Shobha Tandon, 1/E, p. 354

126. Ans: C

Ref: Shobha Tandon, 2/E, p. 459

P AND SD

127. Ans: A

Ref: Soben Peter, 3/E, p. 368

128. Ans: A

Ref: Soben Peter, 3/E, p. 302

129. Ans: A

Ref: Soben Peter, 3/E, p. 209

Explanation

- Fluorosis index developed by Thylstrup A-Fejerskov O in 1978
- To assess prevalence and severity of dental fluorosis original criteria – scoring

Score	Criteria
0	Normal translucency of enamel remains after prolonged air drying
1	Narrow white lines located corresponding to the perikymata
2	Smooth surfaces

130. Ans: B

Ref: Park, 20/E, p. 583

Explanation

- *Family* – is a group individuals who are biologically related and living together and in a common kitchen
- *Community* – a group of people living in a contiguous geographic area, having centres of interest and functioning together in the chief concerns of life
- *Culture* – may be defined as a shared and organized body of customs, skills and ideas and values which is transmitted socially from one generation to another

131. Ans: B

Ref: Soben Peter, 3/E, p. 253

132. Ans: B

Ref: Soben Peter, 3/E, p. 390

Explanation

- ART was pioneered in the mid 1980s in Tanzania

133. Ans: B

Ref: Soben Peter, 3/E, p. 304

134. Ans: B

Ref: Soben Peter, 20/E, p. 304

Explanation

- Sentinel Surveillance is a method for identifying the missing cases of infection or disease

135. Ans: C

Ref: Park, 20/E, p. 802,803

136. Ans: C

Ref: Soben Peter, 3/E, p. 169

137. Ans: C

Ref: Park, 20/E, p.584

138. Ans: A

Ref: Soben Peter, 3/E, p. 135

139. Ans: A

Ref: Park, 20/E, p.792 - 793

140. Ans: D

Ref: Soben Peter, 3/E, p. 724

141. Ans:B

Ref: Soben Peter, 3/E, p. 238

142. Ans:C

Ref: Park, 20/E, p. 750

143. Ans: A

Ref: Biostatistics for oral health care, 1/E, p. 7

PROSTHODONTICS

144. Ans: C

Ref: Nallaswamy, 1/E, p. 41

145. Ans: B

Ref: Nallaswamy, 1/E, p. 440

146. Ans: A

Ref: Nallaswamy, 1/E, p. 171

147. Ans: D

Ref: Nallaswamy, 1/E, p. 224

148. Ans: B

Ref: Nallaswamy, 1/E, p. 449

149. Ans: D

Ref: Schillinburg , 3/E, p. 130

150. **Ans: D**

Ref: Rosensteil, 4/E, p. 56

Explanation

- Anterior deprogramming is the process of getting the temporomandibular joint into a relaxed or comfortable neuromuscular position (Centric relation) by interupting or negating the proprioceptors surrounding the teeth in the periodontal ligament
- *It* is accomplished in 10–15 mins by interposing something between the anterior teeth like leaf guage, Lucia jig or sliding guide

151. **Ans: D**

Ref: Nallaswamy, 1/E, p. 57

152. **Ans: B**

Ref: Nallaswamy, 1/E, p. 207

Explanation

- It is also called as Camper's line or Bromer's line

153. **Ans: B**

Ref: Nallaswamy, 1/E, p. 576

154. **Ans: A**

Ref: Rosensteil, 4/E, p. 562

Explanation

- PKT instruments are designed by the Dr. Peter K. Thomas
- No.1 and No.2 are wax addition instruments
- No. 3 is a burnisher for refining occlusal anatomy
- No. 4 and No. 5 are wax carvers

155. **Ans: C**

Ref: Nallaswamy, 1/E, p. 132, 133

156. **Ans: A**

Ref: Nallaswamy, 1/E, p. 382

157. **Ans: C**

Ref: Nallaswamy, 1/E, p. 327

158. **Ans: B**

Ref: Nallaswamy, 1/E, p. 532

PERIODONTICS

159. **Ans: D**

Ref: Carranza, 10/E, p. 657

160. **Ans: A**

Ref: Gururaja Rao, 2/E, p. 143

161. **Ans: C**

Ref: Carranza, 10/E, p. 978

162. **Ans: D**

Ref: Carranza, 10/E, p. 57

163. **Ans: D**

Ref: Carranza, 10/E, p. 47

164. **Ans: B**

Ref: Carranza, 10/E, p. 69

Explanation

The principal fibers	Type I collagen
Reticular fibers	Type IV collagen

165. **Ans: C**

Ref: Carranza, 10/E, p. 356

Explanation

Stage I gingivitis

- Initial lesion
- PMNs

Stage III gingivitis

- Established lesion
- Plasma cells and Lymphocytes

166. **Ans: C**

Ref: Carranza, 10/E, p. 370

Explanation

- Stillman's cleft narrow triangular shaped gingival recession

- Mc call's festoon – rolled, thickened band of gingiva usually seen adjacent to the cuspids when recession approaches the mucogingival junction

167. Ans: C

Ref: Carranza, 10/E, p. 75

168. Ans: A

Ref: Carranza, 10/E, p. 356

169. Ans: D

Ref: Carranza, 10/E, p. 83

170. Ans: B

Ref: Carranza, 10/E, p. 378

Explanation

Drugs causing gingival enlargement

1. *Anticonvulsants:* Phenytoin, ehtotoin, mephenytoin
2. *Immunosuppressants:* Ethosuximide, cyclosporine, Tacrolimus
3. *Ca channel blockers:* Nifedipine, diltiazem, felodipine verapamil

171. Ans: B

Ref: Carranza, 10/E, p. 714

172. Ans: C

Ref: Carranza, 10/E, p. 1222

173. Ans: C

Ref: Carranza, 10/E, p. 622

Explanation

- The likelihood of restoring tooth stability is inversely proportional to the extent to which mobility is caused by loss of supporting alveolar bone

174. Ans: B

Ref: Carranza, 10/E, p. 212

175. Ans: C

Ref: Carranza, 10/E, p. 853

176. Ans: C

Ref: Carranza, 10/E, p. 391

177. Ans: A

Ref: Carranza, 10/E, p. 141

Explanation

- Coaggregation is a cell to cell recognition of genetically distinct partner cell types
- *For example:* Fusobacterium nucleatam with S. sanguis prevotella loeschi with actinomyces viscosus capnocytophaga ochraceus with A. viscosus

178. Ans: C

Ref: Carranza, 10/E, p. 137

CONS AND ENDO

179. An: D

Ref: : Sturdevant's, 4/E, p.172

180. Ans: C

Ref: Ingle, 6/E, p. 1450

181. Ans: C

Ref: Sturdevant's, 5/E, p. 293

182. Ans: D

Ref: Sturdevant's 5/E, p. 101

Explanation

- Turbid dentin is the zone of bacterial invasion and is marked by widening and distortion of the dentinal tubules, which are filled with bacteria
- This zone cannot be remineralized and must be removed before restoration

Zones of dentinal caries

- Zone 1 – Normal dentin
- Zone 2 – Sub transparent dentin
- Zone 3 – transparent dentin
- Zone 4 – Turbid dentin
- Zone 5 – Infected dentin.

183. Ans: C

Ref: Ingle, 6/E, p. 233

184. **Ans: A**

Ref: Grossman,12/E, p. 230

185. **Ans:B**

Ref: : Sturdevant's 5/E, p. 248

186. **Ans: A**

Ref: Sturdavent 5/E, p. 626

187. **Ans: A**

Ref: Ingle, 6/E, p. 444

188. **Ans: C**

Ref: : Sturdevant's 5/E, p. 479

189. **Ans: B**

Ref: Sturdavent 5/E, p. 815

190. **Ans: B**

Ref: Sturdevant's 5/E, p. 297

191. **Ans: B**

Ref: Sturdevant's, 5/E, p. 290

ORAL SURGERY

192. **Ans: B**

Ref: Synopsis of Oral & maxilla facial surgery by ghosh, p. 57

193. **Ans: C**

Ref: Neelima Malik, 2/E, p. 14

194. **Ans: A**

Ref: Killey's 5/E, p. 9

195. **Ans: C**

Ref: Killey's 5/E, p. 37

196. **Ans: A**

Ref: Rowe and Williams ,vol I, p.253

197. **Ans: A**

Ref: Neelima Malik, 2/E, p. 319

Explanation

- Application of ice pack prevents further extravasation of blood

198. **Ans: A**

Ref: Neelima Malik, 2/E, p. 738

199. **Ans: B**

Ref: Neelima Malik, 2/E, p. 356

200. **Ans: A**

Ref: Neelima Malik, 2/E, p. 249

Explanation

- *Transcutaneous electronic nerve Stimulator (TENS):* Interferes with sensation of pain in the brain and increases blood flow to the site

8

KCET 2010

HUMAN ANATOMY

1. The joint between the atlas and axis is

A. Synovial
B. Closely related to the first cervical nerves
C. Allow rotation of the head
D. Supported by the alar ligaments

2. All the cranial nerves provide innervations for the structures in the head and neck except one, that additionally supplies the thorax and abdomen

A. Glossopharyngeal
B. Spinal accessory
C. Vagus
D. Hypoglossal

3. Hypoglossal nerve is

A. Purely sensory
B. Purely motor
C. Mixed
D. Spinal nerve

4. At which stage congenital defects are more pronounced, especially when certain teratogenic agents interfere during the development of embryo?

A. 4 to 8 weeks
B. initiation stage–before 4th week
C. 5th to 6th month of intrauterine life
D. All the above said phases

5. The maxillary sinus drains into

A. Middle meatus
B. Inferior meatus
C. Superior meatus
D. Spheno ethmoidal recess

6. Meckel's cartilage is derived from the

A. 1st Branchial arch
B. 2nd Branchial arch
C. 3rd Branchial arch
D. 4th Branchial arch

PHYSIOLOGY

7. .... is an example for rapidly acting neurotransmitter

A. Somatostatin
B. Calcitonin
C. Substance P
D. Glycine

8. The fluid mosaic model of membrane structure was proposed by

A. Watson and Crick
B. Edward Angle
C. G.V. Black
D. Singer and Nicholson

9. The vitamin k–dependent proteins C and characterized by their ability to inactivate factor

A. VIII a and V a
B. VIII a
C. V a
D. None of the above

10. When P-R interval in a bipolar limb lead Electrocardiograph prolongs beyond 0.20 seconds the patient has

A. Third degree complete block
B. First degree complete block
C. First degree incomplete block
D. Second degree incomplete block

11. The contribution of operation of sodium potassium electrogenic pump for the development of net-90 millivolt of resting membrane potential is

A. –4 millivolt
B. –80 millivolt
C. –70 millivolt
D. +4 millivolt

BIOCHEMISTRY

12. Deficiency of which vitamin causes megaloblastic anemia?

A. Vitamin B-6
B. Vitamin B-12
C. Vitamin K
D. Vitamin D

13. The total number of ATP molecules that are generated per mol of glucose under aerobic conditions is

A. 38
B. 2
C. 36
D. 40

14. "Von Gierke's" disease, a type of glycogen storage disease is caused due to the deficiency of the enzyme

A. Glycogen synthase
B. Glucose 6-phosphatase
C. Muscle phosphorylase
D. cAMP–dependent proteinkinase A

15. The main pathway for "De-Novo" synthesis of fatty acids occurs in

A. Mitochondria
B. Nucleus
C. Cytosol
D. None of the above

GENERAL PATHOLOGY

16. Rodent ulcer is

A. Squamous cell carcinoma
B. Malignant melanoma
C. Sebborhic wart
D. Basal cell carcinoma

17. The major enzyme responsible for oxidative killing mechanism in neutrophils is

A. Antioxidant
B. Lysozyme
C. Hypochloric acid
D. Superoxide

18. Which cells form the myelin sheath in the CNS?

A. Astrocytes
B. Oligodendrocytes
C. Microglia
D. Schwann cells

19. The necrotic tissue and deposits of immune complexes, complement and plasma protein produce a smudgy eosinophilic deposit is termed as

A. Coagulative necrosis
B. Fibrinoid necrosis
C. Caseous necrosis
D. Fatty necrosis

20. The degradation of P53 through ubiquitous–dependent proteolysis by the binding of high-risk HPV protein is

A. E6 and E7
B. E7
C. E6
D. E6, E7 and E8

21. Which of the following cytokines cause bone resorption?

A. IL-1
B. IL-8
C. IFN-gamma
D. IL-4

22. Which of the following influences the ability of osteoclast to resorb bone matrix?

A. Cathepsin K and carbonic anhydrase
B. Alkaline phosphatase
C. Both of the above
D. Matrix metalloproteinase

MICROBIOLOGY

23. Botryomycosis is a .... disease

A. Fungal
B. Bacterial
C. Viral
D. Parasitic

24. Agglutination test for the diagnosis of infectious mononucleosis

A. Widal test
B. Paul Bunnel test
C. Coomb's test
D. Weil Felix test

25. Negative phase is seen in .... immunity

A. Active
B. Passive
C. Herd
D. Local

26. Following are the characteristics of Cryptococcus neoformans EXCEPT

A. Noncapsulated fungus infecting man
B. Causes meningitis
C. Melanin production related to virulence
D. Basidiomycetes yeast

27. The yeast which shows thick gelatinous capsule and positive for mucicarmine is

A. Cryptococcus neoformans
B. Histoplasmosis
C. Blastomycosis
D. Paracoccidiomycosis

PHARMACOLOGY

28. Which of the following is preferred in an elderly women having macrocytic anaemia with early signs of neurological deficit?

A. Folic acid
B. Hydroxycobalamine
C. Erythropoietin
D. Iron dextran

29. Each of the following statement is correct about Metronidazole except that it

A. Is a broad spectrum antiprotozoal drug
B. Active against bacteroides and clostridium
C. An effective alternative for infection caused by aerobic gram positive cocci
D. May cause peripheral neuropathy on prolonged use

30. Which of the following local anaesthetics is active topically?

A. Lidocaine and benzocaine
B. Lidocaine and mepivacaine
C. Mepivacaine and benzocaine
D. Prilocaine and mepivacaine

31. All of the following drugs reduce the gastric acid secretion EXCEPT

A. Ranitidine
B. Sucralfate
C. Misopristal
D. Pantoprazole

32. The beneficial effect of drug neostigmine in the treatment of myasthenia gravis is due to the action

A. It produces more acetylcholine
B. It inhibits the action of cholinesterase
C. It produces more acetylcholine receptors
D. It increases the action of cholinesterase

33. All of the following statements about ketorolac are incorrect EXCEPT

A. An effective analgesic for mild to moderate post operative dental pain
B. Like morphine it interacts with opiod receptors
C. Administered only by intravenous route
D. Safe even in chronic use

GENERAL MEDICINE

34. Risk factors of tuberculosis includes

A. HIV
B. Type I diabetes mellitus
C. Chronic renal failure
D. All of the above

35. Factors precipitating hepatic encephalopathy include all EXCEPT

A. Infection
B. Magnesium trisilicate therapy

C. Hypokalaemia
D. Gastrointestinal bleeding

36. The beneficial effect of oxygen therapy in histotoxic hypoxia is about
A. 0%
B. 50%
C. 100%
D. 30%

37. Nephrotic syndrome is characterized by
A. proteinuria
B. Oedema
C. Serum albumin <30 gm/L
D. All of the above

38. Differential diagnosis of stroke include all EXCEPT
A. Cerebral tumors
B. Subdural hematoma
C. Myocardial infarction
D. Encephalitis

39. Serum alkaline phosphatase levels is found to increase in
A. Fibrous dysplasia
B. Ossifying fibroma
C. Paget's disease
D. None of the above

40. Infective endocarditis is caused by
A. Bacteria
B. Fungi
C. Virus
D. Both A and B

41. A 30 year old patient developed high fever of sudden onset. Peripheral blood smear showed crescent shaped gametocytes. Malaria pigment was dark brown in colour. Which of the following malarial parasites is the causative agent?
A. Plasmodium vivax
B. Plasmodium malariae
C. Plasmodium falciparum
D. Plasmodium ovale

GENERAL SURGERY

42. Collar stud abscess occurs in
A. Cervical TB lymphadenitis
B. Peri tonsillar abscess
C. Pyogenic lymphadenitis
D. Retro pharyngeal abscess

43. The following are true of primary thyrotoxicosis EXCEPT
A. Tremors
B. Warm extremities
C. Diarrhoea
D. Intolerance to cold

44. An antibioma is
A. A powerful antibiotic
B. An antibiotic contaminant
C. A malignant tumour caused by an abscess
D. An excess mass of fibrous tissue around an abscess, persistently treated by excessive or partly sterilized antibiotic

45. Secondary hemorrhage occurs
A. Within 6 hours after surgery
B. 7 to 14 days after surgery
C. As a result of violent recovery after operation
D. Due to blood transfusion line being Discontinued

46. Rule of nine is used in burns for estimation of
A. Fluid required
B. Surface area effected
C. Infection
D. Area to graft

47. Addison's disease is caused by
A. Tuberculosis
B. HIV
C. Metastatic carcinomas
D. All of the above

48. Commonest thyroid carcinoma is
A. Papillary
B. Follicular
C. Medullary
D. Anaplastic

49. **Which of the following will cause post operative hemorrhage?**
   A. Salicylates
   B. Liver cirrhosis
   C. Prolonged antibiotic administration
   D. All of the above

DENTAL MATERIALS

50. **Ability of a material to elicit an appropriate biological response in a given application in the body is called**
   A. Biocompatibility
   B. Biointegration
   C. Antigen-antibody reaction
   D. Sensitization

51. **The process wherein two or more chemically different monomers, each with some desirable property, can be combined to yield specific physical properties of a polymer is known as**
   A. Step-growth polymerization
   B. Addition polymerization
   C. Condensation polymerization
   D. Copolymerization

52. **The forces that hold atoms together are called**
   A. Primary forces
   B. secondary forces
   C. Cohesive forces
   D. Ionic forces

53. **The simplest alloy is a**
   A. Solid solution
   B. Eutectic alloy
   C. Peritectic alloy
   D. Ternary alloy

54. **The first commercially available castable ceramic material for dental use is**
   A. Dicor
   B. IPS empress
   C. In-ceram
   D. Captek

55. **High copper amalgam can be produced**
   A. From smooth atomized particles
   B. From irregular and spherical particles
   C. From lathe cut particles
   D. From traditional alloy particles

56. **BIS-GMA in composites**
   A. Replaced strontium filler particles
   B. Replaced acid soluble glass particles
   C. Replaced silane coupling agents
   D. Replaced methacrylate based matrix

57. **The strength of gypsum products is generally expressed in terms of**
   A. Tensile strength
   B. Wet strength
   C. Green strength
   D. Compressive strength

58. **Slow or soft start polymerization is seen in**
   A. LED light cure units
   B. Laser light cure units
   C. Quartz-Tungsten-Halogen light cure units
   D. PAC light cure units

59. **One bottle system of adhesive resins**
   A. 4th generation bonding agents
   B. Separate etching step not required
   C. Separate etching step is still required
   D. Contains only primer

60. **Delayed expansion is associated with**
   A. Zinc in the amalgam
   B. Low copper amalgam
   C. High copper amalgam
   D. Mercury in the amalgam

61. **Greening occurring when porcelains are fired on silver free alloys may be attributed to**
   A. Vaporization of silver from the walls of contaminated furnaces
   B. Surface diffusion of silver from the marginal metal
   C. More rapid silver diffusion in sodium containing glass
   D. Silver ionization by porcelains with high oxygen potential

62. The most commonly used titanium implant products are

A. Pure Ti
B. Ti-6A L-4V
C. Ti-6A L-4V ELI(Extra low interstitial)
D. All of the above

63. The ranking of tear strength from the lowest top highest of all impression materials generally is as follows

A. Hydrocolloids, silicones, polyether, polysulphide
B. Silicones, hydrocolloids, polyether, polysulphide
C. Polysulphide, hydrocolloids, silicones, polyether
D. Hydrocolloids, polyether, silicones, Polysulphide

64. The ideal temperature for water bath for softening fluid wax is about

A. 51 to 54 degree F
B. 51 to 54 degree C
C. 70 to 75 degree F
D. 70 to 75 degree C

65. Which of the following wires possess 'shape memory' characteristics?

A. Stainless steel
B. Elgiloy
C. Nickel titanium
D. Gold wire

DADH

66. Orifice of the parotid duct opens opposite

A. Upper third molar
B. Upper 2nd molar
C. Lower 2nd molar
D. Lower incisor

67. Gestation period consists of the following EXCEPT

A. Germinal period
B. Embryonic period
C. Fertilization period
D. Foetal period

68. Intermediate cementum is

A. Highly defined cellular zone near cemento dentinal junction
B. Highly defined fibrillar zone near cemento dentinal junction
C. Poorly defined zone near cemento dentinal junction
D. Both A and B

69. The functions of myoepithelial cells may be

A. Initiating contraction
B. Support for the end piece during active secretion of saliva
C. Provide signals to the acinar secretory cells for structural organization
D. All of the above

70. Which of the listed tooth has got four major cusps?

A. Mandibular molar
B. Maxillary 1st molar
C. Maxillary 2nd molar
D. Mandibular 2nd premolar

ORAL PATHOLOGY AND ORAL MEDICINE

71. MCS classification is done for

A. Oncology
B. Medical risk assessment
C. Major salivary glands
D. Mentally challenged subjects

72. SOAP note refers to

A. Confidentiality of patient record
B. Classification of patient
C. Informed consent
D. Classification of problem

73. The most serious complication which can occur following surgery in maxillary incisor region is

A. Iritis
B. Cellulitis
C. Periapical abscess
D. Cavernous sinus thrombosis

74. The first sign of tetanus is

A. Dysphagia
B. Neck stiffness
C. Back pain
D. Trismus

75. Café au lait macules are seen in

A. Von recklinghausen's neurofibromatosis
B. Albright's syndrome and Bloom's syndrome
C. All of the above
D. None of the above.

76. Blue sclera is a feature of

A. Osteogenesis imperfecta
B. Osteopetrosis
C. Paget's disease
D. Hyperparathyroidism

77. Lupus vulgaris is

A. Generalized collagen disease
B. A local collagen disease of the face
C. Syphilitic lesion on the face
D. Tuberculosis lesion (skin) on the face

78. The treatment of tic doloureux include

A. Trichloroethylene administration in all patients
B. Dilantin sodium administration in all patients
C. Carbamazepine administration in all patients
D. Mandibular nerve block in all patients

79. Which of the following is a virus induced epithelial hyperplasia?

A. Molluscum contagiosum
B. Focal epithelial hyperplasia
C. Squamous papilloma
D. All of the above

80. Eagle syndrome is associated with

A. Elongation of stylohyoid ligament
B. Cysts along the mid palatal raphe
C. Exostosis of mandible /palate
D. None of the above

81. Morphological types of supernumerary teeth is/are

A. Conical
B. Supplemental
C. Odontome
D. All of the above

82. Which of the following is a potentially malignant disorder?

A. Leukoplakia
B. Leukoedema
C. Leukokeratosis nicotina palati
D. Papillary atrophy of tongue

83. Bechet's syndrome is characterized by

A. Recurrent oral aphthous and genital ulcers
B. Eye and skin lesions
C. All of the above
D. None of the above

84. James Ramsay Hunt syndrome is a feature of

A. Syphilis
B. Mumps
C. Herpes zoster
D. Chicken pox

85. Ludwig's Angina is usually caused by

A. Streptococci and various mixed anerobes
B. Anaerobic infection by prevotella and fusobacterium
C. Paramyxo virus
D. Candida species

86. Syndromes associated with jaundice include all except

A. Gilbert's syndrome
B. Dubin-Johnson syndrome
C. Gardner's syndrome
D. Rotor's syndrome

87. Snail track ulcers are seen in

A. Primary syphilis
B. Secondary syphilis
C. Latent syphilis
D. Tertiary syphilis

88. Anti convulsants frequently used in management of trigeminal neuralgia are

A. Phenytoin
B. Gabapentin

C. Baclofen
D. All of the above

89. The characteristic alarm clock headache is a feature of
A. Auriculotemporal neuralgia
B. Trigeminal neuralgia
C. Sphenopalatine neuralgia
D. Glossopharyngeal neuralgia

90. Herpetic Whitlow is seen in
A. Fingers
B. Lymph nodes
C. Bone
D. Tongue

91. Denture sore mouth is a .... type of candidiasis
A. Acute pseudomembranous
B. Chronic atrophic
C. Acute atrophic
D. Chronic hyperplastic

92. Following are the characteristics of Vincent"s angina except
A. Ulcerative gingivostomatitis
B. Caused due to malnutrition
C. A symbiotic infection
D. Caused by Leptospira interrogans

93. The presence of Leisegang ring type of calcification is a feature of
A. Calcifying epithelial odontogenic tumor
B. Pindborg tumor
C. Both a and b
D. None of the above

94. Pulp polyp is a feature of
A. Irreversible pulpitis
B. Chronic hyperplastic pulpitis
C. Reversible pupitis
D. Acute pulpitis

95. Which is the most common cyst in the mandibular premolar region?
A. OKC
B. Lateral periodontal cyst
C. Dentigerous cyst
D. Calcifying odontogenic cyst

96. Benign migratory glossitis is also known as
A. Geographic tongue
B. Wandering rash
C. Erythema migrans
D. All of the above

97. Polyarthritis, urethritis, conjunctivitis is characteristically seen in
A. Albright's syndrome
B. Reiter's syndrome
C. Sjogren's syndrome
D. None of the above

98. Xylitol is a low caloric sweetener inhibits the growth of
A. S.mutans
B. S.pyogens
C. Lactobacillus
D. Actinomycosis

99. Giant cell tumour of bone is otherwise called
A. Osteoblastoma
B. Osteosarcoma
C. Osteoclastoma
D. Osteoma

100. Sicca complex is associated with
A. Primary Sjogren's syndrome
B. Secondary Sjogren's syndrome
C. Peutz Jeghers syndrome
D. Plummer Vinson syndrome

101. Pin point haemorrhages on skin are known as
A. Ecchymosis
B. Petechiae
C. Purpura
D. Haematoma

102. The common area of torus mandibularis when present is
A. Lingual, molar area
B. Lingual, canine area
C. Buccal, premolar area
D. Lingual, premolar area

103. Butterfly rash is typically seen in
A. Herpes simplex
B. Systemic lupus erythematosus
C. Scleroderma
D. None of the above

104. Odontogenic keratocyst is currently known as
A. Follicular cyst
B. Keratocystic odontogenic tumour
C. CEOT
D. None of the above

105. Which is not a feature of chondrosarcoma?
A. Most common primary malignant tumor
B. Most common site is anterior part of maxilla
C. Connective tissue origin
D. Drifting and mobility of teeth

ORAL RADIOLOGY

106. The size of periapical film used in adults is
A. 21 × 31 mm
B. 31 × 41 mm
C. 22 × 35 mm
D. None of the above

107. The function of a grid is to reduce the amount of
A. Breaking radiation
B. Scattered radiation
C. Characteristic radiation
D. All of the above

108. The sunray appearance is seen in
A. Ameloblastoma
B. Periapical cemental dysplasia
C. Osteosarcoma
D. Ossifying fibroma

109. Radiographic "Hair on end" appearance is seen in
A. Thalassemia
B. Aplastic anemia
C. Agranulocytosis
D. Neutropenia

ORTHODONTICS

110. Which of the following is not an example of reciprocal anchorage?
A. Closure of midline diastema
B. Buccal movement of a palatally placed premolar
C. Correction of a single tooth posterior crossbite
D. Expansion of the maxillary arch with a jackscrew

111. Treatment of which type of malocclusion requires no post treatment retention
A. Generalized spacing
B. Deep bite
C. Midline diastema
D. Anterior cross bite

112. Which of the following is not a unilateral landmark on the lateral cephalogram?
A. Nasion
B. Anterior nasal spine
C. Gnathion
D. Gonion

113. Hyalinization is a frequent complication of
A. Excessive force application
B. Too less force application
C. Application of optimal force
D. Removable appliances

114. What is the effect of doubling the diameter of a cantilever spring?
A. Strength increases by 4 times, springiness increases by 8 times
B. Strength decreases by 4 times, springiness decreases by 8 times
C. Strength decreases by 8 times, springiness increases by 16 times
D. Strength increases by 8 times, springiness decreases by 16 times

115. Which of the following is not an indication for serial extraction?
A. Arch length deficiency in comparison to total tooth material

B. Patients with straight profile
C. Absence of sufficient growth to overcome the jaw base tooth size discrepancy
D. Class II and Class III malocclusion with skeletal abnormality

116. Which of the following is not associated with complex tongue thrusting activity?
A. Naso-respiratory distress
B. Contraction of the temporalis muscle
C. Contraction of the mentalis and lower lip during swallow
D. Absence of contact of teeth during Swallow

117. Identify the term which indicate teeth or other maxillary structures too low down in the face
A. Attraction
B. Abstraction
C. Distraction
D. Protraction

118. The Broadbent-Bolton cephalometer was devised in
A. 1930
B. 1927
C. 1931
D. 1946

119. What is the optimum force required for the intrusion of a tooth?
A. 10–20 gm
B. 30–40 gm
C. 50–100 gm
D. 450–600 gm

120. Which of the following statement(s) regarding the adjustment of the Adam's clasp for a proper fit is true?
1. Bending the arrowheads very slightly toward the tooth;
2. Bending at a point buccally to where the tag makes contact with the teeth at the contact point;
3. Bending the tag where they emerge from the base plate
A. 1 and 2
B. 2 and 3
C. 1and 3
D. All of the above

PEDODONTICS

121. Rubber dam is particularly adaptable to primary second molar because the
A. Occluso-cervical height favors its retention
B. Cervical constriction of crown favors its retention
C. Mesio-buccal bulge favors its retention
D. Small diameter of crown favors its retention

122. Which part of the body is underdeveloped at birth?
A. Eyes
B. Ears
C. Face
D. Brain

123. Distal shoe was first advocated by whom in 1929?
A. Wilson
B. Willet
C. Wilhem
D. Roche

124. The primary reason for replacing teeth destroyed due to nursing bottle syndrome is
A. Speech and esthetics
B. Form and function
C. Incising and mastication
D. Arch perimeter requirements in the transitional dentition

125. The term rampant caries applies to mouth having
A. 5 or more lesions per year
B. 2 or more lesions per year
C. 12 or more lesions per year
D. 10 or more lesions per year

126. Stainless steel crowns are contraindicated in

A. Medically compromised patient (VSD, ASD)
B. After endodontic therapy
C. Rampant caries
D. Amelogenesis imperfecta

127. Hand over mouth technique was first described by

A. Dr. Evangeline Jordan
B. Addelston and Gold Fried
C. Dr. Goldman
D. Dr. G.V. Black

128. Class II cavity preparation for amalgam restoration in primary teeth requires

A. More bucco-lingual extension
B. More gingival extension
C. More cervical extension
D. More mesio-distal extension

129. How is two year old positioned for an emergency examination of fractured incisor?

A. On the dental assistant's lap
B. On the parents lap
C. On the dental chair
D. In the papoose board

130. Which pulp horn is most likely to be exposed during cavity preparation on primary molars?

A. Mesio-buccal of 1st molar
B. Disto-buccal of 1st molar
C. Mesio-buccal of 2nd molar
D. Disto-buccal of 2nd molar

131. During what stage of development is Peer group identity strongest?

A. Toddler
B. Latency
C. Teenager
D. Prepuberty

132. Most important morphologic or histologic consideration in cavity preparation in primary teeth is

A. Size of primary molars
B. Thickness of enamel and dentin
C. Direction of roots below CEJ
D. Direction of enamel rods cervically

133. Which among the following is NOT a common finding of the deciduous dentition?

A. Tight contacts, absence of spacing
B. Shallow overjet and overbite
C. Flush terminal plane
D. Ovoid arch form

134. Into how many segments the infant gum pad is divided?

A. Two in each quadrant
B. Three in each quadrant
C. Five in each jaw
D. Five in each quadrant

135. Patient with Down syndrome normally have

A. IQ Score above 80
B. Brachycephalic skull
C. Stiff muscles
D. All of the above

P AND SD

136. DMF index is the most universally employed index for measuring

A. Dental plaque
B. Gingivitis
C. Dental caries
D. Periodontal disease

137. Histogram is a

A. Pie diagram
B. Bar diagram
C. Frequency polygon
D. Line diagram

138. Temporary water hardness is removed by

A. Filtration
B. storage
C. Addition of bleaching powder
D. Boiling

139. The recommended age for Knutson's technique is

A. 3 years, 7 years, 11 years and 13 years

B. 2 years, 3 years, 4 years and 5 years
C. 7 years, 8 years, 9 years and 10 years
D. 5 years, 6 years, 7 years and 8 years

140. Retrospective study is also called as
A. Case–control study
B. Cohort–study
C. Randomized controlled trial
D. Non–randomized trials

141. School water fluoridation is considered as the primary preventive service provided by the
A. Community
B. Individual
C. Dental professional
D. None of the above

142. The valuable test for evaluating caries activity in very young children is
A. Lactobacillus colony count test
B. Swab test
C. Alban test
D. Calorimetric Snyder test

143. April 7th is observed as
A. World health day
B. Doctor's day
C. Anti-AIDS day
D. World No-tobacco day

144. Dental hygienist is included under
A. Non-operating auxiliaries
B. Operating auxiliaries
C. Dental specialist
D. Passive dental manpower

145. Pit and fissure sealant used in primary prevention of caries is
A. BIS–GMA
B. Duraphat
C. Fluor protector
D. APF gel

146. The brushing technique indicated for young children is
A. Fones method
B. Modified Stillman technique
C. Modified Bass technique
D. Charter's technique

147. Mass media includes the following
A. Audiovisual aids
B. Panel discussion and group discussion
C. Newspapers and television
D. Symposium and seminar

148. Which of the following is cariostatic
A. Selenium
B. Magnesium
C. Cadmium
D. Molybdenum

149. Hospital wastes should ideally be disposed by
A. Burial
B. Composting
C. Incineration
D. Trench method

150. The optimal fluoride level for water fluoridation is?
A. 1 ppm
B. 0.5 ppm
C. 2 ppm
D. 0.01 ppm

PROSTHODONTICS

151. Functional cusp bevel has to be placed in following cusps except
A. Mesio-palatal cusp
B. Disto-palatal cusp
C. Disto-lingual cusp of mandibular molar
D. Disto-buccal cusp of mandibular molar

152. During recording centric relation, compound occlusion rims with styli in maxillary arch are used in
A. Patterson technique
B. Intra- oral tracer technique
C. Extra- oral tracer technique
D. Needle-house technique

153. Mechanism of action of indirect retainer resembles
A. First-class lever
B. Second-class lever
C. Third-class lever
D. The action of direct retainers

154. Masticatory forces generated by a complete denture prosthesis is about

A. 44–50 pounds
B. 13–16 pounds
C. 13–15 kilograms
D. 70–80 pounds

155. One of the following is NOT a component of fixed partial denture prosthesis

A. Non-rigid connector
B. Split pontic
C. Abutment
D. Partial veneer crown

156. Extraction of a tilted abutment tooth is indicated when the tilt is

A. More than 25–30 degrees
B. More than 10–15 degrees
C. More than 5–10 degrees
D. More than 45–50 degrees

157. A pathologic condition caused due to over-extension of borders is called as

A. Burning mouth syndrome
B. Combination syndrome
C. Epulis fissuratum
D. Denture stomatitis

158. Wing preparation for metal-ceramic restorations helps in

A. Retention and resistance
B. Structural durability
C. Marginal integration
D. Both (A) and (B)

159. The width of the palatal strap major connector should be not less than

A. 4 mm
B. 6 mm
C. 8 mm
D. 10 mm

160. The only one flexible minor connector is

A. That connecting clasp assembly to major connector
B. That connecting indirect retainer to the major connector
C. That joining the denture base to major connector
D. That approach arm of a bar type clasp

161. Tissue stop for distal extension denture base is made by removing .... of relief wax.

A. 2 mm
B. 3 mm
C. 2 sq. mm
D. 3 sq. mm

162. What is a ferrule?

A. Pin retained restorative preparation
B. Secondary retentive feature for amalgam restoration
C. Band encircling external dimension of tooth
D. Preparation design for composite inlay

163. While arranging artificial teeth, the labial surfaces of the maxillary central incisors are usually.............. infront of the posterior border of the incisive papilla.

A. 12–15 mm
B. 5–8 mm
C. 8–10 mm
D. 2–3 mm

164. The limits of hinge movement in terminal hinge position of the mandible is about

A. 19–22 degrees
B. 12–15 degrees
C. 12–15 millimeters
D. 35 degrees

PERIODONTICS

165. Ideal angle for the sharpening stone must form with the face of the blade is

A. 70–80 degrees
B. 90–100 degrees
C. 100–110 degrees
D. 120–130 degrees

166. FDA approved locally delivered minocycline for subgingival placement marketed under trade name

A. Periochip

B. Atridox
C. Arestin
D. Elyzol

167. Stratification specific keratins present in gingival epithelium are

A. K1, K2
B. K10, K12
C. K16, K6
D. K5, K14

168. Which of the following statements are true?

A. Marginal gingiva is stippled
B. Attached gingiva is stippled
C. Both marginal and attached gingiva are stippled
D. Marginal attached gingiva and alveolar mucosa are stippled

169. The abundant glycoprotein in the basement membrane and has binding domain for both ECM and cell–surface receptor is

A. Laminin
B. Fibronectin
C. E–cadherins
D. Tenascin

170. The transmembrane adhesive molecules present in hemi desmosomes which specifically binds to basal lamina glycoprotein laminin are

A. Integrin $\alpha6\ \beta4$
B. The catenins desmoplakin
C. Cadherins desmoglein
D. α and β catenin

171. Which of the following stages of gingivitis characterizes periodontal breakdown?

A. Initial lesion
B. Early lesion
C. Advanced lesion
D. Established lesion

172. According to Horning and Cohen staging of oral necrotizing diseases stage one represents

A. NUG
B. NUP
C. Necrotizing stomatitis
D. Noma

173. Which of the following is the gold standard for testing breath malador (halitosis)?

A. Portable volatile sulfide monitor
B. Self examination
C. Gas chromatography
D. Organoleptic rating by a judge

174. Decalcified freeze dried bone allograft is considered as

A. Osteogenic
B. Osteoinductive
C. Osteoconductive
D. Osteoplastic

175. Vertical or angular defects are found in

A. Suprabony pockets
B. Infrabony pockets
C. Intrabony pockets
D. Both B and C

176. Shelf like thickening of the alveolar margin due to peripheral buttressing is called as

A. Ledge
B. Crater
C. Lipping
D. Swaging

177. Thin spiral interdental brushes are used in which type of embrasures?

A. Type 1
B. Type 2
C. Type 5
D. Type 3

178. Scraping of the gingival wall of periodontal pocket is called as

A. Gingivectomy
B. Curettage
C. Root planing
D. All of the above

179. **Sequential steps for resective osseous surgery are**
   A. Radicular blending, vertical grooving, flattening interproximal bone, gradualizing marginal bone
   B. Vertical grooving, flattening interproximal bone, gradualizing marginal bone, radicular blending
   C. Vertical grooving , radicular blending, flattening interproximal bone, gradualizing marginal bone
   D. Vertical grooving, radicular blending, gradualizing marginal bone, flattening interproximal bone.

CONS AND ENDO

180. **Application of cold or the electric pulp tester can be used**
   A. To test tooth for entrance sealing restoration
   B. To test tooth under treatment for pulp capping
   C. To test tooth under treatment for pulpal anesthesia
   D. To test tooth for restoring occlusal wear

181. **Caries excavation using carisolv**
   A. Conventional preparation design
   B. Clinical separation of sound and carious dentin
   C. Clinical separation of primary and secondary dentin
   D. Conventional rotary method of cavity preparation

182. **Enterococcus faecalis in post treatment periodontitis**
   A. Cultured easily and disinfected
   B. Disinfected with saline and hydrogen peroxide
   C. Tolerate pH up to 11.5
   D. Treated with intra canal medicaments

183. **Concussion implies luxation injury**
   A. Without displacement and normal mobility
   B. Without displacement and increased mobility
   C. Displacement in an apical direction
   D. Displacement in a coronal direction

184. **Primary anatomic structure of concern in posterior mandible periradicular surgery**
   A. Neurovascular bundle coursing through infraorbital canal
   B. Neurovascular bundle near incisive foramen
   C. Neurovascular bundle near palatine foramen
   D. Neurovascular bundle coursing through mandibular canal

185. **Medium thickness of matrix band**
   A. 0.004 inch
   B. 0.008 inch
   C. 0.010 inch
   D. 0.006 inch

186. **Indication for indirect pulp therapy**
   A. No signs or symptoms of pulp degeneration
   B. No response to hot and cold
   C. Presence of pain on percussion
   D. Presence of pulp polyp

187. **Function of water retraction system**
   A. Retracts water whenever spray is stopped
   B. Retracts water whenever spray is active
   C. Used in water booster
   D. Used in air compressor

188. **Interpretation and results of diagnostic tests are obtained from**
   A. Electric pulp test
   B. Heat test
   C. Laser Doppler flowmetry
   D. Gold standard

ORAL SURGERY

189. **A " leaf gauge" is used to assist in**
   A. Locating the musculo-skeletally stable position of the mandible

B. Locating the posterior most position of the condyle in the glenoid fossa
C. Assessment of the inter-occlusal clearance
D. None of the above

190. Success factor for intraligamentary anesthesia

A. Injection under strong forward pressure
B. Injection under strong back pressure
C. Injection over supragingival tissue
D. Injection over buccal labial fold

191. Le Fort I fracture is characterized by

A. Bleeding from ear
B. Bleeding into antrum
C. CSF Rhinorrhoea
D. All of the above

192. Treatment of calculus within the sub-mandibular salivary gland is

A. Removal of sinus
B. Removal of gland
C. Dichotomy
D. Milking of the stone

193. A patient with fibrous dysplasia can be treated by

A. Surgical excision
B. Removal of adjacent teeth
C. Irradiation of the lesion
D. Conservative surgery

194. A patient with ameloblastoma of the jaw can best be treated by

A. Irradiation
B. Excision
C. Enucleation
D. Surgical removal followed by cauterization

195. An inhaled foreign body, most likely to

A. Enter right bronchus
B. Enter left bronchus
C. Enter oesophagus
D. Perforate pleural membrane

196. The suture material most commonly used for intra oral wound closure is

A. Vicryl
B. Silk
C. Nylon
D. Catgut

197. Properties of local anesthetics include all the following except

A. Preferentially binds to sodium channels in open and inactivated state
B. Low affinity for channels in resting state
C. They are weak bases
D. Less effective in an environment with low extracellular pH

198. A patient is in shock with gross comminuted fracture. Immediate treatment is to give

A. Normal saline intravenously
B. Ringer's lactate solution intravenously
C. Blood transfusion
D. Plasma expanders

199. The most common anatomic fracture of mandible is the

A. Body
B. Angle
C. Condyle
D. Symphysis

200. Hilton's method deals with

A. Decompression of cyst
B. Drainage of abscess
C. Biopsy in a pathological lesion
D. Preanaesthetic checkup

ANSWERS

HUMAN ANATOMY

1. **Ans: C**

   Ref: BD Chaurasia, 1/E, p. 311

2. **Ans: C**

   Ref: BD Chaurasia, 1/E, p. 292

   Explanation

   Vagus nerve (Xth CN) is so called because of its extensive (Vague) course through the head, neck, thorax and abdomen

3. **Ans: B**

   Ref: Cunningham's Manual of Practical Anatomy, Vol. III, 15/E, p. 86

4. **Ans: A**

   Ref: Inderbir Singh, 8/E, p. 325

5. **Ans: A**

   Ref: BD Chaurasia,1/E, p. 337

6. **Ans: A**

   Ref: Inderbir Singh, 8/E, p. 107

PHYSIOLOGY

7. **Ans: D**

   Ref: Sembulingam, 4/E, p. 710

8. **Ans: D**

   Ref: Sembulingam, 4/E, p. 5

   Explanation

   Watson and Crick: DNA double helix model
   Edward angle: Classification of malocclusion, E arch appliance, Ribbon arch appliance, Pin and tube appliance, Edge wise appliance
   GV Black: Classification of cavity preparation
   Singer & Nicholson: Fluid mosaic

9. **Ans: A**

   Ref: Ganong's, 23/E, p. 533

   Explanation

   In circulating blood thrombin is a procoagulant that activates factor V & VIII, but when it binds to thrombomodulin, it become an anticoagulant in that the thrombomodulin - thrombin complex activates protein C, Activated protein C along with its cofactor Protein S, inactivates factor V and VIII.

10. **Ans: B**

    Ref: Sembulingam, 4/E, p. 520

11. **Ans: A**

    Ref: Guyton, 11/E, p. 61

BIOCHEMISTRY

12. **Ans: B**

    Ref: U Sathyanarayana and U. Chakrapani, 3/E, p. 155

    Explanation

    Fat soluble:

Vitamin deficiency	*Condition*
Vitamin A	Night blindness, Xerophthal-mia, Bitot's spots, keratomalacia.
Vitamin D	Rickets in chidren Osteomalacia in adults.
Vitamin E	Increased fragility of erythyrocytes.
Vitamin K	Minor neurological symptoms increased blood clotting time.
Water soluble:	
Vitamin deficiency	Condition
Vitamin C	Scurvy
Vitamin B1/	Beri Beri
	Thiamine
Vitamin B2/	Chelosis, glossitis, dermatitis
	Riboflavin

Niacin	Pellagra – 3D's Dermatitis, Diarrhoea, dementia if not treated death (4th D)
Pyridoxine	Neurological symptoms
Biotin	Anaemia, loss of apetite, nausea, dermatitis, glossitis
Pantothenic acid	Not reported in humans
Folic acid	Megaloblastic anaemia
Cobalamine/ Vitamin B12	Pernicious anaemia

13. Ans: A

Ref: U. Sathyanarayana and U. Chakrapani, 3/E, p. 249

14. Ans: B

Ref: U Sathyanarayana and U. Chakrapani, 3/E, p. 269

15. Ans: B

Ref: U Sathyanarayana and U. Chakrapani, 3/E, p. 297

Explanation

1. Fatty acid synthesis: cytosol
2. Fatty acid oxidation
   a. Activation of fatty acids: Cytosol
   b. beta oxidation proper: Mitochondria

GENERAL PATHOLOGY

16. Ans: D

Ref: Robbin's Pathologic Basis of Disease, 7/E, p. 1242

17. Ans: B

Ref: Robbin's Pathologic Basis of Disease, 7/E, p. 61

18. Ans: B

Ref: Robbin's Pathologic Basis of Disease, 7/E, p. 1350

Explanation

1. Astrocytes–form blood brain barrier
2. Oligodendrocytes–forms myelin sheath in CNS.
3. Microglia–phagocytic cells in CNS.
4. Schwann cells–forms myelin sheath in PNS.

19. Ans: B

Ref: Robbin's Pathologic Basis of Disease, 7/E, p. 214

20. Ans: C

Ref: Robbin's Pathologic Basis of Disease, 7/E, p. 302

21. Ans: A

Ref: Robbin's Pathologic Basis of Disease, 7/E, p. 1275

Explanation

- Cytokines that are crucial for bone resorption are IL – 1, IL – 3, IL – 6, IL – 11, and TNF(Tumor necrosis factor)

Granulocyte –macrocyte colony stimulating factor (GM-CSF) and macrophage colony stimulating factor(M-CSF).

MICROBIOLOGY

23. Ans: B

Ref: Ananthanarayan and Panicker's Text, Book of Microbiology, 8/E, p. 608

Explanation

Botryomycosis is caused by Staphylococcus.

24. Ans: B

Ref: Ananthanarayan and Panicker's Text, Book of Microbiology, 8/E, p. 77, 477

Explanation

1. Widal test–typhoid.
2. Paul Bunnel test–infectious mononucleosis.
3. Coomb's test–detection of antibodies–Rh antibodies.
4. Weil Felix test–typhus fever.

25. Ans: A

Ref: Ananthanarayan and Panicker's Text, Book of Microbiology, 8/E, p. 87

26. **Ans: A**

Ref: Ananthanarayan and Panicker's Text, Book of Microbiology, 8/E, p. 610

27. **Ans: A**

Ref: Ananthanarayan and Panicker's Text, Book of Microbiology, 8/E, p. 610

PHARMACOLOGY

28. **Ans: A**

Ref: KD Tripathi, 6/E, p. 589

29. **Ans: C**

Ref: KD Tripathi, 6/E, p. 799

30. **Ans: A**

Ref: Satoskar, 12/E, p. 238 – 239

Explanation

- Topically active local anesthetics are
  1. Lignocaine
  2. Benzocaine
  3. Tetracaine
  4. Oxathiazine
  5. Prilocaine
  6. Dibucaine

31. **Ans: A**

Ref: KD Tripathi, 6/E, p. 636

32. **Ans: B**

Ref: KD Tripathi, 6/E, p. 103

33. **Ans: A**

Ref: KD Tripathi, 6/E, p. 194

GENERAL MEDICINE

34. **Ans: D**

Ref: Davidson, 20/E, p. 695

35. **Ans: B**

Ref: Davidson, 20/E, p. 951

Explanation

Causes/appearance

- Cirrhosis: Clear, straw – coloured or light green
- Malignant disease: Bloody
- Infection: Cloudy
- Biliary communication: heavy bile staining
- Lymphatic obstruction: Milky – white (chylous)

Useful investigations

- *Total albumin (plus serum albumin)*
- *Amylase*
- *White cell count*
- *Cytology*
- *Microscopy and culture*

36. **Ans: D**

Ref: Davidson, 20/E, p. 668

37. **Ans: D**

Ref: Davidson, 20/E, p. 480

38. **Ans: C**

Ref: Davidson, 20/E, p. 1201

Explanation

- Differential diagnosis of stroke.
  1. Epileptic seizures
  2. Structural lesions
     - Subdural hematoma
     - Tumour
  3. Metabolic/toxic
     - Hyponatremia
     - Hypokalemia
     - Hepatic encephalopathy
     - Wernicke - korsakoff syndrome
     - Hypoglycemia
     - Hyperglycemia - MS
     - Alcohol and drugs - hypertensive encephalopathy
     - Head injury - peripheral nerve lesion.
     - Encephalitis
     - Creutz feldt Jakab disease

39. Ans: C

Ref: Davidson, 20/E, p. 1130

40. Ans: D

Ref: Davidson, 20/E, p. 630

Bacteria:

- Streptococci
  - Viridians 30–40%
  - Enterococci 10–15%
  - Others 20–25%
- Staphylococci
  - Aureus 9–27%
  - Coagulase–negative–1 = 3%
- Gram–ve bacilli
  - Haemophilus
  - Anaerobes
- Other organisms:
  - Rickettsiae, fungi – < 2%

41. Ans: C

Ref: Davidson, 20/E, p. 1130

GENERAL SURGERY

42. Ans: A

Ref: S. Das, 5/E, p. 635

43. Ans: D

Ref: S. Das, 5/E, p. 654

44. Ans: D

Ref: S, Das, 5/E, p. 696

45. Ans: B

Ref: S. Das, 5/E, p. 34

Explanation

- Primary haemorrhage – at the time of injury or operation.
- Reactionary haemorrhage–within 24 hours.
- Secondary haemorrhage – within 7 to 14 days.

46. Ans: B

Ref: S. Das, 5/E, p. 52

Explanation

- "Rule of nine" for estimating percentage of body surface involved in burns are as follows:
  1. Head, face and neck: 9%
  2. Right upper extremity: 9%
  3. Left upper extremity: 9%
  4. Right lower: 18% (Thigh – 9%, leg and foot – 9%)
  5. Anterior trunk: 18% (Chest – 9%, Abdomen – 9%)
  6. Posterior trunk: 18% (Upper half 9%, lower half – 9%)
  7. External genitalia: 1%

47. Ans: D

Ref: S. Das, 5/E, p. 685

48. Ans: A

Ref: S. Das, 5/E, p. 664

49. Ans: D

Ref: S. Das, 5/E, p. 34

DENTAL MATERIALS

50. Ans: A

Ref: Philip's, 11/E, p. 171

Explanation

- *Biocompatibility*–Ability of a material to elicit an appropriate biological response in a given application in the body.
- *Sensitization*– exposure to allergen that results in the development of hyper-sensitivity.

51. Ans: D

Ref: Philip's, 11/E, p. 162

Explanation

- *Step growth polymerization*–2 or more molecules producing a simple macromolecular structure with formation of by products.

- *Addition polymerizing*–Monomers add sequentially to the end of a growing chain.
- *Condensation polymerization*–Monomers add forming polymers with release of by products.

52. Ans: C

Ref: Philip's, 11/E, p. 21

53. Ans: A

Ref: Philip's, 11/E, p. 121

54. Ans: A

Ref: Philip's, 11/E, p. 681

55. Ans: B

Ref: Philip's, 11/E, p. 504

56. Ans: D

Ref: Philip's, 11/E, p. 402

57. Ans: D

Ref: Philip's, 11/E, p. 271

58. Ans: C

Ref: Philip's, 11/E, p. 417

59. Ans: C

Ref: Philip's, 11/E, p. 393

60. Ans: A

Ref: Philip's, 11/E, p. 532

61. Ans: A

Ref: Philip's, 11/E, p. 588

62. Ans: D

Ref: Craig, 12/E, p. 395

63. Ans: A

Ref: Craig, 12/E, p. 396

64. Ans: B

Ref: Craig, 12/E, p. 342

65. Ans: C

Ref: Philip's, 11/E, p. 648

DADH

66. Ans: B

Ref: Orban's, 12/E, p. 269

67. Ans: C

Ref: Orban's, 12/E, p. 6

68. Ans: C

Ref: Orban's, 12/E, p. 145

69. Ans: D

Ref: Orban's, 12/E, p. 263

70. Ans: A

Ref: Wheeler's, 8/E p. 312

Explanation

From a developmental view point, all mandibular molars have major cusps whereas maxillary molars have only three major cusps.

ORAL PATHOLOGY AND ORAL MEDICINE

71. Ans: B

Ref: Burkitt, 11/E, p. 12

72. Ans: D

Ref: Burkitt, 11/E, p. 14

73. Ans: A

Ref: Neville, 3/E, p. 139

74. Ans: D

Ref: Shafer's, 6/E, p. 322

75. Ans: C

Ref: Neville, 3/E, p. 636, 530

76. Ans: A

Ref: Shafer's, 6/E, p. 695

77. Ans: D

Ref: Neville, 3/E, p. 196

78. Ans: C

Ref: Burkitt, 11/E, p. 280

79. Ans: D

Ref: Neville, 3/E, p. 367, 369, 371

80. Ans: A

Ref: Shafers, 6/E, p. 853

81. Ans: D

Ref: Shafers, 6/E, p. 46

82. Ans: A

Ref: Shafers, 6/E, p. 89

83. Ans: C

Ref: Shafers, 6/E, p. 667

84. Ans: C

Ref: Shafers, 6/E, p. 346

85. Ans: A

Ref: Shafers, 6/E, p. 508

86. Ans: C

Ref: Shafers, 6/E, p. 47

87. Ans: B

Ref: Shafers, 6/E, p. 323

88. Ans: D

Ref: Burkitt, 11/E, p. 280

89. Ans: C

Ref: Neville, 3/E, p. 869

90. Ans: A

Ref: Neville, 3/E, p. 244

91. Ans: B

Ref: Shafers, 6/E, p. 365

92. Ans: D

Ref: Shafers, 6/E, p. 387

93. Ans: C

Ref: Shafers, 6/E, p. 281

94. Ans: B

Ref: Shafers, 6/E, p. 479

95. Ans: B

Ref: Neville, 3/E, p. 693

96. Ans: D

Ref: Neville, 3/E, p. 779

97. Ans: B

Ref: Neville, 3/E, p. 782

98. Ans: A

Ref: Shafer's, 6/E, p. 464

99. Ans: C

Ref: Shafer's, 6/E, p. 133

100. Ans: A

Ref: Shafers, 6/E, p. 247

101. Ans: B

Ref: Neville, 3/E, p. 305

102. Ans: D

Ref: Neville, 3/E, p. 22

103. Ans: B

Ref: Shafers, 6/E, p. 827

104. Ans: B

Ref: Shafers, 6/E, p. 258

105. Ans: A

Ref: Shafers, 6/E, p. 166

ORAL RADIOLOGY

106. Ans: B

Ref: White & Pharaoh, 6/E, p. 54

Explanation

Size of bitewing film is same as periapical film.

31 × 41 mm: Adult size, commonly used for bitewing view.

24 × 40 mm: Views for anterior teeth.

22 × 35 mm: For small children.

57 × 76 mm: Large film used for occlusal view.

107. Ans: B

Ref: White & Pharaoh, 6/E, p. 63

108. Ans: C

Ref: White and Pharaoh, 6/E, p. 415, Fig 23.9B

Explanation

Sun ray appearance is also seen in Ewing's sarcoma.

109. Ans: A

Ref: White & Pharaoh, 6/E, p. 469 Fig 25–17

Explanation

Hair on end appearance is also seen in sickle cell anaemia

ORTHODONTICS

110. Ans: B

Ref: Bhalaji, 3/E, p. 206

Explanation

Buccal movement of palatally placed premolar is an example of simple anchorage.

111. Ans: D

Ref: Bhalaji, 3/E, p. 465

112. Ans: D

Ref: Bhalaji, 3/E, p. 147–148

113. Ans: A

Ref: Bhalaji, 3/E, p. 185

Explanation

- Mild force–frontal resorption
- Excessive force–Hyalinization undermining or rearward resorption.

114. Ans: D

Ref: Bhalaji, 3/E, p. 289

Explanation

$F = D^4 / L^3$

where

F = Force

D = Diameter of wire

L = Length of wire

By doubling the diameter force increases by 16 times.

By doubling the length force decreases by 8 times.

115. Ans: D

Ref: Bhalaji, 3/E, p. 228

116. Ans: B

Ref: Bhalaji, 3/E, p. 103

Explanation

Characteristics of complex tongue thrust.

- Teeth apart swallow
- Anterior open bite
- Absence of temporal muscle contraction during swallowing
- Contraction of cirum oral muscles during swallowing
- Poor occlusion

117. Ans: B

Ref: Bhalaji, 3/E, p. 77

Explanation

Sagittal/anteroposterior direction	
Protraction	Dental arch or part of it is farther from orbital plane.
Retraction	Closer or more posteriorly placed in relation to the plane.
Transverse direction	
Distraction	Part or whole of the arch is away from midsagittal plane.
Retraction	Part or whole arch is closer to the midsagittal plane.

118. **Ans: C**

Ref: Gurkeerat Singh, 2/E, p. 95

119. **Ans: A**

Ref: Proffit, 4/E, p. 340

120. **Ans: C**

Ref: Gurkeerat Singh, 2/E, p. 439

PEDODONTICS

121. **Ans: B**

Ref: Pinkham, 4/E, p. 343

122. **Ans: C**

Ref: Mc Donald, 8/E, p.584

123. **Ans: B**

Ref: Shobha Tandon, 1/E, p. 396

Explanation

Distal shoe space maintainer is constructed when there is a premature loss of the 2nd primary molar, prior to the eruption of the first permanent molar.

124. **Ans: A**

Ref: Shobha Tandon, 1/E, p. 221

125. **Ans: D**

Ref: Shobha Tandon, 1/E, p. 221

126. **Ans: A**

Ref: Shobha Tandon, 1/E, p. 318

127. **Ans: A**

Ref: Shobha Tandon, 1/E, p. 151

Explanation

Hand over mouth exercise (HOME) was introduced by Dr. Evangeline Jordan in 1920.

128. **Ans: A**

Ref: Shobha Tandon, 1/E, p. 288

Explanation

Due to the presence of broad contact areas, the gingival floor of the proximal box should be wide so as to place the margins in self cleansing areas.

129. **Ans: A**

Ref: Shobha Tandon, 1/E, p. 9

130. **Ans: A**

Ref: Shobha Tandon, 1/E, p. 289

131. **Ans: B**

Ref: Shobha Tandon, 1/E, p. 124

132. **Ans: B**

Ref: Shobha Tandon, 1/E, p. 288

Explanation

- Few factors to be taken into consideration while restoring primary teeth are:
  - The smaller tooth dimension of the deciduous dentition
  - The thin enamel covering the teeth
  - Broad contact areas
  - Proximity of the pulp chamber to the tooth surface
  - Narrow occlusal table.

133. **Ans: A**

Ref: Shobha Tandon, 1/E, p. 107

134. **Ans: D**

Ref: Shobha Tandon, 1/E, p. 53

135. **Ans: B**

Ref: Shobha Tandon, 1/E, p. 540

P AND SD

136. **Ans: C**

Ref: Soben Peter, 3/E, p. 177

137. **Ans: B**

Ref: Soben Peter, 3/E, p. 29

138. Ans: D

Ref: Park, 20/E, p. 636

Explanation

Method of removal of hardness

Temporary	*Permanent*
a. Boiling	a. Addition of Na_2Co_3
b. Addition of lime	b. Base exchange process
c. Addition of $NaHCO_3$	
d. Permutit process	

139. Ans: A

Ref: Soben Peter, 3/E, p. 297

140. Ans: B

Ref: Park, 20/E, pp. 67 and 72

141. Ans: A

Ref: Soben Peter, 3/E, p. 350

142. Ans: B

Ref: Soben Peter, 3/E, p. 362

Explanation

- It was developed by Grainger et al in 1965.

143. Ans: A

Ref: Park, 20/E, p. 817

Explanation

- World health day–April 17th
- Doctors Day–March 30th
- World Anti–AIDS day–December 1st
- World no Tobacco day–May 31st

144. Ans: B

Ref: Soben Peter, 3/E, p. 793

145. Ans: A

Ref: Soben Peter, 3/E, p. 369

146. Ans: A

Ref: Soben Peter, 3/E, p. 438

Explanation

a. Fone's method–young children.
b. Modified Stilman's–gingival recession.
c. Modified Bass–Routine oral hygiene measure.
d. Charter's technique–patients who have periodontal surgery.

147. Ans: C

Ref: Park, 20/E, p. 766

148. Ans: A & D

Ref: Text Book of Preventive & Community Dentistry, 1/E, p. 43

Explanation

Selenium, molybdenum ,vanadium, strontium – these are Cariostatic trace elements because they reduce the acid solubility of calcified dental tissues

149. Ans: C

Ref: Park, 20/E, p. 660

150. Ans: A

Ref: Park, 20/E, p. 636

PROSTHODONTICS

151. Ans: C

Ref: Rosensteil, 4/E, p. 261

Explanation

Functional cusp bevel is given to mandibular buccal and maxillary lingual cusps

152. Ans: D

Ref: Heartwell, 4/E, p. 735

Explanation

Functional methods

- Needle house method–compound occlusal rim
- Patterson's method–wax occlusal rim

153. Ans: B

Ref: Nallaswamy, 1/E, p. 382

Explanation

- Ist order lever–distal extension partial dentures.
- IInd order lever–Indirect retention of RPD.
- IIIrd order lever–does not occur in partial denture.

154. Ans: B

Ref: Zarb & Bolender, 12/E, p. 10

Explanation

- Natural teeth – 44 lb (20 Kg)
- Artificial teeth – 13–16 lb (6–8 kg)

155. Ans: C

Ref: Nallaswamy, 1/E, p. 503

Explanation

Parts of FPD

• Pontic • Retainer • Connector

Abutment is not a part of FPD.

156. Ans: B

Ref: Heartwell, 4/E, p. 263

Explanation

Limits of hinge movement in this position is about 12–15 degree from maximum intercuspation or about 19–20 mm at the incisal edges

157. Ans: B

Ref: Heartwell, 4/E, p. 427

158. Ans: A

Ref: Shillingburg, 3/E, p. 148

Explanation

Features of metal ceramic tooth preparation

Radial shoulder	Periodontal preservations Structural durability
Chamfer	Marginal integrity Periodontal preservation
Axial reduction	Retention and resistance, structural durability
Wing preparation	Retention and resistance preservation of tooth structure
Incisal notch	Structural durability

159. Ans: C

Ref: Nallaswamy, 1/E, p. 330

160. Ans: D

Ref: Nallaswamy, 1/E, p. 363

161. Ans: C

Ref: Nallaswamy, 1/E, p. 343

162. Ans: C

Ref: Rosensteil, 4/E, p. 375

163. Ans: C

Ref: Winkler's, 2/E, p. 202

164. Ans: B

Ref: Nallaswamy, 1/E, p. 111

PERIODONTICS

165. Ans: C

Ref: Carranza, 10/E, p. 788

166. Ans: C

Ref: Carranza, 10/E, p. 808

167. Ans: D

Ref: Carranza, 10/E, p. 52

Explanation

Keratins	*Specific to*
K1, K2 and K10	Epidermal type differentiation to K12 expressed with high intensity in ortho-keratinised epithelium.
K6 and K16	Highly proliferative epithelia.
K5 and K14	Stratification specific cytokeratins.
K19	Parakeratinized areas.

168. Ans: B

Ref: Carranza, 10/E, p. 62

Explanation

- The attached gingiva and the central portion of IDP are stippled, the marginal gingiva is NOT.

169. **Ans: A**

Ref: Carranza, 10/E, p. 57

Explanation

- Fibronectin–found in ground substance binds fibroblasts to the fibres and many other components of intercellular matrix.
- Laminin–found in basal lamina, serves to attach it to epithelial cells.

170. **Ans: A**

Ref: Carranza, 10/E, p. 52

171. **Ans: C**

Ref: Carranza, 10/E, p. 360

Explanation

Stage I	Initial	Subclinical gingivitis
Stage II	Early	Leukocytic infiltration
Stage III	Established	Plasma cell infiltration
Stage IV	Advanced	Periodontal break down

172. **Ans: A**

Ref: Carranza, 10/E, p. 392

173. **Ans: D**

Ref: Carranza, 10/E, p. 334

174. **Ans: B**

Ref: Carranza, 10/E, p. 1135

175. **Ans: D**

Ref: Carranza, 10/E, p. 446

176. **Ans: C**

Ref: Carranza, 10/E, p. 459

177. **Ans: B**

Ref: Carranza, 10/E, p. 737

178. **Ans: B**

Ref: Carranza, 10/E, p. 909

179. **Ans: C**

Ref: Carranza, 10/E, p. 956

CONS AND ENDO

180. **Ans: C**

Ref: Ingle, 6/E, p. 1320, 1322

181. **Ans: C**

Ref: Ingle, 6/E, p. 764

182. **Ans: C**

Ref: Ingle, 6/E, p. 261

Explanation

Enterococcus faecalis shows low sensitivity to antimicrobial agents, including the ability to resist the high pH of antimicrobial agents commonly used, such as calcium hydroxide paste ($Ca(OH)_2$) of pH > 11.5

183. **Ans: A**

Ref: Grossman, 12/E, p. 363

184. **Ans: D**

Ref: Cohen, 9/E, p. 735

185. **Ans: D**

Ref: Sturdevant's, 5/E, p. 834

186. **Ans: A**

Ref: Ingle, 6/E, p. 866

187. **Ans: A**

Ref: Sturdevant's, 5/E, p. 396

188. **Ans: B**

Ref: Ingle, 6/E, p. 533

ORAL SURGERY

189. **Ans: A**

Ref: Jeffrey. P. Okeson , 4/E, p. 271, 273

190. **Ans: B**

Ref: Monheim's, 7/E, p. 57

191. **Ans: B**

Ref: Neelima Malik, 2/E, p. 355

192. **Ans: D**

Ref: Neelima Malik, 2/E, p. 520

193. **Ans: D**

Ref: Neelima Malik, 2/E, p. 506

194. **Ans: D**

Ref: Neelima Malik, 2/E, p. 488

195. **Ans: B**

Ref: Malamed Medical Emergencies, 6/E, p. 191

Explanation

Compared with the left bronchus the right main bronchus takes a more direct path at the bifurcation of the trachea. The right main bronchus branches off the trachea at a 25 – degree angle, whereas the left main bronchus branches off at a 45-degree angle.

196. **Ans: B**

Ref: Neelima Malik, 2/E, p. 64

197. **Ans: B**

Ref: Monheim's, 7/E, p. 126

198. **Ans: B**

Ref: Neelima Malik, 2/E, p. 773

199. **Ans: A**

Ref: Killey's, 4/E, p. 11

200. **Ans: B**

Ref: Neelima Malik, 2/E, p. 592

9

KCET 2011

ANATOMY

1. Philtrum of upper lip develops from

A. Mandibular process
B. Maxillary process
C. Frontonasal process
D. Palatal process

2. Merkel cells are found in which of the following tissues?

A. Epidermis
B. Papillary layer of dermis
C. Reticular layer of dermis
D. Hypodermis

3. The acrosome reaction occurs when the sperm

A. Enters the uterine cavity
B. Comes in contact with zona pellucida
C. Penetrates corona radiata
D. Penetrates cell membrane of oocyte

4. Which of the following muscle is attached to posterior part of pterygomandibular raphe?

A. Lateral pterygoid
B. Buccinator
C. Superior constrictor
D. Medial pterygoid

5. What is the type of joint formed between the tooth and the alveolar socket?

A. Gomphosis
B. Syndesmosis
C. Suture
D. Synovial

PHYSIOLOGY

6. The first heart sound is due to

A. Sudden closure of mitral and tricuspid valve
B. Sudden closure of semilunar valves
C. Ventricular systole
D. Atrial systole

7. Which one of the following is a vasodilator?

A. Bradykinin
B. Norepinephrine
C. Epinephrine
D. Angiotensin II

8. The condition, in which the person can see near objects but not the far objects is

A. Hypermetropia
B. Myopia
C. Presbyopia
D. Astigmatism

9. The male sex hormone testosterone is produced by

A. Sertoli cells
B. Epithelial cells
C. Interstitial cells of the leydig
D. Primitive germ cells

10. Decrease in salivary secretion is known as

A. Asphyxia
B. Xerostomia
C. Aerophagia
D. Achalasia

11. Parathyroid hormone

A. Decrease the intestinal calcium absorption

B. Stimulates bone resorption
C. Stimulates osteoblasts
D. Increases renal excretion of calcium

12. The pH of gastric juice is about

A. 1
B. 6
C. 9
D. 7

BIOCHEMISTRY

13. Ceruloplasmin is a protein containing

A. Iron
B. Copper
C. Manganese
D. Magnesium

14. LDH has following number of isoenzymes

A. 5
B. 3
C. 11
D. 2

15. In prolonged starvation the main source of energy to brain is

A. Glucose
B. Fructose
C. Fatty acids
D. Ketone bodies

GENERAL PATHOLOGY

16. Tigered effect of heart is seen in

A. Fatty change
B. Hyaline change
C. Amyloidosis
D. Atrophy

17. Carcinoembryonic antigen is associated with

A. Hepatocellular carcinoma
B. Medullary carcinoma of thyroid
C. Seminoma
D. Carcinoma of colon

18. Pellagra is seen in deficiency of

A. Riboflavin
B. Thiamine
C. Niacin
D. Pyridoxine

19. The classic karyotype of klinefelter syndrome is

A. 45, XO
B. 47, XXY
C. Trisomy 18
D. Trisomy 21

20. Somatic mutation of PTEN is seen in

A. Retinoblastoma
B. Osteosarcoma
C. Carcinoma breast
D. Endometrial carcinoma

21. Which of the following is NOT a constituent of Virchow's triad?

A. Damage to endothelium due to injury or inflammation
B. Diminished rate of blood flow
C. Increased coagulability of blood
D. Increased venous blood pressure

MICROBIOLOGY

22. Which of the following organisms does NOT react with gram's stain?

A. *Actinomyces israelii*
B. *Candida albicans*
C. *Mycobacterium tuberculosis*
D. *Streptococcus mutans*

23. In which phase of the bacterial growth curve involution form of the bacteria can be observed?

A. Lag phase
B. Log phase
C. Stationary phase
D. Phase of decline

24. Out of the following hypersensitivity reactions in which type a single dose of the antigen can act as both the sensitizing and shocking dose

A. Anaphylaxis
B. Arthus reaction
C. Serum sickness
D. Contact dermatitis

25. Ziehl Nielsen's staining is routinely performed from sputum samples for the detection of

A. *Mycobacterium tuberculosis*
B. *Bacillus anthracis*
C. *Streptococcus pneumonia*
D. *Mycoplasma pneumonia*

26. Western Blot test is a confirmatory test used for the diagnosis of

A. CMV
B. Hepatitis B Virus
C. HIV
D. Epstein Barr virus

27. Name the fungi which are ovoid or spherical in morphology, produces budding cells and pseudohyphae in culture media and in human tissues

A. Histoplasma capsulatum
B. Candida albicans
C. Blastomyces dermatitis
D. Paracoccidioides brasiliensis

PHARMACOLOGY

28. A 50 year old female with end stage renal disease (ESRD) develops pulmonary tuberculosis, which one of the following drugs should be used in a reduced dose?

A. Rifampicin
B. Isoniazide
C. Pyrazamide
D. Ethambutol

29. According to food and drug administration lactation category S* Refers to

A. Safe for nursing infant, medication usually compatible with breast feeding
B. Safe in nursing infants unknown, inadequate literature available
C. Potential for significant effects on nursing infants medication should be given with caution
D. Not safe for nursing infants, medication contraindicated or requires cessation of breast feeding

30. The most common adverse effect associated with phenytoin is

A. Megaloblastic anemia
B. Gum hypertrophy
C. Hirtuism
D. Drowsiness

31. Morphine withdrawal is characterized by all EXCEPT

A. Miosis
B. Yawning
C. Lacrimation
D. Diarrhoea

32. Ethambutol causes

A. Red discolouration of urine
B. Psychosis
C. Optic neuritis
D. Flu like syndrome

33. Ipratropium bromide is used for

A. Renal colic
B. Organophosphorus poisioning
C. Bronchial asthma
D. Miosis

34. Drug used in treatment of malignant hyperthermia is

A. Baclofen
B. Diazepam
C. Dantrolene
D. Halothane

GENERAL MEDICINE

35. Herpes simplex virus binds to epithelium using

A. Chondroitin sulphate
B. Heparin sulphate
C. Hyaluronidase
D. Keratin sulphate

36. Cardiac pain may be transmitted to the jaw due to the overlapping of

A. 5th cranial nerve, third cervical nerve and first thoracic nerve
B. 7th cranial nerve, third cervical nerve and first thoracic nerve

C. 5th cranial nerve, second cervical nerve and first thoracic nerve
D. 7th cranial nerve, second cervical nerve and first thoracic nerve

37. The break-up time test is performed to evaluate the function of
A. Salivary flow
B. Lacrimal gland
C. Thyroid gland
D. Blood flow

38. An 18 years old lady presents with severe sore throat, fever and malaise, she has cervical lymphadenopathy, splenomegaly and scattered petechiae on the soft plate with enlarged tonsils covered with a white exudates. Which of the following investigations is most likely to help guide your management?
A. Fine needle aspiration of a lymph node
B. Hepatitis B surface antigen
C. Heterophile antibody test
D. HIV test

39. A 30 years old known SLE female presents with ankle swelling. Her BP is 170/100 mmHg and she has marked lower limb odema. Urine dip stick discloses 4+ protein with no hematuria, plasma creatinine is 1.4 mg/dl, albumin is 1.5g/dl and urine protein excretion rate is 6 gms for 24 hours. What is the cause of this presentation?
A. Amyloidosis
B. Class II lupus nephritis
C. Class V lupus nephritis
D. Pericardial effusion

40. A patient presents with congestive cardiac failure with depressed ejection fraction. Which drug may be effective in reducing mortality?
A. Digoxin
B. Frusemide
C. Lidocaine
D. Enalapril

41. A 30 year old lady, previous rheumatic heart disease present with 3 months history of fatigue, weight loss, night sweats and dyspnoea on exertion. She is pyrexial with evidence of mitral regurgitation and splincter hemorrhages. ECHO confirms vegetations, blood cultures are taken and a diagnosis of infective endocarditis is made. What is the most likely infecting organisms in this case?
A. Streptococcus viridans
B. Staphylococcus aureus
C. Staphylococcus epidermitis
D. Enterococcus sp

42. A 70 year old male is admitted to the hospital with a left hemiparesis and altered consciousness. He is on aspirin 75mg OD, atrovostatin 10mg OD and glibenclamide 15 mg daily. His wife says he has been unwell for a couple of days and he has been off food, she has however, still been giving him all his medications. Which of the following tests is going to be most useful in finding a immediately reversible cause for his symptoms
A. Blood glucose levels
B. CT brain
C. ECG
D. Troponin levels

43. A young man presents with jaundice and itching. His viral serology showed active Hepatitis E infection. Which of the following is true of Hepatitis EXCEPT
A. Chronic Hepatitis always occurs
B. Hepatitis E can be prevented by passive immunization
C. Transmission is by feco-oral route
D. Coinfection with hepatitis B is required for pathogenicity

44. A patient presents with jaundice, physical examination reveals an enlarged nodular liver. CT of the abdomen shows a cirrhotic liver with a large mass. CT guided biopsy of the mass demonstrates a malignant

tumour derived from hepatic parenchymal cells. Infection with which of the following viruses would most directly related to the development of this tumour?

A. Epstein – Barr virus
B. Human herpes virus type A
C. Human T-lymphocyte virus
D. Hepatitis B virus

45. **A 60 year old male presents with a 2 day history of a severe left ear ache with a burning sensation in the ear and loss of taste. There is left sided weakness of both upper and lower facial muscles. Facial sensation is normal. A few vesicles are seen in the pharynx. What is the most likely diagnosis?**

A. Bell's palsy
B. Acoustic neuroma
C. Diphtheria
D. Ramsay hunt syndrome

GENERAL SURGERY

46. **Pleomorphic adenomas arising from the minor salivary glands can be treated with**

A. Local excision with 2mm margin
B. Local excision with 5 mm margin
C. Radiotherapy
D. Chemotherapy

47. **The cyst which is associated with a non vital tooth is**

A. Stafne bone cyst
B. Solitary bone cyst
C. Radicular cyst
D. Globulo-maxillary cyst

48. **Cylindroma is another name for**

A. Adenoid cystic carcinoma
B. Adenolymphoma
C. Mucoepidermoid carcinoma
D. Pleomorphic adenoma

49. **Which of the following is NOT a feature of Hutchinson's triad**

A. Facial nerve paralysis
B. Mulberry molars
C. Ocular interstitial keratitis
D. Vestibulocochlear nerve paralysis

50. **The quantity of water lost in expired air each 24hrs is about**

A. 200ml
B. 400ml
C. 600ml
D. 800ml

51. **If during blood transfusion reaction develops in the form of incompatibility the first thing to be done is**

A. Stop the transfusion
B. Inj. hydrocortisone to be given stat
C. Inj. chlorpheneramine maleate to be given stat
D. Inj .frusemide to be given

52. **Small round superficial erosions in the mouth which coalesce to form the so called snail track ulcers are seen in**

A. Primary syphilis
B. Secondary syphilis
C. Tertiary syphilis
D. Congenital syphilis

53. **Treatment of choice for basal cell carcinoma of skin is**

A. Surgical excision
B. Radiotherapy
C. Chemotherapy
D. Congenital therapy

54. **According to the "rule of nine" in burns, what is the percentage of burns if both the upper limbs and lower limbs are involved**

A. 24 %
B. 36 %
C. 54 %
D. 72 %

55. **Commonest location of a thyroglossal cyst is**

A. Floor of mouth
B. Suprahyoid
C. Subhyoid
D. In the region of thyroid cartilage

56. The stimulus of parathyroid hyperplasia in secondary hyperparathyroidism is

A. Chronic hypercalcaemia
B. Chronic hypocalcaemia
C. Chronic hypomagnesemia
D. Chronic hypermagnesemia

DENTAL MATERIALS

57. Which glass ionomer cement develops early resistance to water intake on setting?

A. Reinforced auto cure glass ionomer cement
B. Compomer
C. Resin modified glass ionomer cement
D. Ceramic reinforced glass ionomer cement

58. Which one of the following restorative materials is having coefficient of thermal expansion close to that of tooth enamel and dentin?

A. Microfilled composite resins
B. Pure gold
C. Silver amalgam
D. Type II glass ionomer cement

59. Which of the following impression materials is easy to pour and difficult to remove the stone cast from the impression?

A. Addition polysilicone
B. Condensation polysilicone
C. Polyether
D. Polysulfide

60. As per A.D A No.25. minimum amount of setting expansion required for type V gypsum product is

A. 0.05
B. 0.10
C. 0.15
D. 0.20

61. Polyacid modified composites are designated as

A. Compomers
B. Giomers
C. Hybrid ionomers
D. Ormocers

62. Solder and flux used for joining Elgilloy wire are

A. Gold solder and borax flux
B. Gold solder and fluoride flux
C. Silver solder and borax flux
D. Silver solder and fluoride flux

63. Ceramics fired to metals are processed by

A. Heat pressing
B. Machining
C. sintering
D. Slip casting

64. A true eutectic alloys has melting point

A. Above that of low fusing metal
B. Below that of high fusion metal
C. Above the melting point of either metal
D. Below the melting point of either metal

65. All of the following components are present in the liquid composition of the heat cure acrylic resins EXCEPT

A. Glycol dimethacrylate
B. Hydroquinone
C. Methyl methacrylate
D. N.N-dihydroxy ethyl para toluidine

66. Direct filling gold formed by electrolytic precipitation is called by all the terms EXCEPT

A. Crystalline gold
B. Granular gold
C. Mat gold
D. Sponge gold

67. The dominant phase in a well – condensed, low copper dental amalgam is

A. Ag_2Hg_3
B. Ag_3Sn
C. Cu_3Sn
D. Sn_8Hg

DADH

68. **Which of the following teeth have a mesio-distal dimension greater than the cervico incisal dimension?**
   A. Permanent maxillary central incisor
   B. Primary lower central incisor
   C. Primary lower lateral incisor
   D. Primary maxillary central incisor

69. **The functional occlusal force applied to the periodontal tissues during one deglutition is for duration of _______ seconds**
   A. 0.3
   B. 0.5
   C. 1.0
   D. 1.5

70. **Facial occlusal line in the maxillary arch is formed by**
   A. Stamp cusps
   B. Centric holding cusps
   C. Supporting cusps
   D. Non-supporting cusps

71. **"Y" shaped arrangement of central groove is seen on the occlusal surface of**
   A. Permanent maxillary first premolar
   B. Permanent maxillary second premolar
   C. Permanent mandibular first premolar
   D. Permanent mandibular second premolar

72. **The cusp of carabelli of the maxillary first molar is on**
   A. Mesiobuccal cusp
   B. Mesiolingual cusp
   C. Distobuccal cusp
   D. Distolingual cusp

73. **The first sign of tooth development in human being is around**
   A. 2nd week of intrauterine life
   B. 6th week of intrauterine life
   C. 6th week of life
   D. At birth

74. **Dark bands that are present in enamel rods at intervals of 4 μm are**
   A. Neonatal bands
   B. Cross striations
   C. Striae of Retzius
   D. Hunter–Schregar bands

75. **"Von Ebner" salivary glands are serous glands present in association with**
   A. Filiform papilla
   B. Circumvallate papilla
   C. Foliate papilla
   D. Fungiform papilla

76. **In reflected light, dead tracts are seen as**
   A. White zones
   B. Black zones
   C. Purple zones
   D. A combination of white and black zones

77. **Carmalt's Gland are**
   A. Major salivary gland
   B. Minor salivary gland (retromolar)
   C. Minor salivary gland (lingual)
   D. Taste buds

ORAL PATHOLOGY AND ORAL MEDICINE

78. **Kissing disease is also known as**
   A. Scarlet fever
   B. Glandular fever
   C. Acute herpetic gingivostomatitis
   D. Rubella

79. **Shingles is caused by**
   A. Herpes simplex virus
   B. Varicella zoster virus
   C. Herpes Zoster virus
   D. Coxsackie virus

80. **Presence of Bence Jones Proteins is characteristic of**
   A. Non Hodgkin's Lymphoma
   B. Burkitt's Lymphoma
   C. Multiple Myeloma
   D. Chronic lymphocytic Leukemia

81. **General paresis in Neurosyphilis is a feature of**
A. Primary stage of syphilis
B. Latent phase of syphilis
C. Secondary stage of syphilis
D. Tertiary stage of syphilis

82. **Hemophilia B is caused due to deficiency of clotting factor**
A. VII
B. VIII
C. IX
D. X

83. **Kveim test is done for**
A. Tuberculosis
B. Sarcoidosis
C. Herpes simplex
D. Aphthous ulcers

84. **Ivy technique is a test done to measure the**
A. Bleeding time
B. Capillary fragility
C. Prothrombin time
D. Platelet survival time

85. **Montoux' test is done for the diagnosis of**
A. Syphilis
B. Cat scratch disease
C. Tuberculosis
D. Tetanus

86. **Periapical cemento-osseous dysplasia occurs frequently in the**
A. Mandibular posterior region
B. Mandibular anterior region
C. Maxillary posterior region
D. Maxillary anterior region

87. **Acute infection of bacteria which affects the nervous system**
A. Syphilis
B. Meliodosis
C. Tetanus
D. Tularemia

88. **Koplik's spots are commonly seen in**
A. Measles
B. Rubella
C. Chicken pox
D. Small pox

89. **A form of fibrous dysplasia occurring in children is termed as**
A. Monostotic form
B. Polyostotic form
C. Craniofacial form
D. Cherubism

90. **Rh hump is commonly associated with**
A. Iron deficiency anemia
B. Aplastic anemia
C. Erythroblastosis fetalis
D. Sickle cell anemia

91. **Coup de sabre is commonly associated with**
A. Pemphigus
B. Systemic sclerosis
C. Erythema multiforme
D. Systemic lupus erythematous

92. **Histological appearance of "Abtrofung or dropping off" is commonly seen in**
A. Intradermal nevus
B. Junctional nevus
C. Compound nevus
D. Epithelial nevus

93. **The causative agent for "Oculoglandular syndrome of Parinoud" is**
A. Arachnia propionica
B. Bartonella henselae
C. Bifidobacterium denticum
D. Mycobacterium leprae

94. **Salivary peroxidase system is known to be effective against**
A. Actinomyces viscosus
B. Lactobacillus acidophilus
C. Streptococcus mutans
D. Veillonella parvula

95. **Small palpable mass elevated above the epithelial surface is**
A. Papule
B. Macule
C. Plaque
D. Vesicle

ORAL RADIOLOGY

96. Following exposure the x-rays interact with patient tissues within
   A. 10^{-13} second
   B. 10^{+13} second
   C. 10^{-10} second
   D. 10^{+10} second

97. The traditional unit of equivalent dose is
   A. Rem
   B. Rad
   C. Roentgen
   D. Sievert

98. The SI unit of exposure is
   A. Roentgen
   B. Air kerma
   C. Curie
   D. Sievert

99. Penny test is the quality assurance test to detect
   A. Fixer depletion
   B. Unsafe illumination
   C. Machine malfunction
   D. Contaminated solution

100. Identification of gross osseous change from a lateral aspect can be viewed by which projection
   A. Transcranial
   B. Transorbital
   C. Transpharyngeal
   D. Translaryngeal

101. Dilation of the salivary duct secondary to epithelial atrophy as a result of repeated inflammatory or infectious process is
   A. Sialodochitis
   B. Sialadenitis
   C. Sialolithiasis
   D. Mucocele

ORTHODONTICS

102. Concept of lingual orthodontic appliance was introduced by
   A. Atkinson
   B. Myerson
   C. Johnson
   D. Kurz

103. Intermittent forces are applied with the help of
   A. Elastics
   B. Headgear
   C. Removable plates
   D. All of the above

104. Which of the following drugs is better analgesic for patient who is undergoing orthodontic tooth movement?
   A. Acetaminophen
   B. Aspirin
   C. Ibuprofen
   D. Diclofenac sodium

105. Myofunctional appliances are indicated in cases with
   A. A class II skeletal malocclusion with a faulty mandible
   B. A class II skeletal malocclusion with a faulty maxilla
   C. Appliances identify the fault and correct the malocclusion
   D. Severe tooth material excess of 14 mm or more

106. Surface of NiTi wire is
   A. Rougher that beta titanium wire
   B. Rougher than stainless steel wire
   C. Both of the above
   D. None of the above

107. Which of the following is NOT an essential diagnostic aid in orthodontics?
   A. Case history
   B. Clinical examinations
   C. Plaster study casts
   D. Cephalometric X-rays

108. Which form of stainless steel is used to the manufacturing of orthodontic wire?
   A. Austenitic
   B. Martenstitic
   C. Ferritic
   D. All the three forms can be used

109. Catlan's appliance is given for a period NOT more than 6 weeks because it

A. Cause attrition of upper anteriors
B. Cause periodontitis of anteriors
C. Cause gingival recession in lower anteriors
D. Causes over eruption of posterior teeth

110. Bolton's analysis is used to determine the

A. Proportion of mesiodistal width of the mandibular teeth to that of the basal bone
B. Proportion of mesiodistal width of the maxillary teeth to that of basal bone
C. Proportion of mesiodistal width of the maxillary teeth to the transverse width
D. Properties of mesiodistal width of the mandibular teeth to that of the maxillary teeth

111. Who proposed the "trajectory theory of bone formation"

A. An anatomist, Meyer
B. A mathematician, Cullman
C. Both A and B
D. None of the above

112. The first speech sounds produced by developing child is

A. Linguo alveolar
B. Sibilant
C. Linguo dental
D. Bilabial

113. Rotation correction of tooth can be a hazardous process if correction is more then

A. 20°
B. 45°
C. 60°
D. 90°

PEDODONTICS

114. The art of re-enforcing good behaviour displayed by the child with verbal praise applies the

A. Operant conditioning theory
B. Classical conditioning theory
C. Psychoanalytical theory
D. Social learning theory

115. An example of a sex related disease more commonly seen in males is

A. Primary herpetic gingivostomatitis
B. Anorexia
C. Early childhood caries
D. Hemophilia

116. A developmental alteration where a single tooth bud divides incompletely resulting in the formation of a tooth with a bifid crown and single pulp chamber is called

A. Fusion
B. Concrescence
C. Gemination
D. Dens Evaginatus

117. Space regaining is indicated in all of the following EXCEPT

A. One or more permanent teeth have been lost
B. Some space in the arch has been lost due to mesial drift of 1st permanent molar
C. Mixed dentition analysis shows that, once the lost space is gained back, there will not be any arch length tooth material discrepancy
D. 1st molars are in end to end relation due to Class II skeletal base and Prognathic maxilla

118. The first book on child dentistry was published by

A. G.W .Wright
B. Joseph Hurlock
C. Gerauldy
D. Robert bunan

119. A crying two year old child brought to your Dental clinic would be classified under Wright's classification of child behavior as a

A. Potentially cooperative child
B. Uncooperative child
C. Child lacking cooperation
D. Timid child

120. All of the following materials can be used for obturating root canals of primary tooth EXCEPT

A. Zinc oxide eugenol paste
B. Zinc oxide and iodoform paste
C. Gutta Percha
D. Calcium hydroxide and iodoform paste

121. A mother who does not encourage her child to cope up with new situations thereby making him shy and timid is an example of an

A. Overprotective mother
B. Authoritarian mother
C. Under affectionate mother
D. Rejecting mother

122. Which intraoral radiographic technique follows the "Rule of Isometry"?

A. Paralleling technique
B. Occlusal radiographs
C. Bisecting angle technique
D. Cephalometric radiographs

123. A frightened child is exposed to a dental clinic setting which is pleasant, colorful and different from a previous clinic where a painful experience occurred. The child is happy and treatment is completed. The psychological conditioning principle used here is

A. Acquisition
B. Generalization
C. Extinction
D. Discrimination

124. The groove separating the gum pad from the palate is called

A. Gingival groove
B. Dental groove
C. Lateral sulcus
D. Transverse groove

125. Early mesial shift makes use of

A. Incisal liability
B. Primate space
C. Physiologic spaces
D. Leeway space of Nance

126. Which of the following is TRUE regarding voice control during dental treatment of children?

A. It should be a monotonous soothing cement
B. It is a sudden and firm command
C. It is intended to frighten the child
D. It can be used on a two year old child

127. Which topical fluoride agent makes of thixotrophic properties for better penetration into inter proximal areas?

A. Sodium fluoride solution
B. Fluoride foam
C. Acidulated phosphate fluoride gel
D. Fluoride varnish

P AND SD

128. The tobacco preparation mainly used to clean the tooth is

A. Khaini
B. Mawa
C. Masheri
D. Dhumti

129. The concept which views health as 'absence from disease' is called

A. Biomedical concept
B. Ecological concept
C. Psychosocial concept
D. Holistic concept

130. The frequency of a disease or characteristic expressed per unit size of the population or group in which it is observed is

A. Rate
B. Ratio
C. Proportion
D. Average

131. The common first approach to test causal hypothesis is

A. Descriptive study
B. Case-control study
C. Cohort study
D. Randomized controlled trial

132. **The brushing method recommended for individuals with open interdental spaces with missing papillae and exposed root surface is,**
   A. Fones method
   B. Charters method
   C. Bass method
   D. Smith method

133. **The cationic bisbiguanide used as mouthwash which is effective against gram positive and gram negative microorganisms, fungi, yeasts and viruses is**
   A. Chlorhexidine gluconate
   B. Triclosan
   C. Delmophinol
   D. Sanguinarine

134. **The National Cancer Registry program (NCRP) was initiated by the India Council of Medical Research in the year**
   A. 1972
   B. 1982
   C. 1992
   D. 2002

135. **The degree to which the health education message is perceived as trustworthy by the receiver is called**
   A. Setting an example
   B. Comprehension
   C. Credibility
   D. Reinforcement

136. **The Indian Government passed the "cigarettes and other Tobacco products Act" to prohibit advertisement of and regulate the production, supply and distribution of tobacco products in the year**
   A. 1973
   B. 1983
   C. 1993
   D. 2003

137. **The world's first artificial water fluoridation plant was started at**
   A. Culemborg
   B. Grand rapids
   C. Muskegon
   D. Oak Park

138. **The fluoride concentration in 8% stannous fluoride topical application is**
   A. 1000 ppm
   B. 9200 ppm
   C. 19500 ppm
   D. 12300 ppm

139. **Milk fluoridation was introduced by**
   A. Knutson
   B. Bibby
   C. Wespi
   D. Zeigler

140. **The WHO periodontal examination probe weighs**
   A. 5 gms
   B. 10 gms
   C. 15 gms
   D. 20 gms

141. **The ratio between the achievements of program activity and the desired level which the planners had proposed result from the program is called**
   A. Effectiveness
   B. Efficiency
   C. Appropriateness
   D. Adequacy

142. **The dye used in the salivary Reductase test is**
   A. Bromocresol green
   B. Diazo resorcinol
   C. Methylene blue
   D. Basic fuschin

PROSTHODONTICS

143. **For strength and rigidity, the vertical height of a finished lingual bar should be at least**
   A. 6mm
   B. 7mm
   C. 4mm
   D. 5mm

144. A reliable guide for positioning maxillary anterior teeth in complete dentures is

A. Rugae
B. Incisive papilla
C. Maxillary ridge
D. Fovea palatini

145. Average masticatory load for natural teeth is around

A. 10 kg
B. 20 kg
C. 30 kg
D. 40 kg

146. Articulated diagnostic casts help in the following except

A. Diagnostic wax up to evaluate outcome
B. Detailed analysis of occlusal plane and occlusion
C. Fabrication of wax patterns for casting
D. Performing mock tooth preparation

147. Least hygienic pontic

A. Sanitary
B. Bullet
C. Spheroidal
D. Saddle

148. Advantage of a palatal strap

A. Increased rigidity with less bulk
B. Reduction of bulk
C. Better stimulation of the underlying tissues
D. Easy manipulation

149. Relief under a maxillary major connector

A. Is generally not required
B. Is required
C. May be used
D. May not be used

150. .... major connector is a poor choice for distal extension RPD

A. Single palatal strap
B. Complete palatal coverage
C. Horse shoe shaped or U shaped MC
D. Anterior posterior of Double Palatal bar

151. Recommended convergence between opposing axial walls which optimize retention is

A. 6 degree
B. 30 degree
C. 15 degree
D. 45 degree

152. In case of a hard median suture line and an inoperable torus the major connector of choice is

A. Single palatal strap
B. Complete palatal coverage
C. Horse shoe shaped or U shaped MC
D. Anterior posterior or double palatal bar

153. Height of contour is a term coined by

A. Kennedy
B. Cummer
C. Devan
D. Applegate

154. The first person to employ mechanical device to determine the relative parallelism of tooth surface was

A. Fortunati
B. Ney
C. Applegate
D. Kratochvil

155. Prognosis is

A. Most likely cause of the disease
B. Least likely cause of the disease
C. Estimation of the likely course of the disease
D. None of the above

156. Occlusal offset in an anterior partial veneer crown may generally be necessary to provide

A. Retention
B. Conservation of tooth surface
C. Esthetics
D. Structural durability

PERIODONTICS

157. Ideal thickness of a free gingival graft obtained from the palate is

A. 0.5–1 mm
B. 1–1.5 mm
C. 1.5–2.0 mm
D. 2.0–2.5 mm

158. Fusion of Cementum and alveolar bone with the obliteration of periodontal ligament is called

A. Avulsion
B. Extrusion
C. Ankylosis
D. Luxation

159. Flaps which accomplish the double objectives of pocket elimination and increasing the width of attached gingiva is

A. Apically displaced flap
B. Coronally displaced flap
C. Papilla preservation flap
D. Undisplaced flap

160. The sixth complication of diabetes mellitus is

A. Retinopathy
B. Renal failure
C. Ischemic heart disease
D. Periodontitis

161. A drug that exerts anticollagenase activity

A. Penicillin
B. Metronidazole
C. Erythromycin
D. Tetracycline

162. The function of Langerhan's cells is

A. Melanin synthesis
B. Protein synthesis
C. Antigen presentation to neutrophils
D. Antigen presentation to lymphocytes

163. A replacement drug used as substitute for cyclosporine exhibiting less severe gingival enlargement is

A. Methotrexate
B. Tacrolimus
C. Nifedipine
D. Bleomycin

164. Stage IV of ANUG according to Horning and Cohen is characterized by

A. Necrosis of the tip of interdental papilla
B. Necrosis extending to the attached gingiva
C. Necrosis exposing alveolar bone
D. Necrosis perforating skin of cheek

165. The lactoperoxidase thiocyanate system present in saliva is against

A. *A. actinomycetemcomitans*
B. *Streptococcus*
C. *P. gingivalis*
D. *Actinomyces*

166. In a biofilm the capacity of bacteria to communicate with each other is called

A. Quorum sensing
B. Conjugation
C. Transformation
D. Transmission

167. Which of the following acute infection is contagious?

A. Acute gingival abscess
B. Necrotizing ulcerative gingivitis
C. Primary herpetic gingivostomatitis
D. Acute pericoronitis

168. No surgical procedure should be performed in patients with thrombocytopenia unless the platelet count is

A. >60,000
B. >70,000
C. >80,000
D. >50,000

169. All of the following organisms can be detected by BANA analysis EXCEPT

A. Tanneralla forsythia
B. Porphyromonas gingivalis
C. Capnocytophaga
D. Actinomycetemcomitans

170. **An example of vertical method of tooth brushing**
   A. Leonard's method
   B. Fones method
   C. Smith's method
   D. Bass method

171. **Which of these drugs can be given safely to a patient with renal disease?**
   A. Phenacetin
   B. Tetracycline
   C. Aminoglycoside
   D. Diazepam

CONS AND ENDO

172. **One of the following statements regarding HIV is NOT true**
   A. When used properly, all disinfectants except some quaternary ammonium compounds are said to inactivate HIV in less than 2 minutes
   B. HIV is killed by all methods of sterilization
   C. Aerosols produced during dental treatments have been found to transmit HIV infection
   D. HIV has been transmitted by blood contaminated fluids that have been heavily spattered of splashed

173. **Whenever the caries cone in enamel is larger or at least the same size as that in dentin, it is called as**
   A. Residual caries
   B. Recurrent caries
   C. Forward caries
   D. Backward caries

174. **"Right rear" operator position refers to**
   A. 1 O' clock
   B. 5 O' clock
   C. 7 O' clock
   D. 11 O' clock

175. **The disadvantage of winged rubber dam retainer is that is interferes with the placement of**
   A. Matrix bands
   B. Dental floss
   C. Rubber dam frame
   D. Rubber dam sheet

176. **Discolored areas seen through the enamel in the teeth that have amalgam restorations are known as**
   A. Amalgam tattoos
   B. Amalgam overhands
   C. Amalgam blues
   D. Amalgam ditching

177. **Which of the following item in the dental operatory cannot be classified as a semi-critical item?**
   A. Suction tip
   B. Hand piece
   C. Endodontic file
   D. Water syringe tip

178. **One of the following statement regarding pin retained restoration is NOT true**
   A. Pinholes should never be prepared at different levels on the tooth
   B. A minimum of 0.5 mm clearance should be provided around the circumference of the pin for adequate condensation of the amalgam
   C. Pinhole should be located on a flat surface that is perpendicular to the proposed direction of the pinhole
   D. The pinhole should be positioned no closer than 1 mm to DEJ and no closer than 1.5 mm to external surface

179. **All of the following surface tests are used to determine the status of the pulp EXCEPT**
   A. Heat test
   B. Cold test
   C. Electric pulp test
   D. Anesthetic test

180. **A peeso reamer is used for**
   A. Preparation of post space in the root canal for receiving a post
   B. Enlarging the canal orifices during access cavity preparation

C. Removal of the lingual shoulder to improve the access in anterior teeth
D. Cleaning and shaping of the cervical third of the root canal

181. In chronic hyperplastic pulpitis pulp response to vitality tests will be
A. Normal response
B. Hyper response
C. Reduced response
D. Normal to hyper response

182. The advantage of silver point as obturating material is that it
A. Can be used in fine tortuous canals
B. Is easier to retrieve if retreatment becomes necessary
C. Gives a perfect seal at the apical 1/3rd of the root canal
D. Provides better adaptation of canal walls compared to Gutta Percha

183. If a tooth has abnormal mobility, but is not displaced from the socket it is termed as
A. Concussion
B. Subluxation
C. Extrusive luxation
D. Partial avulsion

184. The type of root resorption seen after bleaching is
A. Cervical root resorption
B. Lateral root resorption
C. Apical root resorption
D. Internal root resorption

185. In an endodontic file, D2 will be
A. At the tip of the instrument
B. At 2mm from the tip of the instrument
C. At 3 mm from the tip of the instrument
D. At 16 mm from the tip of the instrument

ORAL SURGERY

186. You are managing a cardiac arrest, which drug is to be given for ventricular fibrillation after unsuccessful defibrillation
A. 1 mg Atropine
B. 1 mg epinephrine
C. 1 mg/kg $NaHCO_3$
D. 1 mg/kg lidocaine

187. The 'Hanging drop' sign if visualized in the water's projection of the traumatized face indicates
A. Nasal bone fracture
B. Orbital floor
C. Zygomatic arch fracture
D. Le fort I fracture

188. Felypressin is
A. Vasoconstrictor: predominate effect on venous system
B. Vasodilator: predominant on arterial system
C. Vasoconstrictor: predominant effect on arterial system
D. Vasodilator: predominant effect on venous system

189. Highest percentage of clinical failures are seen with which nerve block
A. Buccal nerve block
B. Inferior alveolar nerve block
C. Mental nerve block
D. Incisive nerve block

190. Oxygen as an emergency drug is contraindicated in
A. Anaphylaxis
B. Asthma
C. Hyperventilation
D. COPD

191. Rhytidectomy is
A. Removal of skin wrinkles
B. Alteration of nasal septum position
C. Salivary gland excision
D. Cheek augmentation

192. Trans osseous wiring in an example of
A. IMF with osteosynthesis
B. Osteosynthesis with IMF
C. IMF
D. None of the above

193. A morbid patient unlikely to survive 24 hours with or without surgery is classified as

A. ASAI
B. ASA III
C. ASA V
D. ASA VII

194. A direct connection between living bone and load bearing Endosseous implant at the light microscopic level

A. Osteosynthesis
B. Osteogenesis
C. Osseointegration
D. Osseoinduction

195. Antibiotic that achieves high concentration in Hard tissue, because of its molecular size is

A. Ceftum
B. Ciprofloxacin
C. Clindamycin
D. Erythromycin

196. Garre's sclerosing osteomyelitis is also known as

A. Proliferative periostitis
B. Infantile osteomyelitis
C. Chronic sclerosing oseomyelitis
D. Necrosis

197. Marx-University of Miami protocol for osteoradionecrosis is related to

A. High dose antibiotic therapy
B. Hyperbaric oxygen therapy
C. Both A and B
D. None of the above

198. The most important reason for placing an alveolar graft in cleft palate patient is

A. Improve pronounciation
B. Improve breathing efficiency
C. Make eruptive pathway of permanent canine
D. Improve feeding efficiency

199. The orthognathic surgery that is commonly carried out for correction of mandibular prognathism is

A. Sagittal split osteotomy
B. Le fort I osteotomy
C. Vertical Ramus osteotomy
D. Genioplasty

200. The weakest part and most vulnerable part for fracture in the mandible is

A. Ramus of mandible
B. Condylar neck
C. Angle of the mandible
D. Region of the canine tooth

ANSWERS

ANATOMY

1. Ans: C

   Ref: Inderbir Singh, 8/E, pg.128

2. Ans: A

   Ref: Di Fiore's Atlas of Histology, 11/E, pg.213

3. Ans: B

   Ref: Inderbir Singh, 6/E, p.35

4. Ans: C

   Ref: BD Chaurasia, 1/E, p.327

5. Ans: A

   Ref: Text Book of Anatomy by Inderbir Singh, 4/E, p. 246

PHYSIOLOGY

6. Ans: A

   Ref: Sembulingam, 4/E, p.501

7. Ans: A

   Ref: Sembulingam, 4/E, p.415

8. Ans: B

   Ref: Sembulingam, 4/E, p.902

9. Ans: C

   Ref: Sembulingam, 4/E, p.425

10. Ans: B

    Ref: Sembulingam, 4/E, p.202

11. Ans: B

    Ref: Sembulingam, 4/E, p.372

12. Ans: A

    Ref: Sembulingam, 4/E, p.206

BIOCHEMISTRY

13. Ans: B

    Ref: U. Sathyanarayana, U. Chakrapani, 3/E, p. 186

14. Ans: A

    Ref: U. Sathyanarayana, U. Chakrapani, 3/E, p. 110

15. Ans: D

    Ref: U. Sathyanarayana, U. Chakrapani, 3/E p. 294

GENERAL PATHOLOGY

16. Ans: A

    Ref: Robbin's Pathologic Basis of Disease, 7/E, p. 36

17. Ans: D

    Ref: Robbin's Pathologic Basis of Disease, 7/E, p. 339

18. Ans: C

    Ref: Harsh Mohan, 3/E, p.93

19. Ans: B

    Ref: Harsh Mohan, 3/E, p.65

20. Ans: D

    Ref: Robbin's Pathologic Basis of Disease, 7/E, p.1087

21. Ans: D

    Ref: Robbin's Pathologic Basis of Disease, 7/E, p.130

MICROBIOLOGY

22. Ans: C

    Ref: Ananthanarayan and Panicker's Text, Book of Microbiology, 8/E, p.348

23. Ans: D

Ref: Ananthanarayan and Panicker's Text, Book of Microbiology, 8/E, p. 24

24. Ans: C

Ref: Ananthanarayan and Panicker's Text, Book of Microbiology, 8/E, p. 121

25. Ans: A

Ref: : Ananthanarayan and Panicker's Text, Book of Microbiology, 8/E, p.353

26. Ans: C

Ref: Ananthanarayan and Panicker's Text, Book of Microbiology, 8/E, p. 578

27. Ans: B

Ref: Ananthanarayan and Panicker's Text, Book of Microbiology, 8/E, p.615

PHARMACOLOGY

28. Ans: D

Ref: KD Tripathi, 6/E, p.742

Explanation

Ethambutol is a commonly used antitubercular drug. It is excreted in urine by glomerular filtration and tubular secretion. Hence caution is required in its use in patients with renal disease

29. Ans: C

Ref: KD Tripathi, 6/E,p.912

30. Ans: B

Ref: KD Tripathi, 6/E, p.404

31. Ans: A

Ref: KD Tripathi, 6/E, p.457

32. Ans: C

Ref: K.D Tripathi,6/E, p. 742

33. Ans: C

Ref: K.D Tripathi, 6/E, p. 217

34. Ans: C

Ref: KD Tripathi, 6/E, p. 347

GENERAL MEDICINE

35. Ans: B

Ref: Harrison, Vol. I ,17/E, p. 1079

36. Ans: A

Ref: Harrison, Vol. I, 17/E, p. 87

37. Ans: B

Ref: Harrison, Vol. II,17/E, p. 2107

38. Ans: C

Ref: Davidson, 20/E, p. 307

39. Ans: C

Ref: Davidson, 20/E, p. 515,

40. Ans: D

Ref: Davidson, 20/E, p. 550

41. Ans: A

Ref: Davidson, 20/E, p. 630

42. Ans: A

Ref: Davidson, 20/E, p. 829

43. Ans: C

Ref: Davidson, 20/E, p. 968

44. Ans: D

Ref: Davidson, 20/E, p. 966

45. Ans: D

Ref: Davidson, 20/E, p. 305

GENERAL SURGERY

46. Ans: B

Ref: Bailey and Love, 25/E, pp. 752, 753

47. Ans: C

Ref: S. Das, 3/E, p. 566

48. **Ans: A**

Ref: S Das, 3/E, p. 609

49. **Ans: A**

Ref: S. Das, 3/E, p.73

50. **Ans: B**

Ref: S.Das, 3/E, p. 20

51. **Ans: A**

Ref: S.Das, 3/E, p. 41

52. **Ans: B**

Ref:S .Das, 3/E, p. 72

53. **Ans: A**

Ref: S Das, 3/E, p. 103

54. **Ans: C**

Ref: S .Das, 3/E, p. 52

55. **Ans: C**

Ref: S .Das, 3/E, p. 669

56. **Ans: B**

Ref: S .Das, 3/E, p. 675

DENTAL MATERIALS

57. **Ans: C**

Ref: Phillip's, 11/E, p. 482

58. **Ans: D**

Ref: Phillip's, 11/E, p. 55

59. **Ans: C**

Ref: Phillip's, 11/E, p. 222

60. **Ans: B**

Ref: Phillip's, 11/E, p. 273

61. **Ans: A**

Ref: Phillip's, 11/E, p. 485

62. **Ans: D**

Ref: Phillip's, 11/E, p. 643

63. **Ans: C**

Ref: Phillip's, 11/E, p. 656

64. **Ans: D**

Ref: Phillip's, 11/E, p. 131

65. **Ans: D**

Ref: Phillip's, 11/E, pp. 723, 735

66. **Ans: B**

Ref: Phillip's, 11/E, p. 550

67. **Ans: A**

Ref: Phillip's, 11/E, p. 502

DADH

68. **Ans: D**

Ref: Wheeler's, 9/E, p. 50

69. **Ans: C**

Ref: Wheeler's, 9/E, p. 271

70. **Ans: D**

Ref: Wheeler's, 8/E, p. 460

71. **Ans: D**

Ref: Wheeler's, 8/E, p. 260

72. **Ans: B**

Ref: Wheeler's, 8/E, p. 264

73. **Ans: B**

Ref: Orban's , 12/E, p. 22

74. **Ans: B**

Ref: Orban's, 12/E, p. 49

75. **Ans: B**

Ref: Orban's, 12/E, p. 237

76. **Ans: A**

Ref: Orban's, 12/E, p. 98

77. **Ans: B**

Ref: Michael Miloro and Sterling R Schow, p. 435

ORAL PATHOLOGY AND ORAL MEDICINE

78. Ans: B

    Ref: Shafer, 5/E, p. 1065

79. Ans: B

    Ref: Shafer, 5/E, p. 480

80. Ans: C

    Ref: Shafer, 5/E, p. 261

81. Ans: D

    Ref: Burkit's, 11/E, pg.490

82. Ans: C

    Ref: Shafer's, 6/E, p. 785

83. Ans: B

    Ref: Shafer's, 6/E, p. 669

84. Ans: A

    Ref: Burket's, 11/E, p. 414

85. Ans: C

    Ref: Shafer's, 6/E, p. 316

86. Ans: B

    Ref: Burkit's, 11/E, p. 144

87. Ans: C

    Ref: Burkit's, 11/E, p. 491

88. Ans: A

    Ref: Shafer's, 6/E, p. 341

89. Ans: D

    Ref: Shafer's, 6/E, p. 711

90. Ans: C

    Ref: Shafer's, 6/E, p. 764

91. Ans: B

    Ref: Shafer's, 6/E, p. 831

92. Ans: B

    Ref: Shafer's, 6/E, p. 85

93. Ans: B

    Ref: Neville, 3/E, pp. 205, 206

94. Ans: B

    Ref: Shafer's, 6/E, p.428

95. Ans: A

    Ref: Burkit's, 11/E, p. 42

ORAL RADIOLOGY

96. Ans: A

    Ref: White and Pharaoh, 6/E, p. 18

97. Ans: A

    Ref: White and Pharoah, 6/E, p. 16

98. Ans: B

    Ref: White and Pharoah, 6/E, p. 16

99. Ans: B

    Ref: White and Pharoah, 6/E, p. 102

100. Ans: A

     Ref: White and Pharoah, 6/E, pp. 477,479

101. Ans: A

     Ref: Dental Radiographic Diagnosis, Kavas. H. Thunthy, 1/E, p. 518

     Explanation
     It is also called as sialoangitis or sialoductitis

ORTHODONTICS

102. Ans: D

     Ref: Gurkeerat Singh, 2/E, p. 491

103. Ans: D

     Ref: Bhalaji, 3/E, p. 201

104. Ans: A

     Ref: Profitt, 4/E, p. 348

105. Ans: A

Ref: Bhalaji, 3/E, p. 333

106. Ans: C

Ref: Bhalaji, 3/E, p. 315

107. Ans: D

Ref: Bhalaji, 3/E, pp. 115, 116

108. Ans: A

Ref: Bhalaji, 3/E, p. 315

109. Ans: D

Ref: Bhalaji, 3/E, p. 429

110. Ans: D

Ref: Bhalaji, 3/E, p. 178

111. Ans: C

Ref: Bhalaji, 3/E, p. 53

112. Ans: D

Ref: Proffit,4/E, p. 85

113. Ans: B

Ref: Orthodontics for Dental Students, Thomas White & James Holmes, 3/E, p. 273

PEDODONTICS

114. Ans: A

Ref: Pinkham, 4/E, p. 195

115. Ans: D

Ref: Pinkham, 4/E, p. 78

116. Ans: C

Ref: Pinkham, 4/E, p. 64

117. Ans: D

Ref: Shobha Tandon, 2/E, p. 470

118. Ans: B

Ref: Shobha Tandon, 2/E, p. 4

119. Ans: C

Ref: Shobha Tandon, 2/E, p. 143

120. Ans: C

Ref: Shobha Tandon, 2/E, p. 417

121. Ans: A

Ref: Shobha Tandon, 2/E, p. 147

122. Ans: C

Ref: Shobha Tandon, 2/E, p. 20

123. Ans: D

Ref: Shobha Tandon, 2/E, p. 126

124. Ans: A

Ref: Shobha Tandon, 2/E, p. 57

125. Ans: B

Ref: Shobha Tandon, 2/E, p. 112

126. Ans: B

Ref: Shobha Tandon, 2/E, p. 153

127. Ans: C

Ref: Shobha Tandon, 2/E, p. 283

P AND SD

128. Ans: C

Ref: Soben Peter, 3/E, pp. 457,460

129. Ans: A

Ref: Soben Peter, 3/E, p. 2

130. Ans: A

Ref: Soben Peter, 3/E, p. 80

131. Ans: B

Ref: Soben Peter, 3/E, p. 101

132. Ans: B

Ref: Soben Peter, 3/E, p. 437

133. Ans: A

Ref: Soben Peter, 3/E, p. 444

134. Ans: B

Ref: Soben Peter, 3/E, p. 388

135. Ans: C

Ref: Soben Peter, 3/E, p. 525

136. Ans: D

Ref: Park, 20/E, p. 388

137. Ans: B

Ref: Soben Peter, 3/E, p. 335

138. Ans: C

Ref: Soben Peter, 3/E, p. 304

139. Ans: D

Ref: Joseph John,1/E, p. 211

140. Ans: A

Ref: Soben Peter, 3/E, p. 169

141. Ans: A

Ref: Soben Peter, 3/E, p. 622

142. Ans: B

Ref: Soben Peter, 3/E, p. 364

PROSTHODONTICS

143. Ans: C

Ref: Nallaswamy, 2/E, p. 337

144. Ans: B

Ref: Winkler, 2/E, p. 209

145. Ans: B

Ref: Zarb and Bolender, 12/E, p. 10

146. Ans: C

Ref: Zarb and Bolender, 12/E, p. 291

147. Ans: D

Ref: Nallaswamy, 2/E, p. 510

148. Ans: A

Ref: Mc Cracken, 11/E, p. 48

149. Ans: A

Ref: Nallaswamy, 2/E, p. 329

150. Ans: C

Ref: Nallaswamy, 2/E, p.332

151. Ans: A

Ref: Rosensteil, 4/E, p.229

152. Ans: C

Ref: McCracken, 11/E, p. 52

153. Ans: A

Ref: McCracken, 11/E, p. 84

154. Ans: A

Ref: Nallaswamy, 1/E, p. 307

Explanation

The surveyor is a parallelometer, an instrument used to determine the relative parallelism of surfaces of teeth or other areas on a cast. Dr.A.J.Fortunati (1918) was the first person to use a surveyor.

155. Ans: C

Ref: Rosensteil, 4/E, p. 106

156. Ans: D

Ref: Rosensteil, 4/E, p. 291

PERIODONTICS

157. Ans: B

Ref: Carranza, 10/E, p. 1009

158. Ans: C

Ref: Carranza, 10/E, p. 79

159. Ans: A

Ref: Carranza, 10/E, pp. 926, 927

160. Ans: D

Ref: Carranza, 10/E, p. 320

161. Ans: D

Ref: Carranza, 10/E, p. 803

162. Ans: D

Ref: Carranza, 10/E, p. 52

163. Ans: B

Ref: Carranza, 10/E, p. 378

164. Ans: B

Ref: Carranza, 10/E, p. 392

165. Ans: B

Ref: Carranza, 10/E, p. 349

166. Ans: A

Ref: Carranza, 10/E, p. 150

167. Ans: C

Ref: Carranza, 10/E, p. 398

168. Ans: A,B, C & D

Ref: Carranza, 10/E, p. 668

169. Ans: D

Ref: Carranza, 10/E, p. 591

170. Ans: A

Ref: Carranza, 10/E, p. 733

171. Ans: D

Ref: Carranza, 10/E, p. 661

CONS AND ENDO

172. Ans: C

Ref: Sturdevant, 5/E, p. 369

173. Ans: C

Ref: Sturdevant, 5/E, p. 289

174. Ans: D

Ref: Sturdevant, 5/E, p. 450

175. Ans: A

Ref: Sturdevant, 5/E, p. 466

176. Ans: C

Ref: Sturdevant, 5/E, p. 423

177. Ans: C

Ref: Sturdevant, 5/E, p. 386

178. Ans: A

Ref: Sturdevant, 5/E, p. 819

179. Ans: D

Ref: Grossman, 12/E, p. 70

180. Ans: A

Ref: Grossman, 12/E, p. 232

181. Ans: C

Ref: Grossman, 12/E, p. 89

182. Ans: A

Ref: Grossman, 12/E, p. 281

183. Ans:B

Ref: Grossman, 12/E, p. 363

184. Ans: A

Ref: Grossman, 12/E, p. 352

185. Ans: D

Ref: Grossman, 12/E, p. 226

ORAL SURGERY

186. Ans: B

Ref: Peterson, 4/E, p. 27

187. Ans: B

Ref: Balaji, 1/E, p. 636

188. Ans: A

Ref: Malamed, 5/E, p. 50

189. Ans: B

Ref: Malamed, 5/E, p. 228

190. Ans: C

Ref: Peterson, 4/E, pp. 30, 31

191. Ans: A

Ref: Peterson, 4/E,p. 606

192. **Ans: A**

Ref: Killey's, 5/E, p.84

193. **Ans: C**

Ref: Peterson, 4/E, p. 10

Explanation

ASA I: A normal healthy patient

ASA II: A patient with mild systemic disease or significant health risk factor

ASA III: A patient with severe systemic disease that is not incapacitating

ASA IV: A patient with severe systemic disease that is a constant threat to life

ASA V: A moribund patient who is not expected to survive without the operation

ASA VI: A declared brain – dead patient whose organs are being removed for donor purposes

194. **Ans: C**

Ref: Peterson, 4/E, p. 308

195. **Ans: C**

Ref: Peterson, 4/E, p. 377

196. **Ans: A**

Ref: Neelima Malik, 2/E, p. 656

197. **Ans:B**

Ref: Neelima Malik, 2/E, p. 667

198. **Ans: C**

Ref: Peterson, 4/E, p. 636

199. **Ans: A**

Ref: Neelima Malik, 2/E, p. 297

200. **Ans: B**

Ref: Neelima Malik, 2/E, p. 406